Clinical Companion

EDITION

Foundations *of* Maternal–Newborn Nursing

Sharon Smith Murray, M.S.N., R.N.,C.
Professor, Health Professions
Golden West College
Huntington Beach, California

Emily Slone McKinney, M.S.N., R.N.,C.
Baylor Healthcare System
Dallas, Texas

Trula Myers Gorrie, M.N., R.N.,C.
Professor Emeritus
Golden West College
Huntington Beach, California

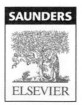

SAUNDERS

ELSEVIER

SAUNDERS
ELSEVIER

11830 Westline Industrial Drive
St. Louis, Missouri 63146

CLINICAL COMPANION FOR FOUNDATIONS OF   ISBN-13: 978-1-4160-0143-0
MATERNAL-NEWBORN NURSING, FOURTH EDITION   ISBN-10: 1-4160-0143-3

NOTICE

Knowledge and best practice in this field are constantly changing. As new
research and experience broaden our knowledge, changes in practice,
treatment, and drug therapy may become necessary or appropriate.
Readers are advised to check the most current information provided
i) on procedures featured or ii) by the manufacturer of each product to be
administered, to verify the recommended dose or formula, the method and
duration of administration, and contraindications. It is the responsibility
of the practitioner, relying on his or her own experience and knowledge
of the patient, to make diagnoses, to determine dosages and the best
treatment for each individual patient, and to take all appropriate safety
precautions. To the fullest extent of the law, neither the Publisher nor the
Authors assumes any liability for any injury and/or damage to persons or
property arising from or related to any use of the material contained in
this book.

ISBN-13: 978-1-4160-0143-0
ISBN-10: 1-4160-0143-3

Acquisitions Editor: Catherine Albright Jackson
Senior Developmental Editor: Laurie K. Gower
Publishing Services Manager: Jeff Patterson
Project Manager: Anne Konopka
Cover Design: Teresa McBryan
Interior Design Direction: Paula Ruckenbrod

Working together to grow
libraries in developing countries

www.elsevier.com | www.bookaid.org | www.sabre.org

ELSEVIER BOOK AID International Sabre Foundation

Printed in the United States of America

Last digit is the print number: 9 8 7 6 5 4 3 2

Preface

PURPOSE

This Clinical Companion was written for nursing students and practicing nurses. Its handy size makes it a portable reference book that can easily be carried to the clinical area where information that relates to hands-on practice is most useful. Although the authors briefly explain essential background information and describe expected medical interventions, the focus is on nursing assessments and interventions. This Clinical Companion complements the fourth edition of *Foundations of Maternal-Newborn Nursing* by Murray and McKinney but it also can be used alone by nurses who need only a review. Trula Myers Gorrie contributed to the previous edition, *Clinical Manual for Foundations of Maternal-Newborn Nursing.*

CONTENT AND ORGANIZATION

The manual is divided into seven sections. Section One provides an overview of the antepartum period. It includes a brief review of reproductive anatomy and physiology and the hereditary and environmental factors that affect care. This section briefly covers the physiologic and psychosocial adaptations to pregnancy and common complications of the antepartum period.

Section Two addresses the intrapartum period and briefly describes the components and processes of normal and complicated childbirth. Intrapartum nursing care, including pain management and support for the family during labor, is outlined.

Section Three outlines adaptation of the normal newborn and presents necessary nursing assessments and care. In addition, this section addresses therapeutic management and nursing considerations of the most common complications of the neonatal period.

Section Four briefly describes adaptations and nursing care required during normal and complicated postpartum periods. Major areas of concern include teaching self care and infant care, including nutrition of the infant.

Section Five deals with women's health care as well as reproductive issues such as family planning and infertility. Health maintenance is emphasized, as well as the most common benign and malignant disorders of the woman's reproductive system.

Section Six presents step-by-step guides for some of the most common procedures in maternal-newborn nursing and drug guides for specific medications.

Section Seven provides drug guides for medications that are commonly given for women during pregnancy and childbearing and for newborns. Drugs used for pain relief during the intrapartum period are summarized in a table.

Three appendices are included in this Clinical Companion. Appendix A includes normal laboratory values for tests that are often done during the childbearing or nonpregnancy periods. Appendix B provides similar information for laboratory values during the newborn period. Appendix C provides one table containing basic information about the safety and effectiveness of drugs that may be used during pregnancy or lactation. A second table in Appendix C provides information about the use of botanical or herbal preparations including the known risks for use during pregnancy and lactation and in women's health.

Acknowledgments

The Clinical Companion was a group effort and we sincerely thank several people at Saunders. Catherine Jackson, Acquisitions Editor, was always available and encouraging. Laurie Gower, Senior Developmental Editor, assisted the authors to improve organization and contents of the companion book to accompany *Foundations of Maternal-Newborn Nursing,* 4th edition and kept the project moving.

Sharon Smith Murray
Professor, Health Professions
Golden West College
Huntington Beach, California

Emily Slone McKinney
Baylor Healthcare System
Dallas, Texas

Trula Myers Gorrie
Professor Emeritus
Golden West College
Huntington Beach, California

Contents

Section 1

Antepartum

REPRODUCTIVE ANATOMY AND PHYSIOLOGY
SEXUAL DEVELOPMENT
Prenatal Development
- Genetic sex determination.
  - Fertilizing spermatozoon bears an X chromosome: female results
  - Fertilizing spermatozoon bears a Y chromosome: male results
- Reproductive systems of males and females are undifferentiated during the first 6 weeks of prenatal life.
- As the prenatal female's ovaries secrete estrogen, female internal sex organs and external genitalia develop.
- As the prenatal male's testes secrete testosterone, male internal sex organs and external genitalia develop.
- After birth, the sex glands of females and males are quiet until puberty because the hypothalamus suppresses any estrogen or testosterone secreted.

Sexual Maturation. Puberty, the time when reproductive organs become fully functional, begins in late childhood and early adolescence. Puberty includes development of:

- Primary sex characteristics, such as development of ova in the female's ovaries and sperm in the male's testes.
- Secondary sex characteristics, such as development of the breasts in the female and growth of facial and chest hair in the male.

Initiation of Sexual Maturation
- Hypothalamus allows increasing secretion of estrogen and testosterone; sex organs mature.

- Hypothalamus secretes more gonadotropin-releasing hormone (GnRH), which stimulates the anterior pituitary to release its hormones.
- Anterior pituitary secretes:
  — Follicle-stimulating hormone (FSH).
  — Luteinizing hormone (LH).
- FSH and LH, in turn, stimulate:
  — Ovaries to develop ova and secrete sex hormones, primarily estrogens and progesterone.
  — Male testes to develop sperm and secrete sex hormones, primarily testosterone.

Female Puberty
- Ovaries secrete estrogen and progesterone, causing other puberty changes.
- Breasts exhibit the earliest signs of sexual maturation.
  — Nipples enlarge and protrude.
  — Glandular tissue and milk ducts grow and develop.
- Fat deposits increase in the hips and breasts.
- Height increases at about the time of breast development.
- Bony pelvis widens.
- Pubic and axillary hair appears.
- Internal sexual organs and the external genitalia mature.
- Menarche (first menstrual period) occurs about 2 to 3 years after breast development begins.

Male Puberty
- Testes secrete testosterone, causing other puberty changes.
- Testes grow, followed by growth and lengthening of the penis.
- Nocturnal emissions ("wet dreams") occur.
- Pubic, axillary, facial, and chest hair appears.
- Muscle mass increases.
- Height increases. The male growth spurt begins later than the female's, but lasts longer, resulting in a greater average male height at maturity.
- Voice deepens

Decline in Fertility. Female produces less estrogen, gradually ceases to produce ova, and has her last menstrual
period (menopause) in her late 40s to early 50s. Males have
a gradual decline in testosterone and sperm production, but
no distinct marker such as menopause.

FEMALE REPRODUCTIVE ANATOMY
EXTERNAL FEMALE REPRODUCTIVE ORGANS

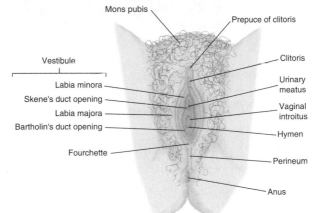

Figure 1-1 External female reproductive structures.

INTERNAL FEMALE REPRODUCTIVE ORGANS

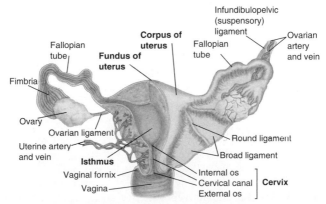

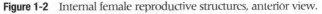

Figure 1-2 Internal female reproductive structures, anterior view.

- Vagina: Tube of muscular and membranous tissue that connects the uterus with the exterior
- Uterus: Muscular organ that houses and nourishes the developing baby, then contracts to expel the fetus during labor; has three divisions and three layers
  - Divisions of the uterus
    - Corpus: Upper body of the uterus; the *fundus* is the part above where the fallopian tubes enter
    - Isthmus: Narrower zone between the corpus (above) and the cervix (below)
    - Cervix: Tubular "neck" of the uterus, about 2 to 3 cm long
- Layers of the uterus
  - Perimetrium: Outer layer that covers most of the uterus
  - Myometrium: Thick muscular layer containing three types of muscle fibers
    - Longitudinal fibers are found mostly in the fundus; they contract during labor to expel the fetus.

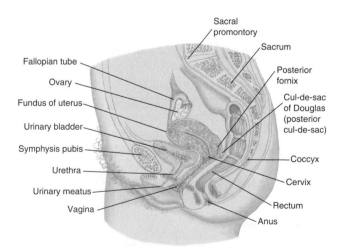

Figure 1-3 Internal female reproductive structures, midsagittal view.

- – Interlacing fibers in the middle layer contract around bleeding vessels after placental separation to control blood loss.
- – Circular fibers surround the entry point of the fallopian tubes and the internal cervical os to prevent reflux of menstrual products into the tubes and to retain the fetus until the time of birth.
- — Endometrium: Inner layer of the uterus that responds to cyclic variations of estrogen and progesterone during the female reproductive cycle
- Fallopian tubes: Pathway to allow the ovum released from the ovary to reach the uterus
- Ovaries: Female gonads, or sex glands
  - — Produce female sex hormones
  - — Mature an ovum during each female reproductive cycle

FEMALE SUPPORT STRUCTURES

- Pelvis: Group of bones at the end of the spine, forming a "basin"; the lower pelvis (below the linea terminalis) is the most important in childbirth.
- Muscles: Paired muscles provide support for pelvic organs.
  - — Levator ani muscles: Pubococcygeus, also called *pubovaginal, puborectal,* and *iliococcygeus* muscles, support internal pelvic structures and resist increases in intraabdominal pressure
  - — Ischiocavernosus muscles: Extend from the clitoris to the ischial tuberosities
  - — Transverse perineal muscles: Extend from perineum to the ischial tuberosities
- Ligaments: Paired ligaments stabilize the internal reproductive organs.
  - — Broad ligaments extend from each side of the uterus to the lateral pelvic walls. Blood vessels, lymphatics, and the ovarian ligaments lie within each broad ligament.
  - — Cardinal ligaments extend from the side walls of the cervix and vagina to the side walls of the pelvis.
  - — Ovarian ligaments connect the ovaries to the lateral uterine walls.

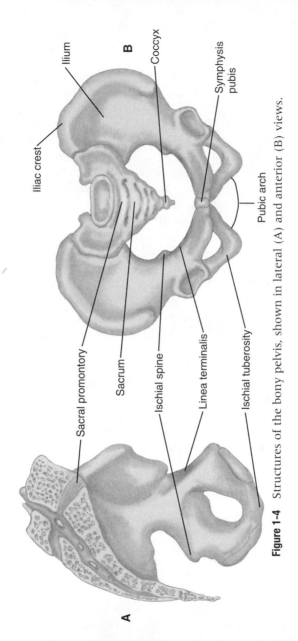

Figure 1-4 Structures of the bony pelvis, shown in lateral (A) and anterior (B) views.

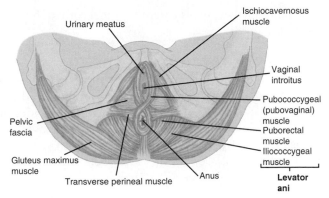

Figure 1-5 Muscles of the female pelvic floor.

— Infundibulopelvic (suspensory) ligaments connect the lateral ovary and distal fallopian tubes to the pelvic side walls.

— Round ligaments connect the upper uterus to the connective tissue of the labia majora to maintain the uterus in the normal anteflexed position.

— Pubocervical ligaments connect the cervix to the interior surface of the symphysis pubis.

— Uterosacral ligaments support the posterior uterus by connecting it with the sacrum.

BLOOD SUPPLY

- Uterus
  — Uterine arteries branch from the internal iliac artery.
  — Uterine veins drain into the internal iliac veins.
- Ovaries
  — Ovarian arteries branch from the abdominal aorta.
  — Left ovarian vein drains into the left renal vein.
  — Right ovarian vein drains into the inferior vena cava.

NERVE SUPPLY

Functions of the reproductive system are controlled by the autonomic nervous system. Sensory and motor nerves for the reproductive organs enter the spinal cord at the T-12 through L-2 levels.

FEMALE REPRODUCTIVE CYCLE

The female reproductive cycle involves regular and recurrent changes in the anterior pituitary hormones, which, in turn, cause cyclic changes in the ovaries, the uterine endometrium, and the cervical mucus. The cycle averages 28 days, with a range of 20 to 45 days. Significant variations from regular 28-day cycles are associated with reduced fertility.

OVARIAN CYCLE

- GnRH from the hypothalamus causes a woman's anterior pituitary to secrete FSH and LH, which stimulate maturation of an ovum and preparation of the uterine endometrium for implantation of a fertilized ovum.
- Follicular phase: The time during which an ovum matures, beginning with the first day of the menstrual period and ending about 14 days later. Several ovarian follicles begin maturation, but one outgrows the others.
- Ovulation: A surge of LH about 2 days before ovulation, accompanied by a slight decrease in estrogen, causes full maturation of one ovum within its follicle. The ovum is released from the surface of the ovary and is picked up by the fringed (fimbriated) end of the fallopian tube.
- Luteal phase: LH causes cells from the old follicle (corpus luteum) to persist for about 12 days and secrete large amounts of estrogen and progesterone to enrich the uterine lining in preparation for a fertilized ovum. If fertilization does not occur, the corpus luteum regresses and the woman has her menstrual period.

ENDOMETRIAL CYCLE

The endometrial cycle also consists of three phases.

- Proliferative phase: The endometrium proliferates, and endometrial glands and tiny endometrial spiral arteries and endometrial veins grow; it lasts about the first 14 days of the cycle.

- Secretory phase: The endometrium further thickens, and substances are secreted to nourish a fertilized ovum; it lasts about 12 days after ovulation.
- Menstrual phase: Occurs when the corpus luteum regresses because an ovum was not fertilized. Vasospasm of endometrial vessels occurs, causing the endometrium to become ischemic and necrotic, resulting in the menstrual period.

CERVICAL MUCUS

- During most of the female reproductive cycle, the cervical mucus is thick and sticky.
- Near ovulation, it becomes clear, thin, and elastic to promote passage of sperm into the uterus and fallopian tubes to promote fertilization.

FEMALE BREAST

- Nipple: Sensitive erectile tissue that responds to sexual stimulation; it and the areola are more darkly pigmented than surrounding skin.

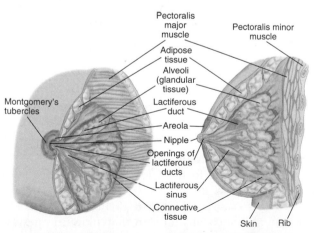

Figure 1-6 Structures of the female breast.

- Areola: Flattened area surrounding the nipple that contains Montgomery's tubercles, which secrete a moisturizing substance during pregnancy and lactation.
- Glandular tissue: Arranged like spokes of a wheel around a hub. Fifteen to 20 lobes comprise the glandular tissue.
- Alveoli: Small sacs that secrete milk, which drains into the lactiferous ducts.
- Lactiferous sinuses: Widened portions of each duct that lie under the areola.

MALE REPRODUCTIVE ANATOMY AND PHYSIOLOGY
EXTERNAL MALE REPRODUCTIVE ORGANS

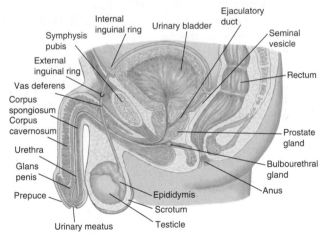

Figure 1-7   Structures of the male reproductive system, midsagittal view.

- Penis: An organ containing erectile tissue
  — Deposits sperm in the female's vagina during sexual intercourse
  — Provides passage for urine to drain from the bladder
- Scrotum: A pouch of thin skin that allows the testes to remain cooler than the core body temperature, promoting proper sperm production

INTERNAL MALE REPRODUCTIVE ORGANS

- Testes have two functions.
  - — Secretion of male sex hormones, primarily testosterone, within the *Leydig cells*.
  - — Production and maturation of sperm within the seminiferous tubules; *Sertoli cells* nourish and support sperm during maturation.
- Accessory ducts and glands
  - — Epididymis carries sperm into the vas deferens, which joins the ejaculatory duct before it then joins the urethra.
  - — The seminal vesicles, prostate, and bulbourethral glands secrete seminal fluid.
    - – Nourish sperm
    - – Protect sperm from the acidic environment of the female's vagina
    - – Enhance the motility of sperm
    - – Wash all sperm out of the urethra to ensure that the maximum number are available for fertilization

GENETIC AND ENVIRONMENTAL INFLUENCES ON CHILDBEARING
CHROMOSOMES

- There are 46 paired chromosomes in the nucleus of each somatic (body) cell, other than mature erythrocytes, which do not have a nucleus.
- There are 23 single chromosomes in every germ cell (sperm or ovum).
- Studied by analyzing living cells.
  - — White blood cells
  - — Skin fibroblasts
  - — Bone marrow cells
  - — Fetal cells from chorionic villi or amniotic fluid
- Care of specimens for chromosome analysis
  - — No temperature extremes
  - — Blood should not clot
  - — Only approved preservatives

- The chromosome analysis is abbreviated by a combination of numbers and letters.
  — First number: The total number of chromosomes
  — Sex chromosomes: XY (male) or XX (female)
  — Normal male: 46, XY
  — Normal female: 46, XX
  — Additional notations describe any abnormalities, for example, Down syndrome female: 47, XX, +21 (the extra chromosome that is present in each body cell)
- Chromosome abnormalities
  — Numerical
    – Trisomy: Entire single chromosome added in each body cell, for example, trisomy 21 (Down syndrome)
    – Monosomy: Entire single chromosome missing in each body cell, for example, monosomy X (Turner's syndrome)
    – Polyploidy: One or more added full sets of chromosomes
  — Structural
    – Part of a chromosome missing or added in each body cell
    – Rearrangements of material within a chromosome
    – Two abnormally joined chromosomes

SINGLE GENE INHERITANCE

- Autosomal dominant traits
  — Characteristics
    – Single copy of the gene can produce the trait.
    – Males and females are equally likely to have the trait.
    – Often appear in every generation of a family, but people who have the trait may have widely varying manifestations
    – May have multiple and seemingly unrelated effects on body structure and function
  — Transmission of trait from parent to child
    – Parent with the trait has a 50% (1 in 2) chance of passing the trait to a child.

- Trait may arise as a new mutation from an unaffected parent
- Autosomal recessive traits
  - Characteristics
    - Two autosomal recessive genes are required to produce the trait.
    - Males and females are equally likely to have the trait.
    - If multiple family members are affected, they are usually full siblings.
    - Consanguinity (blood relationship) of the parents increases the likelihood that the trait will appear.
    - Disorders are more likely to occur in groups isolated by geography, culture, religion, or other factors.
    - Some autosomal recessive disorders are more common in specific ethnic groups.
  - Transmission of trait from parent to child
    - Unaffected parents carry an abnormal recessive trait.
    - Each child of two carrier parents has a:
      - 25% (1 in 4) chance of receiving both copies of the defective gene and having the disorder.
      - 50% (1 in 2) chance of receiving only one copy of the defective gene and being a carrier like the parents.
      - 25% (1 in 4) chance of receiving two normal genes and being neither a carrier nor affected.
- X-linked recessive traits
  - Characteristics
    - Gene for the trait is carried on the X chromosome
    - One copy is enough to produce the trait in a male because males have a single X chromosome, with no compensating X that does not have the trait.
    - Females carry the trait, but usually are not adversely affected.
    - Affected males are related to each other through carrier females.
    - Affected males do not transmit the trait to their sons because they give the Y chromosome to a son.

— Transmission of trait from parent to child
  – Males who have the disorder transmit the gene to 100% of their daughters.
  – Sons of carrier females have a:
    - 50% (1 in 2) chance of being affected.
    - 50% chance of being unaffected.
  – Daughters of carrier females have a:
    - 50% (1 in 2) chance of being carriers.
    - 50% of being neither affected nor carriers.
  – An abnormal X-linked recessive gene may also arise by mutation.

MULTIFACTORIAL DISORDERS

- These disorders result from an interaction among genetic factors and environmental influence.
- Characteristics
  — Present and detectable at birth
  — Usually single, isolated defects, although the primary defect can cause secondary defects
- Risks of occurrence or recurrence vary. Factors that can alter the risk are:
  — Number of affected close relatives.
  — Severity of the disorder in affected family members.
  — Sex of affected person(s).
  — Geographic location.
  — Seasonal variations.
- Infants who have several major and/or minor defects that are not directly related probably *do not* have a multifactorial defect, but have another syndrome, such as a chromosome abnormality.

TERATOGENS

- Environmental agents that may harm the fetus include:
  — Maternal infectious agents.
  — Drugs and other substances, including therapeutic agents, illicit drugs, tobacco, and alcohol.
  — Pollutants, chemicals, and other substances.
  — Ionizing radiation.

— Maternal hyperthermia.
— Effects of maternal disorders such as diabetes mellitus or phenylketonuria.
- Avoiding fetal exposure to teratogens
  — Avoid maternal immunization for infections such as rubella at least 28 days (1 month) before pregnancy. Immunization during the immediate postpartum period is offered to nonimmune women.
  — Avoid situations that are more likely to result in infection.
  — Avoid all unnecessary drugs, or use the least harmful drug that will have the desired effect.
  — Stop smoking.
  — Ingest no alcohol.
  — Avoid high-heat areas such as hot tubs or saunas.
  — Delay nonurgent radiologic procedures until the first 2 weeks after the menstrual period begins.
  — Maintain proper diet and drug therapy for metabolic conditions such as diabetes or phenylketonuria.
- Maintain adequate folic acid intake at 400 mcg before conception and continue during pregnancy. Increased doses may be recommended for the fetus with a higher risk for neural tube defect.

PRENATAL DEVELOPMENT
PRE-EMBRYONIC PERIOD
- The first 2 days of development occur in the fallopian tube. The zygote enters the uterus by 4 days after conception.
- Implantation begins about 6 days after conception and is complete on the 10th day, usually in the uterine fundus.
- The zygote secretes human chorionic gonadotropin (hCG) to signal the woman's body that a pregnancy has begun, allowing uninterrupted estrogen and progesterone secretion from the corpus luteum to maintain the uterine endometrium until the placenta takes over secretion.

EMBRYONIC PERIOD
- The embryonic period extends from the beginning of the third week through the eighth week after conception.

- The embryo is vulnerable to damage from teratogens at this time because all organ systems are developing rapidly.

FETAL PERIOD

- The fetal period begins 9 weeks after conception and ends with birth.
- Growth and refinement of all systems occur.
- Teratogens may damage already formed structures, but are less likely to cause major structural damage. The central nervous system is vulnerable to damage during the entire pregnancy, however.
- During prenatal development, the relative proportions of body segments change. At 9 weeks, the head is about 50% of the total fetal length and has the largest circumference compared with the circumferences of the chest or abdomen. At 38 weeks, the head is about 25% of the total fetal length, and the head and abdominal circumferences are about equal.

TIMETABLE OF PRENATAL DEVELOPMENT

This timetable is based on *fertilization age*, about 2 weeks less than the *gestational age*, which is based on the woman's last menstrual period. CRL = crown-rump length

3 WEEKS (1.5 mm [0.06 Inch] CRL)

- Heart consists of two parallel tubes that begin beating.
- Three germ layers that will evolve into all body tissues develop.

4 WEEKS (4 mm [0.16 Inch] CRL)

- Neural tube (future brain and spinal cord) closes. Failure to close results in defects such as anencephaly or spina bifida.
- Eyes begin as an outgrowth of the forebrain.
- Heart tubes begin partitioning into four chambers; complete by 6 weeks.
- Upper limbs are like flippers. Lower limb buds appear.

6 WEEKS (13 mm [0.52 Inch] CRL)
- Ears begin developing in the neck.
- Lung lobes (3 right and 2 left) develop.
- Most of the intestines are in the umbilical cord.
- Male and female gonads look identical.
- Fingers are webbed; feet develop slightly later.
- Primary tooth buds begin.

8 WEEKS (30 mm [1.2 Inches] CRL)
- Ears have their final form, but are still low-set.
- Heartbeat can be detected with ultrasound.
- Male and female genitalia begin to look different.

10 WEEKS (61 mm [2.4 Inches] CRL; WEIGHT 14 g [0.5 oz])
- Intestines are now contained within the abdominal cavity.
- All parts of digestive tract are connected and patent from mouth to anus.
- Male and female genitalia are more differentiated, but still easily confused.
- Fingernails begin development.
- Tooth buds for permanent teeth form below those for primary teeth.

12 WEEKS (87 mm [3.5 Inches] CRL; WEIGHT 45 g [1.6 oz])
- Nose and mouth are developed; palate is intact.
- Sucking reflex is present.
- Male and female genitalia can be distinguished easily.
- Lanugo hair appears.
- Heartbeat detectable with Doppler.

16 WEEKS (140 mm [5.6 Inches] CRL; WEIGHT 200 g [7 oz])
- Lungs and pulmonary circulation are developing rapidly.
- Fetus swallows amniotic fluid and produces meconium in intestinal tract.
- Urine is excreted into amniotic fluid.
- Woman may begin to feel movement.
- Fingerprints are developing.

20 WEEKS (160 mm [6.4 Inches] CRL; WEIGHT 460 g [ABOUT 1 lb])

- Myelination of nerves begins and continues through the first year after birth.
- Heartbeat is detectable with fetoscope.
- Testes begin descent toward scrotum in males. Follicles of ovary begin developing in females.
- Mother feels fetal movements, and they may be palpable to the observer.
- Skin is covered with vernix.

24 WEEKS (230 mm [9.2 Inches] CRL; WEIGHT 820 g [1.8 lb])

- Surfactant production begins in the lungs.
- Fetal activity more noticeable to woman.
- Fingerprints and footprints developed.
- Brows and lashes present.

28 WEEKS (270 mm [10.8 Inches] CRL; WEIGHT 1300 g [About 3 lb])

- Erythrocyte production shifts completely to bone marrow.
- Sufficient alveoli, capillary network, and surfactant allow respiratory function, although respiratory distress syndrome is common in infants born at this time.
- Skin becomes smoother as subcutaneous fat is deposited.

32 WEEKS (300 mm [12 Inches] CRL; WEIGHT 2100 g [4.7 lb])

- Testes enter the scrotum.
- Fingernails reach fingertips.
- Lanugo is disappearing.

38 WEEKS (360 mm CRL [14.4 Inches]; 3400 g [7.6 lb])

- Testes are palpable in scrotum.
- Fetus has plump appearance with smooth skin.
- Vernix remains only in creases.
- Lanugo on upper back and shoulders.

- Fingernails extend beyond fingertips.
- Ear cartilage is firm.

AUXILIARY STRUCTURES
PLACENTA

- Maternal component
  — Eighty to 100 spiral arteries arise from the uterine lining and carry oxygenated and nutrient-bearing blood into the intervillous spaces.
  — Endometrial veins drain deoxygenated blood and waste products from the placenta.
- Fetal component: Chorionic villi are tiny projections into the intervillous space that contain a fetal artery and vein to release waste products and pick up oxygen and nutrients from maternal blood.
- Theoretically, fetal and maternal blood do not mix within the placenta.

UMBILICAL CORD

- Two arteries carry deoxygenated blood and waste products to the placenta.
- One vein carries oxygenated blood and nutrients to the fetus.
- Wharton's jelly cushions the cord vessels.

FETAL MEMBRANES AND AMNIOTIC FLUID

- Two membranes contain the amniotic fluid and provide some barrier against infection.
  — Amnion (inner membrane)
  — Chorion (outer membrane)
- Functions of amniotic fluid are to:
  — Cushion fetus against impacts to the maternal abdomen.
  — Maintain stable temperature.
  — Allow symmetrical development.
  — Keep the membranes from adhering to the developing fetus.
  — Allow room and buoyancy for fetal movement.

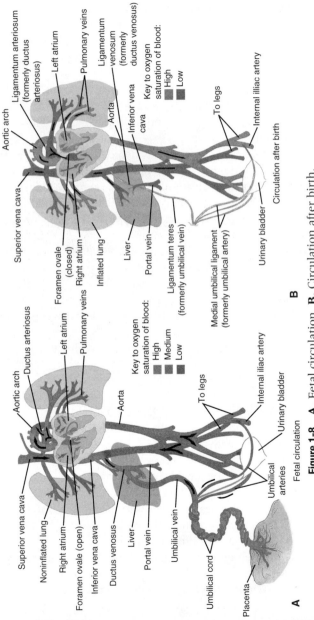

Figure 1-8 **A,** Fetal circulation. **B,** Circulation after birth.

ANTEPARTUM ADAPTATION
OVERVIEW
The average duration of pregnancy, based on the menstrual cycle, is 40 weeks or 280 days. The date on which the baby is expected, called the estimated date of delivery (EDD) or estimated date of birth (EDB), is calculated from the first day of the last menstrual period (LMP).

TERMS TO REMEMBER
- Gravida: A woman who is or has been pregnant, regardless of duration or outcome
- Multigravida: A woman who has been pregnant more than once
- Multipara: A woman who has given birth more than once at 20 or more weeks of gestation
- Nullipara: A woman who has never completed a pregnancy beyond a spontaneous or elective abortion
- Para: Number of pregnancies that reach 20 or more weeks of gestation at delivery, whether the infant is born alive or dead; refers to the number of pregnancies, not the number of fetuses
- Primigravida: A woman who is pregnant for the first time
- Primipara: A woman who has given birth once after a pregnancy of at least 20 weeks
- Trimester: Division of pregnancy into time segments of about 13 weeks

PHYSIOLOGIC ADAPTATIONS TO PREGNANCY
Although the greatest changes occur in the reproductive system, all body systems must adapt to pregnancy (Table 1-1).

DIAGNOSIS OF PREGNANCY
The diagnosis of pregnancy is based on presumptive indications (subjective signs observed by the woman), probable indications (objective signs observed by examiner), and positive indications (those that can be caused only by pregnancy).

Text continued on p. 28

Table 1-1	Physiologic Adaptations to Pregnancy

Significant Changes	Reasons for Changes
	Reproductive System
	Uterus
Grows in a predictable pattern (see Figure 1-9). Note that uterine height is lower at 40 weeks than at 36 weeks.	Hypertrophy and hyperplasia occur and the muscle fibers stretch in all directions to accommodate the growing fetus. The fetal head drops into the pelvis near term, resulting in less pressure on the diaphragm (lightening) and easier breathing.
	Cervix and Vagina
Become bluish purple (Chadwick's sign) and softer (Goodell's sign). Mucus plug forms in cervix.	Tissue is congested with blood, and connective tissue softens as collagen fibers become less concentrated. Cervical mucus increases as cervical glands proliferate.
	Ovaries
Corpus luteum secretes progesterone until the placenta is developed. Ovulation ceases.	Adequate progesterone is necessary to maintain pregnancy. Placenta secretes high levels of estrogen and progesterone, inhibiting follicle-stimulating and luteinizing hormones.

Breasts

Increase in size and become highly vascular. Nipples become larger and more pigmented; tubercles of Montgomery become more prominent; colostrum is often present by the second trimester.

Estrogen and progesterone promote growth of mammary ducts and lobes; tubercles of Montgomery secrete a substance that lubricates the nipples.

Cardiovascular System

Blood Volume

Plasma increases by about 50% over prepregnancy level.

Increased plasma is needed to transport nutrients and oxygen to the placenta and expanded maternal tissue and to compensate for blood lost at childbirth.

Red blood cells (RBCs) increase 25%-33%.

Extra RBCs are needed to carry oxygen; increase is less and occurs later than that in plasma volume, resulting in hemodilution and the physiologic anemia of pregnancy.

Leukocytes (white blood cells or WBCs) increase up to 12,000/mm³ and up to 25,000 in labor.

WBCs increase during pregnancy and as a result of exertion during labor.

Blood pressure remains within normal limits.

Peripheral vascular resistance decreases due to progesterone, vasodilation, the uteroplacental unit, and prostaglandins causing maternal resistance to vasoconstrictors.

Clotting factors (especially fibrin and fibrinogen) increase. Fibrinolytic activity decreases.

Clotting factors increase to prevent postpartum hemorrhage, but also increase the risk of thrombus formation.

Continued

Table 1-1	Physiologic Adaptations to Pregnancy—cont'd
Significant Changes	**Reasons for Changes**
	Respiratory System
The ribs flare, the substernal angle widens, and the chest circumference expands. Some women experience shortness of breath in late pregnancy.	Tidal volume (air exchanged in quiet respirations) increases. Progesterone causes decreased airway resistance and slight hyperventilation with mild alkalosis. The uterus lifts the diaphragm and limits lung expansion.
	Gastrointestinal System
The gums become hyperemic and bleed easily. Gastrointestinal tone and motility decrease, causing heartburn, bloating, abdominal distention, and constipation.	These effects are due to elevated levels of estrogen. Progesterone relaxes all smooth muscles; the enlarging uterus displaces the stomach and intestines.
Bile becomes thicker, which predisposes to formation of gallstones.	The gallbladder is hypotonic and emptying time is decreased as a result of progesterone.
	Urinary System
Urinary frequency and urgency.	These effects are from pressure of the uterus on the bladder, hormones, and glomerular filtration increases.

The woman is at increased risk for urinary tract infection; nocturia may occur.

Progesterone causes stasis of urine and increased capacity of bladder and ureters resulting from decreased muscle tone. Sodium and water are excreted more during the night.

Integumentary System

Activity of the sweat and sebaceous glands increases; acne; diaphoresis. Increased pigmentation such as melasma and linea nigra.

Activity is encouraged by the increased circulation to the skin. Pigmentation from estrogen, progesterone, and elevated melanocyte-stimulating hormone.

Striae gravidarum ("stretch marks") may develop on breasts, buttocks, abdomen.

Due to linear tears in connective tissue; fade to silvery lines after childbirth.

Musculoskeletal System

Softening of pelvic cartilage and connective tissue, resulting in wide stance, waddling gait, and lordosis.

The hormones relaxin and progesterone cause softening; increasing uterine size forces the woman to lean backward to maintain her balance.

Abdominal wall muscles separate (diastasis recti).

This occurs when muscles are stretched beyond their capacity in the third trimester.

Endocrine System

Pituitary

Follicle stimulating hormone and luteinizing hormone are suppressed.

Suppression is due to high levels of estrogen and progesterone during pregnancy.

Continued

Table 1-1	Physiologic Adaptations to Pregnancy—cont'd
Significant Changes	**Reasons for Changes**
Prolactin is released from the anterior pituitary. Oxytocin from the posterior pituitary induces uterine contractions and the milk-ejection reflex.	Prolactin prepares the breasts for lactation. This action is inhibited by high levels of progesterone during pregnancy.
	Thyroid
Total thyroxine increases, slight increase in size of thyroid; basal metabolic rate increases up to 25%.	Hyperplasia and increased vascularity increases size. Increased basal metabolic rate results from fetal metabolic activity.
	Parathyroid
Parathyroid hormone level low normal or slightly decreased.	Level remains high enough for stable calcium levels to meet fetal and maternal needs.
	Pancreas
Hypoglycemia may occur; insulin production increases in second half of pregnancy.	Continuous fetal draw of glucose may cause hypoglycemia; human placental lactogen, prolactin, estrogen, progesterone,

and cortisol cause resistance of maternal cells to insulin and increased insulin production.

Adrenal Glands

Cortisol increases.	Result of estrogen and decreased metabolism of cortisol; necessary for accelerated protein and carbohydrate metabolism.
Aldosterone increases.	Increase overcomes the salt-wasting effects of pregnancy and maintains expanded blood volume.

Placental Hormones

Human chorionic gonadotropin (hCG) is produced by trophoblastic cells and causes positive pregnancy tests.	hCG maintains the corpus luteum, which produces progesterone during the first weeks of pregnancy.
Estrogen level increases.	Estrogen stimulates uterine and breast development, increases blood to the uterus, and causes hyperpigmentation.
Progesterone level increases.	Progesterone maintains uterine lining, relaxes all smooth muscles, promotes fa- deposits, and helps prepare the breasts for lactation.
Human placental lactogen is produced.	Human placental lactogen (hPL) increases glucose for the fetus by being antagonistic to insulin; stimulates metabolism of fatty acids for energy.
Relaxin is produced by the corpus luteum and placenta	Relaxin softers muscles and joints of the pelvis, inhibits uterine activity, and softens cervical tissue.

Text continued from p. 21

PRESUMPTIVE INDICATIONS
- Amenorrhea
- Nausea and vomiting
- Fatigue
- Urinary frequency
- Breast and skin changes
- Cervical color changes
- Quickening

PROBABLE INDICATIONS
- Abdominal enlargement
- Cervical softening
- Changes in the uterus (consistency, ballottement, Braxton Hicks contractions, palpation of fetal outline)
- Pregnancy tests, based on detection of human chorionic gonadotropin in blood or urine

POSITIVE INDICATIONS
- Auscultation of fetal heartbeat
- Fetal movement felt by examiner
- Visualization by ultrasound

ESTIMATED DATE OF DELIVERY (EDD)

Nägele's rule is used to compute EDD. Subtract 3 months and add 7 days to the first day of the last normal menstrual period (LNMP), and correct the year.

> For example: LMP June 30, 2006
> Subtract 3 months = March 30, 2006
> Add 7 days = April 6, 2006
> Correct the year = April 6, 2007

A pregnancy wheel may also be used. Ultrasound performed early in pregnancy can accurately determine gestational age.

PSYCHOSOCIAL ADAPTATIONS

Psychosocial adaptations to pregnancy occur gradually as the focus shifts from the self to the fetus as a separate, though entirely dependent, human (Table 1-2).

Table 1-2	**Psychosocial Adaptations to Pregnancy**	
First Trimester	**Second Trimester**	**Third Trimester**
Emotional Response		
Uncertainty, ambivalence, focus on self, emotional lability	Increased focus on fetus, narcissistic, introverted, concerned about changes in her body and sexuality	Vulnerability, increased dependence; acceptance that fetus is separate but totally dependent
Physical Validation		
Little change in body contour or size; no obvious signs of fetal growth; ultrasound may be performed	Enlarging abdomen, quickening, audible fetal heart rate, ultrasound of fetus	Obvious fetal growth, discomfort, decreased maternal activity
Role		
Seeks "safe passage" for self and fetus by prenatal care, cultural expectations	Seeks acceptance of the fetus and her role as mother from family and significant others	Prepares for birth; internalizes a view of how a "good" mother behaves and sets up expectations for self
"Self" Statement		
"I am pregnant."	"I am going to have a baby."	"I am going to be a mother."

INITIAL ANTEPARTAL ASSESSMENT
HISTORY

- History of family, individual, and partner with particular attention to:
  - Chronic diseases such as asthma, diabetes, hypertension, or heart disease.
  - Medications (prescribed or over the counter), complementary or alternative therapies used, chemical dependency (including tobacco or alcohol use).
  - Previous illnesses or surgeries, episodes of sexually transmitted diseases such as herpes.
  - Occupation and workplace hazards, including exposure to teratogenic substances.
  - Religious and cultural practices and influences.
- Reproductive history including:
  - Menstrual and contraceptive history.
  - Gravida, para, preterm births, living children, abortions, stillbirths.
  - Type of births (vaginal or cesarean), hours of labor, condition and weight of infant, complications of labor or postpartum.

PHYSICAL EXAMINATION

- Vital signs, including auscultation of maternal heart sounds
- Height, weight, and preconception weight
- Inspection and palpation of the breasts and abdomen
- Palpation of the fundus (Figure 1-9)
- Brachial and patellar reflexes for hyperreflexia, which suggests preeclampsia
- Pelvic examination, including external and internal genitalia, cervical cultures, Pap smear, and measurement of pelvic dimensions to estimate whether size seems adequate for vaginal birth
- Current pregnancy status including:
  - Confirmation of pregnancy by presumptive, probable, and positive signs of pregnancy.
  - Confirmation of gestational age by noting (a) abdominal enlargement; (b) measurement of fundal height

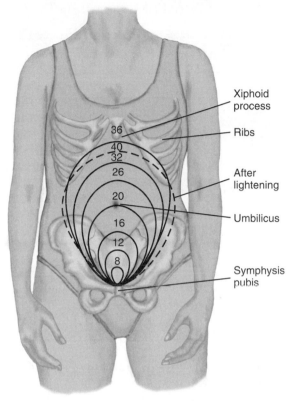

Figure 1-9 Uterine growth pattern during pregnancy.

(Figure 1-10); (c) sonography that can accurately determine fetal age early in pregnancy.

— Fetal heartbeat that can be detected with a Doppler by 10 weeks of gestation and much earlier by ultrasound examination.

— EDD based on LNMP and confirmed by fundal height or sonography.

• Antepartum laboratory screening (Table 1-3) and Appendix A.

• Nutrition assessment.

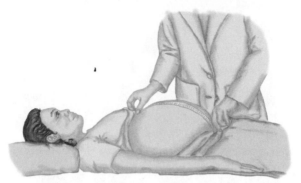

Figure 1-10   Measurement of fundal height.

PSYCHOSOCIAL ASSESSMENT

Psychosocial assessment focuses on:

- Progressive acceptance of mother (and father) of pregnancy.
- Availability of adequate resources and support system.
- Changes in sexual practices and concerns.
- Educational needs that change over time; relief of nausea and vomiting in early pregnancy, how to care for a newborn during the last weeks.
- Language barriers.
- Cultural beliefs or practices that may affect the pregnancy.

SCHEDULE OF ANTEPARTAL ASSESSMENTS

Ideally, a woman with an uncomplicated pregnancy should begin prenatal care in the first trimester and then should be evaluated every:

- 4 weeks until 28 weeks.
- 2 to 3 weeks until 36 weeks.
- 1 week thereafter until birth.

Text continued on p. 36

Table 1-3	Antepartum Tests and Procedures
Test	**Purpose**
	Initial Visit
Blood grouping	To determine blood type and Rh factor to identify possible incompatibility with the fetus
Complete blood count (CBC)	To detect infection, anemia, or cell abnormalities
Rh factor and antibody screen	For possible maternal-fetal blood incompatibility
Indirect Coombs'	Performed if mother is Rh-negative and father is Rh-positive to determine if mother is sensitized; if negative, repeated at 28 weeks; if positive, repeated more often to determine rising antibody titers
Serologic test for syphilis (RPR, VDRL)	To screen for syphilis
Rubella antibody titer	To determine maternal immunity
Hemoglobin electrophoresis	To screen for sickle cell trait if client is of African-American descent
Hepatitis B screen.	To detect presence of antigens in maternal blood
Human immunodeficiency virus (HIV) screen	Voluntary test encouraged at first visit to detect HIV antibodies
Tuberculin skin test	To screen for tuberculosis
Urinalysis	To detect renal disease or infection; testing for presence of protein, glucose, ketones, and bacteria repeated throughout pregnancy; culture performed if infection is suspected

Continued

Table 1-3	Antepartum Tests and Procedures—cont'd
Test	**Purpose**
Papanicolaou (Pap) test	To screen for cervical neoplasia
Cervical culture	To detect sexually transmitted diseases such as gonorrhea and chlamydia
	Subsequent Tests
Multiple marker screen (16-18 weeks): maternal serum alpha-fetoprotein, human chorionic gonadotropin (hCG), and estriol; may include other tests such as inhibin A	Abnormal results may indicate neural tube defects or chromosomal defects; if abnormal, additional tests, such as amniotic fluid alpha-fetoprotein or amniocentesis for other diagnostic purposes may be recommended.
Hemoglobin (Hgb) or hematocrit (Hct)	To detect anemia; often checked several times during pregnancy
50-g glucose challenge test (24-28 weeks)	To screen for gestational diabetes (<140 mg/dL generally considered normal; some use a lower level)
3-hour 100-g glucose tolerance test	Recommended if glucose screening test levels are 140 mg/dL or greater
Cervical culture for group B *Streptococcus*	Colonization in late pregnancy is treated by intrapartum chemoprophylaxis
Counting fetal movements ("kick counts")	Fetal activity indicates fetal well-being

Additional Tests for High-Risk Pregnancies

Ultrasonography (1st trimester)	To confirm pregnancy; to determine fetal number, age and viability; to identify some abnormalities; and to assess fetal growth and development
(2nd and 3rd trimesters)	To confirm fetal presentation, position, viability, and age; evaluate fetal anatomy; locate the placenta; guide other procedures, such as amniocentesis; to assess fetal movements and amount of amniotic fluid
Amniocentesis	To identify chromosomal abnormalities, determine fetal lung maturity, or to evaluate fetal condition in Rh isoimmunization
Nonstress test (NST)	To screen for fetal well-being by determining if the fetal heart accelerates normally; to be reactive or reassuring there must be two accelerations peaking at least 15 bpm above baseline, lasting 15 seconds, and occurring within 20 minutes
Vibroacoustic stimulation	To confirm nonreactive NSTs and shorten time to obtain reactive NSTs
Contraction stress test (CST)	To determine how the fetal heart responds to the stress of uterine contractions; decelerations with 50% of contractions are abnormal
Biophysical profile	Measures fetal breathing movements, gross fetal movements, fetal muscle tone, and amniotic fluid volume by ultrasonography and fetal heart rate reactivity as demonstrated by NST

Text continued from p. 32

SUBSEQUENT ANTEPARTAL ASSESSMENTS

• Vital signs

Measure blood pressure while the woman is sitting with the arm supported in a horizontal position at heart level. Use the same arm each visit and document position, pressure, and whether Korotkoff's fourth (muffling) or fifth (disappearance of sound) phase was used. Vital signs should remain near prepregnancy levels. Diastolic blood pressure may decrease slightly from 24 to 32 weeks of gestation and returns to baseline by term. Deviations should be reported.

• Weight and pattern of weight gain (see p. 44)
• Urinalysis

Test urine for protein, glucose, ketones, and bacteria.

• Fundal height

To be accurate, this measurement must be taken when the bladder is empty (see Figure 1-10). Fundal height corresponds to weeks of gestation (particularly between 16 and 38 weeks of gestation) within 3 cm. For instance, 22 cm suggests 22 weeks of gestation.

• Leopold's maneuvers

These maneuvers provide a systematic method for palpating the fetus through the abdominal wall to determine presentation and position. See Section VI, Procedure: Leopold's Maneuver, p. 437.

• Fetal heart rate

Normal parameters are 110 to 160 beats per minute.

• Fetal activity
• Signs of labor

Asking about signs of labor helps identify preterm labor and prepare the woman for the onset of labor.

HIGH-RISK FACTORS IN PREGNANCY

A *high-risk pregnancy* is defined as one in which the mother or fetus is more likely than the low-risk population to experience complications. A variety of medical, obstetric, or social factors may increase the risk to a childbearing family (Table 1-4).

Table 1-4	Summary of High-Risk Factors in Pregnancy
Factors	**Implications**
Demographic Factors	
<16 years or >35 years	Increased risk for preterm labor, preeclampsia, congenital anomalies
Low socioeconomic status or dependent on public assistance	Increased risk for preterm labor, low-birth-weight infants
Nonwhite race	Incidence of infant and maternal death higher than that of whites
Multiparity: >4 pregnancies	Increasing parity increases risk of pregnancy loss, antepartum or postpartum hemorrhage, and cesarean birth
Social-Personal Factors	
Low prepregnancy weight	Associated with low-birth-weight infants
Obesity	Increased risk for preeclampsia, difficult labor and delivery, large-for-gestational-age infant, diabetes, and cesarean birth
Height <152 cm (5 feet)	Increased incidence of cesarean birth due to cephalopelvic disproportion
Smoking	Associated with increased infant mortality, low-birth-weight infants, intrauterine growth restriction, preterm birth, preterm labor, spontaneous abortion, and placental problems
Use of alcohol or unprescribed drugs	Increased risk of congenital anomalies, neonatal withdrawal syndrome, and fetal alcohol syndrome

Continued

Table 1-4	**Summary of High-Risk Factors in Pregnancy—cont'd**

Obstetric Factors

Birth of previous infant >4000 g (8.8 lb)	Increased need for cesarean birth; increased risk for infant birth injury, neonatal hypoglycemia, and maternal gestational diabetes
Previous fetal or neonatal death	Maternal psychological distress
Rh sensitization	Fetal anemia, erythroblastosis fetalis, kernicterus

Existing Medical Conditions

Diabetes mellitus	Increased risk of preeclampsia, cesarean birth, infant either small or large for gestational age, neonatal hypoglycemia, fetal or neonatal death, congenital anomalies
Thyroid disorder Hypothyroidism	Increased incidence of spontaneous abortion, congenital anomalies, congenital hypothyroidism
Hyperthyroidism	Maternal risk of preeclampsia, thyroid storm, or postpartum hemorrhage; neonatal risk of thyrotoxicosis
Cardiac disease	Maternal risk for cardiac decompensation and increased death rate; increased risk for fetal and neonatal death
Renal disease	Maternal risk for renal failure and preterm delivery; fetal risk for intrauterine growth restriction
Concurrent infections	Severe fetal implications (heart disease, blindness, deafness, bone lesions) if maternal disease occurred in the first trimester, increased incidence of spontaneous abortion or congenital anomalies associated with some infections

Table 1-5	Danger Signs of Pregnancy

Danger Sign	Possible Cause
Vaginal bleeding with or without discomfort	Placental abnormalities, lesions of cervix or vagina, "bloody show" (sign of labor onset)
Escape of fluid from vagina	Premature rupture of membranes
Swelling of fingers or face	Excessive edema
Continuous pounding headache	Chronic hypertension or preeclampsia
Visual disturbances (blurred vision, dimness, flashing lights, spots before the eyes)	Worsening preeclampsia
Persistent or severe abdominal or epigastric pain	Ectopic pregnancy (if early), worsening preeclampsia, or abruptio placentae
Fever or chills	Infection
Painful urination	Urinary tract infection
Persistent vomiting	Hyperemesis gravidarum
Change in frequency or strength of fetal movement	Fetal compromise or death
Uterine contractions, cramps, constant or irregular low backache, pelvic pressure before 38 weeks	Preterm labor

DANGER SIGNS OF PREGNANCY

The pregnant woman and at least one other person in the family must be instructed about signs that indicate a problem that should be reported at once (Table 1-5).

NURSING INTERVENTIONS
TEACHING HEALTH PROMOTION

- Bathing
  — Recommend daily showers or tub baths; caution the woman to take precautions to prevent falls during the third trimester, when her balance has changed.
  — Suggest avoiding hyperthermia especially in early pregnancy because it is associated with fetal anomalies. She should stay in a hot tub no more than 10 minutes and

keep her head and chest out of the water; a sauna no more than 15 minutes.

- Douching
  — Emphasize that there is no hygienic need for douching, despite increased vaginal discharge.
  — Explain that douching increases the risk of infection and preterm labor.
- Breast care
  — Instruct the woman to wash her breasts and nipples with clear water and to avoid soap that removes the natural lubricant.
  — Advise her to wear a good support bra with wide straps that distribute the weight evenly across the shoulders.
  — Emphasize avoidance of breast stimulation that may cause uterine contractions if a history of preterm labor or signs of preterm labor are present.
- Exercise
  — Recommend moderate exercise 30 or more minutes daily but suggest she avoid:
    – Beginning strenuous exercise or intensifying training.
    – Exercise where there is a risk of falling or abdominal trauma.
    – Vigorous exercise in hot or humid weather.
    – All exercises in supine position after the first trimester (increases risk of supine hypotensive syndrome).
  — Emphasize the importance of taking adequate fluids before and after exercising and to stop exercises that cause undue fatigue.
  — Stress the importance of following her health care provider's advice about taking her pulse during exercise and keeping it within a certain range.
  — Instruct her to stop exercise and seek medical advice if she has chest pain, dizziness, headache, decreased fetal movement, or signs of labor.
  — Suggest she include warm-up and cool-down periods and stretching exercises.
- Sleep and rest
  — Instruct her to use pillows to support the abdomen and back during the last trimester.

— Recommend that she rest in a lateral position to prevent hypotension that may occur as a result of lying in a supine position.
- Employment
  — Suggest that she work out a schedule for frequent rest periods with her feet elevated to prevent undue fatigue.
  — Assist her to plan ways to change positions or to walk briefly to stimulate circulation.
  — Recommend she avoid heavy lifting and curtail jobs that require balance during the last trimester when the center of gravity shifts and she is at greater risk for falls.
- Avoiding teratogens
  — Advise the woman to investigate her specific situation to determine possible exposure to toxic substances. Groups at risk include hairdressers, painters, printers, nurses, and laundry and dry-cleaning workers.
  — Emphasize the ill effects of exposure to passive smoking. If she smokes, help her to make a plan for smoking cessation and provide referral, encouragement, and follow-up.
  — Explain the harmful effects of alcohol and illicit drugs.
- Over-the-counter drugs, complementary and alternative therapy
  — Advise her to consult her health care provider or pharmacist before taking any over-the-counter drugs or complementary and alternative therapy.
  — Suggest that she tell the health care provider and pharmacist she is pregnant if she routinely takes prescribed medications.
- Sexual activity
  — Reassure the couple that sexual intercourse does no harm to the fetus or healthy pregnant woman.
  — Suggest that they alter the position during the last trimester, when supine hypotensive syndrome may result from a male-superior position.
  — Advise them to curtail all sexual activity if the woman is at risk for preterm labor, if the membranes have ruptured, or if there is vaginal bleeding.

- Travel
  - Recommend that she validate that medical care is available at the destination.
  - Remind her to fasten the seat belt snugly with the lap belt under the abdomen and the shoulder belt in place.
  - Counsel her to stop frequently to empty her bladder and walk around.
- Immunizations
  - Remind her that live virus vaccines such as those for measles, rubella, and mumps are contraindicated during pregnancy.
  - Counsel her to consult with her health care provider before taking any immunization during pregnancy.

HOW TO OVERCOME THE COMMON DISCOMFORTS OF PREGNANCY

- Nausea and vomiting
  - Eat crackers or dry toast before arising in the morning, then get out of bed slowly.
  - Eat dry crackers every 2 hours to prevent an empty stomach or eat five or six small meals a day rather than three full meals.
  - Drink fluids separately from meals.
  - Avoid fried, high-fat, greasy, or spicy foods and foods with strong odors.
  - Eat a protein snack at bedtime.
  - Try ginger, peppermint, or tart and salty food combinations.
- Heartburn
  - Avoid spicy or fatty foods.
  - Eat small, frequent meals; avoid overeating or eating at bedtime.
  - Remain upright after eating to reduce reflux; sleep with an extra pillow.
  - Avoid smoking and coffee, which increase acids.
  - Breathe deeply and sip water to relieve burning sensation.
  - Avoid antacids that are high in sodium.

- Backache
  - Maintain correct posture with shoulders and neck straight, back flattened, and pelvis tucked under.
  - Avoid high-heeled shoes.
  - Squat, rather than bend from the waist, to pick up objects.
  - Use foot supports, arm rests, and pillows to support the back.
  - Strengthen the back by doing exercises such as tailor sitting, shoulder circling, and pelvic rocking.
  - A maternity back binder may be helpful.
- Round ligament pain
  - Avoid stretching and twisting at the same time.
  - Bend toward the pain, squat, or flex the knees to the chest to relax the ligament.
  - Use a heating pad.
- Urinary frequency and loss of urine
  - Void when the urge occurs.
  - Maintain daytime fluid intake.
  - Use Kegel exercises (contracting the muscles around the vagina for 10 seconds, relaxing 10 seconds) 30 times daily.
- Varicosities
  - Avoid constricting clothing or crossing the legs at the knees, which impedes blood return from the legs.
  - Take frequent rest periods with legs elevated above the level of the hips.
  - Wear support hose or elastic stockings to prevent blood pooling in the legs.
  - Walk for a few minutes at least every 2 hours to stimulate circulation and relieve discomfort.
- Hemorrhoids
  - Avoid straining when having a bowel movement.
  - Drink plenty of water, eat high-fiber foods, and exercise regularly.
  - Take frequent, tepid baths; apply cool witch hazel compresses or use anesthetic ointments to relieve existing hemorrhoids.

— Lie on the side with the hips elevated on a pillow to promote drainage of blood from swollen hemorrhoids.
— Push hemorrhoids back into the rectum if necessary. Use a clean glove and lubricate the index finger. Maintain pressure for 1 to 2 minutes.
— Notify physician or midwife if there is persistent pain or bleeding.
- Constipation
  — Establish a regular pattern of bowel elimination.
  — Drink at least 8 glasses of water each day in addition to any caffeinated drinks.
  — Consume foods high in fiber, such as unpeeled fresh fruit, whole grain cereals and bread, and vegetables.
  — Restrict consumption of cheese, which can cause constipation, and sweets, which increase bacterial growth in the intestine and cause flatulence.
  — Continue iron supplementation and consult health care provider if constipation persists. A stool softener may be prescribed.
  — Walk briskly for at least 1 mile daily to stimulate peristalsis.
- Leg cramps
  — Dorsiflex the foot and extend the leg to relieve cramp.
  — Elevate the legs frequently to improve circulation.
  — Avoid excessive intake of phosphorus; ask provider about supplemental calcium or magnesium.

NUTRITION FOR PREGNANCY AND LACTATION
WEIGHT GAIN AND PATTERN OF WEIGHT GAIN

The recommended weight gain for pregnancy is 11.5 to 16 kg (25 to 35 lb). Weight gain should follow a predictable pattern of approximately 1.6 kg (3.5 lb) in the first trimester and a weekly gain of 0.4 kg (0.88 lb) in the second and third trimesters. The amount is greater for women who are under their ideal weight for height or who carry more than one fetus, and it is lower for obese women.

NUTRIENT NEEDS

On average, pregnant women need:

- No added calories during the first trimester, 340 additional calories during the second trimester, and 452 added calories during the third trimester.
- Approximately 71 g of protein (an increase of 25 g).
- Additional vitamins (B_6, D, E, and folic acid).
- Additional minerals (iron, calcium, zinc, and magnesium).

FOOD SOURCES TO MEET NUTRIENT NEEDS

During pregnancy, the increased need for most nutrients may not be met unless the additional calories are selected carefully. The pregnant woman should include each day:

- Seven servings of grains (bread, cereal, pasta, rice) with at least half from whole grains.
- Two cups (4 servings) of fruits and 2½ cups (5 servings) of vegetables. The woman should include 3 cups dark green vegetables (broccoli, spinach), 2 cups orange or dark yellow vegetables (carrots, sweet potatoes), 3 cups legumes (pinto beans, lentils, tofu), 3 cups starchy vegetables (white potatoes, corn, green peas), and 6½ cups of other vegetables (tomatoes, green beans) each week.
- Three servings of dairy products (nonfat or low-fat milk, cottage cheese, hard cheese).
- Seven ounces of protein foods (meat, fish, poultry, eggs, tofu). Although legumes are included in both the vegetable and protein groups, a serving should be counted in only one group.
- Oils, fats, and concentrated sugars, which should be taken sparingly; 2 tablespoons unsaturated fats is adequate. Saturated fats and *trans* fatty acids should be avoided.

NUTRITIONAL RISK FACTORS

- Poverty: Carbohydrate foods are less expensive than meats, dairy products, fresh fruits, and vegetables. Therefore, low-income women may have a diet that is high in calories and deficient in protein, vitamins, and minerals. Referral to food supplement programs such as Women, Infants, and Children (WIC) may be needed.

- Adolescence: The adolescent must consume enough nutrients to support her own growth and maturation as well as that of the fetus. Diets are often low in vitamins C and A, folic acid, calcium, iron, and zinc.

- Vegetarian diets: Vegetarian diets are often high in fiber and low in calories and may not meet the energy needs of pregnancy. Vegans who avoid all animal products may get inadequate calcium, iron, zinc, and vitamins D and B_{12}. Diets may also be low in protein.

- Lactose intolerance: Women with a deficiency of the enzyme lactase are unable to absorb lactose and experience nausea, bloating, flatulence, diarrhea, and cramping when they consume milk products. As a result, they may be deficient in calcium unless they eat other foods high in calcium, such as salmon or sardines with bones, dark green vegetables (broccoli, kale, collards), or tofu. They may also take lactase, which decreases their problem with milk products.

- Anemia: A hemoglobin level of less than 11 g/dL during the first and third trimesters or less than 10.5 g/dL during the second trimester is considered anemia. These women may need help in choosing foods high in iron and encouragement to take iron supplements.

- Pica: Women with pica eat nonnutritive substances such as ice, clay, or cornstarch in amounts that may decrease their intake of essential nutrients. An understanding, matter-of-fact approach is necessary in discussing nutrition with these women.

- Multiparity and multifetal pregnancy: Women who have closely spaced pregnancies may begin a new pregnancy with inadequate nutrient stores to meet their own needs and fetal requirements. The woman with a multifetal pregnancy must provide enough calories to meet the needs of each fetus without depleting her own stores.

Suggested weight gain for a woman with twins is 4.5 to 9 kg (10 to 20 lb) more than for a woman with a single pregnancy.

- Substance use: Smoking and use of alcohol and illicit drugs may interfere with the intake of nutrients and their availability to the fetus. Smoking cessation programs and referral to other sources of help may be necessary.

SUPPLEMENTATION

- Supplementation should not be used as a substitute for eating a good diet because supplements do not contain all nutrients needed during pregnancy.
- Iron (30 mg per day) is often prescribed for women during the second and third trimesters because it is difficult to obtain adequate amounts through normal food intake. The dose is higher (60 to 120 mg per day) for women who have been diagnosed with iron deficiency anemia. Recommend that these women:
  - Take iron with food, if necessary, to decrease the nausea that some women experience.
  - Eat foods high in fiber (fresh fruits and vegetables) and drink at least 8 glasses of water a day to prevent constipation.
  - Avoid taking iron with calcium supplements, milk, tea, coffee, or antacids, which interfere with iron absorption.
  - Get plenty of vitamin C (in citrus fruits, tomatoes, melons, and berries) and heme iron (in meats) to increase absorption of iron.
  - Expect stools to be black or dark green, a side effect of iron supplementation.
- Folic acid (400 mcg per day) is recommended for all women of childbearing age to prevent neural tube defects in the fetus. Intake during pregnancy should be 600 mcg daily.
- Additional prenatal vitamins and minerals are recommended when there is reason to believe the diet may not be adequate.

EDUCATION FOR CHILDBEARING

Some of the most common educational programs offered to the childbearing family are:

- Early pregnancy classes: Provide information about how the body adapts to pregnancy and how to deal with common discomforts.
- Exercise classes: Should be preceded by warm-up, should be low impact, and should avoid excessive heart rate elevation.
- Childbirth preparation classes: Describe what to expect during labor and birth and focus on self-help measures for the couple. Classes include information about phases and stages of labor, pharmacologic and non-pharmacologic methods of pain relief, and supervised practice of relaxation and coping strategies.
- Breastfeeding classes: Explain the importance of breastfeeding and include information on techniques and common problems and solutions.
- Parenting classes: Provide instruction in care of the newborn.

THE CHILDBEARING FAMILY WITH SPECIAL NEEDS
ADOLESCENT PREGNANCY

Implications for Maternal Health. Pregnancy presents significant health risks for adolescents.

- Preeclampsia
- Anemia
- Inappropriate weight gain (too much or too little)
- Urinary tract infections
- Depression
- Nutritional deficiencies, particularly vitamins A and C, folic acid, calcium, iron, and zinc

Socioeconomic Implications
- Pregnancy is often unplanned and may be unwanted.
- Developmental tasks of adolescence (identity, independence) are incomplete.

- May become more dependent on parents.
- Interference with education may limit employment opportunities.
- May become more motivated to finish school and change poor lifestyles.
- May be upset about physical changes of pregnancy.
- Fathers unready for pregnancy and may or may not be supportive.

Implications for Fetal-Neonatal Health. An infant born to a teenage mother is at higher risk for two major complications.

- Prematurity and the resulting consequences
- Low birth weight (<2500 g)

Impact on Parenting. Adolescent mothers are at risk of becoming non-nurturing parents. They may exhibit:

- Immature or punitive responses to the infant due to life stresses.
- Fewer instances of mutual gazing, verbal interaction, and touching.
- Little understanding of normal development and unrealistic expectations of the infant.

Assessment. Assessment of pregnant teenagers is similar to that of older patients and should include a thorough health and family history. In addition, the assessment should focus on the following specific areas:

- Compliance with recommended prenatal care (keeping prenatal appointments, taking vitamin and iron supplementation, attending recommended prenatal classes)
- Signs of complications such as anemia, preeclampsia, or sexually transmitted diseases (STDs).
- Lifestyle behaviors such as poor nutrition, smoking, or alcohol or drug use
- Screening for physical or sexual abuse

- Cognitive development and ability to make long-term plans
- Knowledge of infant needs
- Family support

Nursing Diagnoses
- Risk for Ineffective Health Maintenance related to lack of knowledge of measures to promote health during pregnancy and increased family stress
- Disturbed Body Image related to perceived negative effects of pregnancy
- Situational Low Self-Esteem related to feelings of rejection by family
- Risk for Impaired Parenting related to deficient knowledge about infant needs
- Risk for Delayed Growth and Development related to conflict between identity development and maternal tasks of pregnancy
- Imbalanced Nutrition: Less Than Body Requirements related to lack of knowledge of nutritional needs
- Imbalanced Nutrition: More Than Body Requirements related to frequent consumption of fast foods and high-fat snacks
- Interrupted Family Processes related to integration of infant into existing family structure

Antepartum Nursing Interventions
- Eliminate barriers to health care
  — Determine the most convenient time and location for appointments.
  — Find ways to maintain positive attitudes of health care workers when adolescents do not comply with recommendations for prenatal care.
- Apply appropriate principles of teaching-learning.
  — Recognize the importance of peer groups.
  — Form small groups with like concerns.
  — Encourage questions and repeat material as needed.
  — Use audiovisual aids, which may be more helpful than reading material for this age-group.

- — Maintain open, friendly posture and convey empathy.
- Allow time to counsel about specific problems such as stress reduction.
- Use ultrasound and listening to the fetal heartbeat to increase maternal attachment to the fetus.
- Provide instructions about infant growth and development, with particular emphasis on infant cues and signals that require prompt, gentle response.
- Promote family support and discuss such topics as:
  - — Who will help care for the infant.
  - — Plans for returning to school.
  - — Financial assistance from the infant's father and family.
- Refer to appropriate national and community resources.
  - — Well-baby clinics
  - — Programs for school-age mothers offered by high schools
  - — Social services assistance programs
  - — Women, Infants, and Children (WIC)
  - — Church and community organizations

Nutrition for the Pregnant Adolescent
- Emphasize the benefits of good nutrition for the health of both the mother and infant.
- Reinforce the value of nutritional supplements, such as iron and vitamins, particularly folic acid.
- Explain the importance of breakfast and suggest nontraditional foods if she doesn't like breakfast foods.
- Provide information about the best food choices, such as milk and milk products, chicken, lean meats, fish, fruits, vegetables, whole grain products.
- Explain that foods that are broiled, roasted, or barbecued are lower in fats than foods that are fried.
- Recommend curtailing salty foods, such as olives, pickles, and chips, to prevent or decrease fluid retention.
- Suggest cutting down on fried foods (french fries, onion rings) and substituting baked potatoes with broccoli, cheese, or meat fillings.
- Consider snacks and fast foods, which provide about one fourth of a teenager's calories, when planning nutrition.

— Recommend yogurt, fresh fruit, peanuts, or cheese and crackers for nutritional snacks.
— Suggest adding cheese, tomatoes, and lettuce to hamburgers and avoiding dressings that are high in fat and calories.
— Point out that a milk shake provides more nutrition than carbonated beverages, which are high in sodium and phosphorus.

Intrapartal Care. Supportive nursing interventions are particularly necessary for adolescents, who often have a fear of hospitals and inadequate information about the birth process. Interventions include:

• A nurturing attitude that includes frequent physical contact, reassurance that she will not be left alone, and involvement of the father or other family members.
• Acknowledgment of feelings and concerns.
• Ongoing information about the labor and delivery process.
• Demonstrations of relaxation and breathing techniques.
• Attention to physical comfort and pain relief.
• Frequent encouragement and reassurance.

Postpartum Interventions. The adolescent mother requires the same nursing care as an adult woman. However, her developmental level may make it necessary to focus more on the following interventions:

• Self-care measures (breast and perineal care, comfort measures)
• Measures to promote maternal role acquisition
— Provide extended contact with the newborn.
— Instruct in safe and effective parenting skills (feeding, bathing, diapering, and dressing).
— Teach how to protect the infant from accidents; teach the signs and symptoms of illness that should be reported (see p. 99).
— Remind the mother that crying indicates a need, and a consistent gentle response will not spoil the infant.

— Emphasize that in addition to food, sleep, and comfort, infants also need appropriate stimulation (cuddling, hearing the parents' voices, looking at their faces).
— Teach that infants also signal when they have had enough stimulation (gaze aversion, yawning, splaying the fingers, hiccoughing, etc.).
— Help to identify support system to assist with child care.
— Emphasize the importance of follow-up appointments and immunizations.
— Include the grandparents or significant other in teaching.

DELAYED PREGNANCY
MATERNAL-FETAL IMPLICATIONS

Women who delay childbirth until 35 years or older are increasingly common. Although most mature gravidas have normal pregnancies, there is a higher risk for:

- A delay in becoming pregnant due to normal aging of the ovaries and the increased incidence of reproductive tract disorders.
- Chromosomal abnormalities, particularly trisomy 21.
- Complications due to preexisting diseases, such as hypertension, diabetes mellitus, and uterine myomas (fibroids).
- Obstetric complications such as preeclampsia, gestational diabetes, placenta previa, vaginal bleeding, preterm labor, dysfunctional labor, cesarean birth, and multiple gestation.
- Small-for-gestational-age infant.

ADVANTAGES OF DELAYED PREGNANCY

Most women older than 35 years of age who become pregnant have planned the pregnancy after careful thought. They often have resources that include:

- Psychosocial maturity.
- Self-confidence.
- A high level of empathy and flexibility in childrearing attitudes.

- Problem-solving skills.
- Financial security.

DISADVANTAGES OF DELAYED PREGNANCY
- Need more time to recover from childbirth
- Have less energy than younger counterparts
- May lack family and peer support
- Experience a feeling of social isolation during early post-partum weeks

NURSING CONSIDERATIONS
Because the fetus of a mature primigravida is at increased risk for chromosomal abnormalities, the mother will need information about available diagnostic tests. Although only professionals with special preparation in genetics should provide genetic counseling, all nurses must be prepared to reinforce and clarify information that has been provided. Testing may include:

- Chorionic villus sampling.
- Amniocentesis.
- Ultrasonography.

Test results may not be known for several days or weeks. Nurses provide information and support and an opportunity for the woman and her family to express their concerns.

First-time mothers older than the age of 35 years are especially receptive to prenatal classes of all types and printed materials describing growth and development and infant care.

SUBSTANCE ABUSE
When a pregnant woman takes a substance, by drinking, smoking, snorting, or injecting it, the fetus receives the same substance and experiences the same effects. The fetus, however, is unable to metabolize the drug as efficiently as the expectant mother and experiences more severe effects for a longer period of time. Table 1-6 summarizes the maternal, fetal, and neonatal effects of specific drugs. Although five highly abused substances are presented separately, it must be

Text continued on p. 58

Table 1-6	Effects of Commonly Abused Substances
Maternal Effects	**Fetal/Neonatal Effects**
Caffeine	
Stimulates CNS and cardiac function, causes vasoconstriction and mild diuresis, half-life triples during pregnancy	Crosses placental barrier and stimulates fetus; teratogenic effects are undocumented
Tobacco	
Nicotine causes vasoconstriction; reduces placental perfusion: carbon monoxide inactivates hemoglobin, resulting in hypoxia; decreased appetite; increase in spontaneous abortions and preterm labor	Prematurity; LBW; delayed neurologic and intellectual development; hyperactivity, shorter attention span, increased SIDS
Alcohol	
Increased incidence of second trimester abortions; intoxication; decreased maternal appetite	Fetal alcohol syndrome (specific craniofacial dysmorphic features, prenatal and postnatal growth restriction, CNS impairment); prematurity; LBW; mental retardation and long-term learning problems

Continued

Table 1-6	Effects of Commonly Abused Substances—cont'd
Maternal Effects	**Fetal/Neonatal Effects**
Marijuana	
Maternal anemia, inadequate weight gain; often paired with other drugs such as cocaine and alcohol	Unclear, may exhibit hyperirritability, tremors, sensitivity to light, sleep problems
Cocaine	
Hyperarousal state, generalized vasoconstriction, hypertension, cardiovascular complications (stroke, heart attack), seizures, increased STDs, stimulates uterine contractions, increased spontaneous abortion, preterm labor, precipitous delivery, abruptio placentae	Fetal tachycardia and decreased heart rate variability, stillbirth, LBW, prematurity, IUGR, irritability, decreased ability to interact with environmental stimuli, poor feeding reflexes, vomiting, learning problems, prune-belly syndrome, increased risk for SIDS
Sedatives	
Lethargy, drowsiness, CNS depression, spontaneous abortion, IUGR	Neonatal abstinence syndrome, seizures, delayed lung maturity, possible teratogenic effects

Amphetamines and Methamphetamines

Vasoconstriction, hypertension, tachycardia, malnutrition	IUGR, fetal death, intravascular hemorrhage, abnormal sleep patterns, agitation, vomiting

Opioids

Physical addiction, poor general health, increased incidence of STDs, HIV exposure, hepatitis, malnutrition, spontaneous abortion, PROM, preterm labor	Intrauterine hypoxia, IUGR, perinatal asphyxia, intellectual impairment, neonatal abstinence syndrome (tremors, jitteriness, seizures, hypertonicity and continuous crying, uncoordinated sucking and swallowing reflexes, vomiting, and diarrhea), neonatal infections, SIDS, child abuse and neglect

CNS, Central nervous system; *HIV,* human immunodeficiency virus; *IUGR,* intrauterine growth restriction; *LBW,* low birth weight; *PROM,* premature rupture of membranes; *SIDS,* sudden infant death syndrome; *STDs,* sexually transmitted diseases.

Text continued from p. 54

remembered that it is rare for only one drug to be used. Multiple substance use is common.

ASSESSMENT

All women must be assessed for substance abuse because it occurs in all ages and all socioeconomic groups. Women who use one substance often use others as well.

Signs and Symptoms. Although any of these signs and symptoms may occur in women who have never abused drugs, the most common signs and symptoms indicating drug use are:

- Seeking prenatal care late in pregnancy.
- Failing to keep appointments.
- Inconsistent follow-through with recommendations.
- Poor grooming, inadequate weight gain.
- Needle punctures, thrombosed veins, cellulitis.
- Defensive or hostile behaviors.
- Anger or apathy regarding the pregnancy.

History. The medical and obstetric history should focus on:

- Previous episodes of medical problems such as depression, seizures, hepatitis, pneumonia, cellulitis, STDs, hypertension, or suicide attempts.
- Current problems such as insomnia, panic attacks, exhaustion, and heart palpitations.
- Previous obstetric problems such as spontaneous abortions, premature births, abruptio placentae, and stillbirths.
- Current obstetric problems such as STDs, vaginal bleeding, an inactive or hyperactive fetus, fundal height inconsistent with gestational age.
- All forms of drug use, including cigarettes, over-the-counter drugs, prescribed medications, alcohol, and illicit drugs.
- Pattern of drug use, which can range from occasional binges to daily dependence.

Toxicology Screening. Screening for metabolites of drugs may be indicated for pregnant women, new mothers, and newborn infants.

NURSING DIAGNOSES
- Ineffective Health Maintenance related to inability to manage stress without the use of drugs
- Risk for Imbalanced Nutrition: Less Than Body Requirements, related to anorexia and lifestyle that does not emphasize nutrition
- Risk for Infection related to lifestyle that involves exposure to pathogens
- Ineffective Coping related to physiologic and psychological demands of pregnancy and childbirth

ANTEPARTUM MANAGEMENT
Effective interventions for substance abuse require the combined efforts of nurses, physicians, social workers, law enforcement agencies, and numerous community and federal agencies.

- Examine own reactions to reduce feelings of anger or judgmental behavior.
- Maintain feelings of concern, empathy, and helpfulness.
- Allow time to get acquainted with the expectant mother to learn what stressors may contribute to the pattern of substance abuse.
- Provide accurate information about the effects of substances such as tobacco, alcohol, and illicit drugs.
- Help the woman identify personal and family strengths.
- Acknowledge her actions when she abstains from drugs for even a short time.
- Focus on helping the woman remain drug free day by day.
- Describe how the newborn benefits when the woman abstains from drugs.
- Verify compliance with recommended treatment regimens, such as chemical-dependence referral programs.
- Coordinate care among various service providers, such as group therapy and prenatal classes.

INTRAPARTUM MANAGEMENT

Nurses who work in labor and delivery units must become skilled at recognizing drug-induced signs and symptoms.

ASSESSMENT
Signs of Recent Use of Cocaine

- Physical signs
  - Profuse sweating
  - Hypertension
  - Irregular respirations
  - Lethargic response
  - Dilated pupils
  - Increased body temperature
  - Sudden onset of severely painful contractions
- Emotional signs
  - Angry, caustic, or abusive reactions
  - Emotional lability
  - Paranoia
- Fetal signs
  - Tachycardia
  - Excessive fetal activity

Signs of Recent Use of Heroin

The pregnant woman addicted to heroin often comes to the delivery unit intoxicated from a recent drug administration. When the drug begins to wear off, withdrawal symptoms may be observed.

  - Yawning
  - Diaphoresis
  - Rhinorrhea
  - Restlessness
  - Excessive tearing of the eyes

NURSING INTERVENTIONS

Nursing interventions focus on preventing injury to mother and fetus during labor and childbirth.

- Assign two nurses to admit the woman to the unit: one nurse provides physical care, while the other acts as communicator.
- Set limits (no smoking, must remain in bed or may only walk in her room after membranes rupture, etc.).
- Initiate seizure precautions (keep bed locked in lowest position, pad side rails to prevent injury, ensure suction and oxygen equipment are working).
- Reduce environmental stimuli as much as possible.
- Maintain a therapeutic pattern of communications; acknowledge feelings; avoid confrontations.
- Provide pain control.
  - Provide prescribed pain medication as needed.
  - Avoid drugs, such as butorphanol, that may cause acute withdrawal symptoms.
  - Use nonpharmacologic nursing interventions such as sacral pressure, back rubs, and continuous support.
- Administer methadone to prevent withdrawal during labor in women who usually receive methadone at a chemical-dependence center.

POSTPARTUM MANAGEMENT
See Section 3, pp. 271-272 for care of the infant and helping the mother bond with the newborn.

BIRTH OF AN INFANT WITH CONGENITAL ANOMALIES
Congenital anomalies may be discovered during pregnancy when the mother has an ultrasound, or the abnormality may not be identified until the infant is born. Whenever they become aware of the fact that their infant will not be normal, parents are often overwhelmed with feelings of shock and disbelief. Before they can form attachment with the newborn, they must grieve for the perfect infant they expected.

MANAGEMENT
Physicians and nurses are aware that the timing and manner of being told of the anomalies influences the emotional response of parents.

- Tell (and show) the parents as soon as possible.
- Remain with the parents during the initial phase of shock and denial.
- Maintain an atmosphere that encourages families to express their feelings.
  - Listen carefully and reflect the content and feelings expressed.
  - Be aware that cultural and religious beliefs affect expressions of grief.
- Promote bonding and attachment.
  - Communicate acceptance of the infant by handling gently and presenting the infant as precious.
  - Emphasize the normal aspects of the infant.
  - Allow long periods of uninterrupted time between parents and infant (as the infant's condition permits).
- Provide accurate information about follow-up treatments or procedures that may be necessary.
- Answer questions as honestly as possible; seek answers to questions if unsure of information.
- Encourage communication between family members. Include fathers (and grandparents if desired) in discussions and demonstrations of care.
- Teach necessary home care (e.g., how to feed an infant with a cleft palate).
- Help parents prepare siblings for changes the newborn will make in family functioning.
- Refer to community and national resources such as the March of Dimes or the disabled children's services of the public health department.

PREGNANCY LOSS

Death of an infant at any time during pregnancy or the neonatal period is devastating for families. All staff must be sensitive to the family's needs at this time.

MANAGEMENT

- Use a symbol on the door of the mother's room and chart to make all staff aware of the loss.

- Acknowledge the basic rights of the baby:
  — To be recognized as a person who was born and died.
  — To be named.
  — To be seen, touched, and held by the family.
  — To have life-ending acknowledged.
  — To be put to rest with dignity.
- Bring the infant and parents together while the infant is still warm and soft if possible.
  — Wash the infant and apply baby lotion or powder if necessary.
  — Wrap the infant in a soft, warm blanket.
  — Keep the infant in a warmed incubator if necessary. If this is not possible, tell the parents the infant's skin will feel cool.
  — Prepare the parents for the infant's appearance.
- Encourage parents to keep the infant as long as they wish, and make them feel free to unwrap the infant.
- Permit parents to progress at their own speed when inspecting the infant.
- Allow as much privacy and time as the parents and other family members need to be together.
- Prepare a "memory packet" that might include a photograph, footprints, the identification bracelet, a crib card with the infant's name, weight, and length, blanket used for the baby, and a lock of hair.
- Keep the memory packet on file if the parents do not want to take it home at this time.
- Offer to call clergy if the parents wish.
- Explain the normal grieving process and the effect on all family members.
- Refer to groups designed to help parents after loss: Resolve through Sharing, Aiding Mothers and Fathers Experiencing Neonatal Death (AMEND), Source of Help in Airing and Resolving Experiences (SHARE), and Helping After Neonatal Death (HAND).

RELINQUISHMENT FOR ADOPTION

The woman who will relinquish her baby for adoption also needs special attention before and after birth.

MANAGEMENT
- Before the birth, determine the woman's wishes about contact with the infant and the adoptive parents.
- Ensure that all staff are aware of the woman's decision.
- Encourage the mother to see and hold her infant to help her with the grieving process.
- Use therapeutic communication to help the woman express her feelings.
- Teach the adoptive parents how to care for the newborn.

INTIMATE PARTNER VIOLENCE
Physical abuse occurs in a cycle that consists of three phases.

- A tension-building phase, during which the man engages in increasingly hostile behaviors such as throwing objects, pushing, or threatening.
- A battering phase, when the man explodes in violence to hit, beat, or rape the woman.
- A honeymoon phase, when the batterer is contrite and remorseful and promises never to do it again. This phase may decrease or disappear over time.

SIGNS OF PHYSICAL ABUSE
- Nonverbal signs: Facial grimacing, slow and unsteady gait, vomiting, abdominal tenderness, absence of facial response
- Injuries: Welts, bruises, swelling, lacerations, burns, vaginal or rectal bleeding; evidence of old or new fractures of the nose, face, ribs, or arms
- Vague somatic complaints: Anxiety, depression, panic attacks, sleeplessness, anorexia
- Discrepancy between history and type of injuries; wounds do not match the woman's story; multiple bruises in various stages of healing; bruising on the arms (which she may have raised to protect herself); old, untreated wounds

ASSESSMENT
Every woman should be asked about violence at various times during and after pregnancy. Asking shows the woman

that help is available even if she is not ready to seek it yet. However, introducing the subject of violence in the presence of the man places the woman in danger. It is essential to:

- Separate the woman from the man for the interview.
- Explain that all women are asked about intimate partner violence.
- Reassure the woman that confidentiality will be absolute.
- Include standard screening questions such as:
  — Have you been threatened, hit, slapped, kicked, choked or otherwise physically hurt by anyone within the last year?
  — Has this happened since you have been pregnant?
  — Within the last year, has anyone forced you to have sexual activities?
  — Are you ever afraid of anyone?
- Ask direct questions as appropriate ("Did you get these injuries from being hit?").
- Evaluate and document all signs of injury, past and present.
- Be alert for nonverbal cues of physical abuse.
- Keep in mind that the woman may fear for her life because abusive episodes tend to escalate.

MOST COMMON NURSING DIAGNOSES
- Fear related to possibility of severe injury to herself and/or her children
- Acute Pain related to injuries received during violent episode
- Post-Trauma Response related to assault
- Rape-Trauma Syndrome related to repeated physical and sexual abuse

MANAGEMENT
- Help the woman make concrete plans to protect her own and her children's safety if she returns to the shared home.
  — Recommend keeping car and house keys, personal information, and necessities packed and hidden until needed.

— Emphasize the importance of locating the nearest safe house or shelter and making specific plans for going there when the cycle of violence begins.
— Help her devise a code word to use with a trusted person who will respond by calling the police.
— Suggest memorizing the number of a shelter and hotline such as 1-800-799-SAFE.
- Reinforce that she is not to blame for violence against her.
- Teach basic family processes.
— Violence is not normal.
— Physical abuse is against the law.
— Violence usually escalates and is repeated.
— Battered women have alternatives.
- Refer to community agencies that are available to help the victim (police departments, community shelters, counseling agencies, and social services).
- Accept the decisions of the battered woman and acknowledge that she must act on her own timetable.
- Inform her that resources are available for her partner, but he must admit abuse and seek assistance before help can be offered. Initiating referrals before he asks for help will increase the danger to the woman if her partner feels he has been betrayed.

COMPLICATIONS OF PREGNANCY

Only those complications that have a strong clinical component are presented. The reader is referred to a reference book, such as *Foundations in Maternal-Newborn Nursing*, second edition, for information about less common conditions or those that respond primarily to medical management.

ANEMIAS

Anemia is a condition in which there is a hemoglobin concentration of less than 10.5 to 11 g/dL (Kilpatrick & Laros, 2004). The most common types of anemia observed during pregnancy are anemias caused by iron deficiency, folic acid deficiency, sickle cell disease, and thalassemia.

IRON-DEFICIENCY ANEMIA

Most women do not have iron stores that meet the needs of pregnancy. Furthermore, it is difficult to meet pregnancy needs by diet alone, and iron supplementation with ferrous sulfate, is generally required. For additional information about supplementation, see page 47.

FOLIC ACID-DEFICIENCY (MEGALOBLASTIC) ANEMIA

A deficiency in folic acid results in a reduction in the rate of DNA synthesis and mitotic activity of individual cells, resulting in large, immature erythrocytes (megaloblasts). Folate deficiency is associated with increased risk of spontaneous abortion, abruptio placentae, and fetal anomalies such as neural tube defects. It is now recommended that all women of childbearing age take 400 mcg (0.4 mg) of folic acid daily, increasing their intake to 600 mcg (0.6 mg) when pregnancy is confirmed. Greater folic acid supplementation is recommended for women who have had a child with a neural tube defect.

SICKLE CELL ANEMIA

Sickle cell anemia occurs when a defect in hemoglobin causes erythrocytes to be shaped like a sickle, or crescent. Pregnancy can bring on sickle cell crisis that may include cessation of bone morrow function, massive erythrocyte destruction resulting in hyperbilirubinemia, and severe pain caused by infarctions in the joints and major organs.

Management is based on the knowledge that dehydration, hypoxemia, extremes in temperature, exertion, and infection stimulate the sickling process. Some specific measures include:

- Frequent evaluations of hemoglobin, blood count, serum iron, total iron binding capacity, and serum folate.
- Fetal surveillance studies, such as ultrasonography and biophysical profiles.
- Maintenance of adequate hydration.
- Recommendation to dress warmly in cold weather and to avoid exertion in hot weather.

- Folic acid supplementation to increase erythrocyte production.
- Rest periods throughout the day, as well as good hygienic practices and avoidance of people with infectious illnesses.
- Testing for infections such as sexually transmitted disease, HIV, tuberculosis, and hepatitis. Immunizations for other diseases such as hepatitis B, varicella, pneumonia, or influenza.
- Prompt treatment for fever or other signs of infection.
- Administration of oxygen continuously during the intrapartum period.

BLEEDING COMPLICATIONS OF PREGNANCY
ABORTION

Abortion is the loss of pregnancy before the fetus is capable of living outside the uterus (approximately 20 weeks of gestation or 500 g). Abortion may be spontaneous, usually called "miscarriage" by laypeople and many health professionals, or induced by medical termination of pregnancy.

Etiology and Predisposing Factors. The primary causes of spontaneous abortion or miscarriage are:

- Abnormal embryonic development.
- Chromosomal defects.
- Endocrine imbalances such as type 1 diabetes mellitus, hypothyroidism, or inadequate progesterone.
- Immunologic factors such as antiphospholipid antibodies.
- Infections such as syphilis, listeriosis, toxoplasmosis, brucellosis, rubella, and cytomegalovirus, or intraabdominal infections.
- Systemic disorders such as lupus erythematosus.
- Anomalies of the reproductive tract, such as bicornuate uterus.

Types of Spontaneous Abortion. Spontaneous abortion is divided into six categories

- Threatened: Vaginal bleeding occurs, but the products of conception are not expelled.

- Inevitable: Abortion cannot be stopped when there is rupture of membranes and dilation of the cervix.
- Incomplete: Some, but not all, products of conception are expelled from the uterus.
- Complete: All products of conception are expelled.
- Missed: The fetus dies, but the products of conception are retained.
- Recurrent: Three or more consecutive pregnancies end in spontaneous abortion.

Signs and Symptoms
- Vaginal bleeding
- Rhythmic uterine cramping
- Backache or feeling of pelvic pressure
- Rupture of membranes
- Dilation of the cervix
- Decline in placental hormone production

Management
- Evaluation by ultrasound to determine if a fetus is present and alive
- Reassurance that bed rest does not improve the prognosis for a threatened abortion
- Analgesia as necessary
- Evacuation of the remaining products of conception if abortion is incomplete
- Administration of oxytocin, prostaglandin, or methylergonovine to stimulate uterine contraction and control bleeding
- Intravenous fluids and blood replacement as necessary to maintain fluid and electrolyte balance
- Prophylactic $Rh_o(D)$ immune globulin (RhoGAM) for all unsensitized Rh-negative mothers
- When fetal death is confirmed in a missed abortion, the usual management is to evacuate the uterus. Antimicrobial therapy will be started if infection has occurred.
- Two major complications of missed abortion: uterine infection and disseminated intravascular coagulation (DIC) (see p. 77)

- Examination of the cervix and uterus to identify anatomic defects that may be the cause of recurrent abortion
- Studies to identify and treat immunologic factors, autoimmune disorders, infections, or other systemic diseases
- Genetic screening for factors that might increase the risk of recurrent abortion
- Suturing of the cervix (cerclage) to keep it closed and thus maintain the pregnancy if there is a history of recurrent pregnancy loss related to painless cervical dilation

ECTOPIC PREGNANCY

The term *ectopic pregnancy* refers to implantation of a fertilized ovum in an area outside the uterine cavity, usually in the fallopian tube. This is a life-threatening event because of massive bleeding that can occur if the tube ruptures.

Etiology and Predisposing Factors. Ectopic pregnancy is most likely to occur when transport of the fertilized ovum through the fallopian tube is hampered. The primary predisposing factors are:

- Pelvic infection, often caused by *Chlamydia* or *Neisseria gonorrhoeae*.
- Previous ectopic pregnancy.
- Tubal ligation.
- Intrauterine device.
- Delayed or premature ovulation or reduced tubal motility

Signs and Symptoms
- Missed menstrual period and other presumptive signs of pregnancy, such as breast tenderness and nausea
- Abdominal pain
- Pelvic mass
- Vaginal "spotting"
- Signs of internal hemorrhage such as increasing pulse, falling blood pressure, vertigo, shoulder pain due to irritation of phrenic nerve

Management. Following diagnosis, which is usually made by transvaginal ultrasound examination and assay of the beta subunit of human chorionic gonadotropin (beta-hCG), management depends on whether the tube is intact or ruptured. If it is intact, initial care may include:

- Administration of methotrexate, a chemotherapeutic agent to stop cell reproduction in the tube.
- An incision into the tube and removal of the products of conception (lineal salpingostomy). The goal of this procedure is to preserve the tube and to prevent hemorrhage that occurs when the tube ruptures.

If the tube is ruptured, management focuses on measures to control bleeding and to prevent hypovolemic shock. These measures include:

- Administration of intravenous fluids and blood as necessary to maintain hemodynamic status.
- Removal of the tube (salpingectomy).
- Recognition of the family's feelings, which include grief at pregnancy loss and concern about the chances for future pregnancies.

GESTATIONAL TROPHOBLASTIC DISEASE (HYDATIDIFORM MOLE)

Gestational trophoblastic disease refers to an abnormal growth of trophoblastic cells that attach the fertilized ovum to the uterine wall. The proliferating trophoblasts fill the uterus with vesicles that resemble a cluster of grapes. Malignant change (choriocarcinoma) may follow gestational trophoblastic disease.

Types of Gestational Trophoblastic Disease
- Complete: No fetal tissues are present. Believed to occur when the ovum is fertilized by a sperm that duplicates its own chromosomes while the chromosomes of the ovum are inactivated.

- Partial: Fetal tissues or membranes are present. The maternal chromosome contribution is present, but the paternal chromosome contribution may be double. Possible karyotypes include 69,XXY, or 69,XYY.

Etiology and Predisposing Factors. The cause of gestational trophoblastic disease is unknown. Recognized risk factors include:

- Asian or Asian descent
- Age at the youngest and oldest ends of reproductive life
- History of previous molar pregnancy

Signs and Symptoms
- Elevated levels of beta-hCG
- Characteristic ultrasonographic pattern that shows the vesicles and the absence of a fetal sac or fetal heart activity in a complete molar pregnancy
- A uterus that is larger than one would expect based on the duration of the pregnancy
- Vaginal bleeding, which varies from dark brown spotting to profuse hemorrhage
- Excessive nausea and vomiting (hyperemesis gravidarum), which may be related to high levels of hCG from the proliferating trophoblasts
- Early development of preeclampsia, which is rarely diagnosed before 24 weeks in an otherwise normal pregnancy

Management. Management includes two phases: (1) immediate evacuation after diagnosis by ultrasound examination, and (2) follow-up to detect malignant changes of the remaining trophoblastic tissue. Immediate care includes:

- Imaging to detect metastatic disease.
- Complete blood count, coagulation tests, blood typing and screening or crossmatching.
- Replacement of fluids and blood as necessary.
- General or regional anesthesia.

- Vacuum evacuation, followed by curettage of the uterus.
- Laboratory evaluation of tissue to identify benign or malignant cytology.
- Intravenous oxytocin to reduce blood loss following evacuation of the uterus.

Follow-up care protocol includes:

- Evaluation of serum hCG levels for at least a year.
- Advice to avoid pregnancy for at least a year. Oral contraceptives are often prescribed.
- Response to feelings of sadness at loss of pregnancy and concern about the need for long-term follow-up.

PLACENTA PREVIA
In placenta previa, the placenta implants in the lower uterine segment and infringes on or covers the cervical os. Placenta previa may be marginal (extends only to the cervical os), partial (covers part of the os), or complete (extends over the entire cervical os).

Etiology and Predisposing Factors. The direct cause is unknown, but factors that have been associated with a higher incidence of placenta previa include:

- Multiparity.
- Increasing maternal age.
- Prior placenta previa.
- Previous cesarean birth or medical termination of pregnancy.

Signs and Symptoms
- Ultrasound examination that identifies low placental implantation
- Painless uterine bleeding in the latter half of pregnancy
- Subsequent episodes of heavier bleeding
- Bleeding that occurs when labor begins (heavier and brighter than "bloody show")

Management

- Delay vaginal examinations until the location of the placenta is determined
- Ultrasound examination to locate the position of the placenta
- Electronic monitoring to determine the condition of the fetus
- Evaluation of mother for signs of hypovolemia (increasing pulse, falling blood pressure, pallor, etc.)
- Laboratory examination for signs of anemia and infection (CBC, Hg, Hct) and type and crossmatch to replace whole blood as necessary
- Bed rest and careful monitoring of fetus, maternal vital signs, and vaginal bleeding if initial bleeding was scant or moderate, and if the fetus is immature and shows no signs of compromise
- Assistance for the family, who must plan for long-term bed rest, and instructions in how to monitor the mother and fetus
- Criteria for home care include:
  - No evidence of active bleeding.
  - No signs or symptoms of preterm labor.
  - Home no more than 15 to 20 minutes from the hospital.
  - Emergency support systems in place for emergency transport to the hospital.
  - The presence of a responsible adult at all times.
- Preparation for cesarean delivery when fetal lungs are mature or if bleeding is excessive regardless of fetal maturity

ABRUPTIO PLACENTAE

Abruptio placentae, also called placental abruption or premature separation of the placenta, occurs when a normally implanted placenta separates from the uterine wall prior to the birth of the infant. The bleeding that occurs may dissect upward toward the fundus, resulting in concealed hemorrhage, or extend downward toward the cervix, resulting in external or obvious bleeding. The major dangers for the woman are hemorrhage, hypovolemic shock, and clotting disorders (disseminated intravascular coagulation [DIC]). The major dangers for the fetus are anoxia as placental blood flow is compromised, blood loss, or delivery before the fetus is mature.

Etiology and Predisposing Factors
- Cocaine use
- Smoking
- Multiparity, often accompanied by advanced maternal age
- Maternal hypertension
- Previous abruptio placentae
- Preterm rupture of membranes
- Short umbilical cord
- Abdominal trauma

Signs and Symptoms
- Persistent abdominal or low back pain that may be aching or dull; possible sudden and severe pain
- Uterine tenderness that may be localized at the site of abruption
- Uterine irritability with frequent contractions and poor relaxation between the contractions
- Persistent high uterine resting tone evident on fetal monitor
- Bleeding that may be evident vaginally but may be concealed behind the placenta
- Signs of hypovolemic shock, with or without external bleeding

Management. Management is a collaborative process that involves nurses and physicians whose major goals are to prevent hypovolemic shock and to deliver a healthy infant safely. Interventions include:

- Monitor hemodynamic status of mother.
- Initiate electronic fetal monitoring to detect signs of fetal hypoxia, such as tachycardia or late decelerations.
- Insert an indwelling catheter to assess urine output accurately.
- Observe for uterine hyperactivity such as contractions that have a persistent prolonged duration (over 90 to 120 seconds) or inadequate rest interval (shorter than 30 seconds) or a palpable uterine tone that remains tense and irritable.

- Administer intravenous fluids, blood, plasma, cryoprecipitate, and platelets as necessary.
- Prepare for rapid delivery to prevent fetal compromise and to control bleeding.
- Keep family informed about interventions that must often be performed quickly.
- Acknowledge the family's concern for the mother and the fetus and offer reassurance when possible.

Conservative management is occasionally used if the fetus is very preterm and in no distress and if abruption is minimal.

Nursing Considerations. Vaginal bleeding is frightening for the family members, who are usually concerned about the safety of the mother as well as the fetus. Moreover, bleeding is often accompanied by pain and loss of the pregnancy. Nurses usually try to:

- Confirm pregnancy and determine length of gestation according to prenatal records or history taken at initial contact.
- Evaluate vital signs, skin color and temperature, capillary return, urinary output, and level of consciousness to determine hemodynamic status.
- Evaluate the amount of bleeding and obtain a description of the location and severity of pain.
- Monitor the condition of the fetus.
- Collaborate with physician to administer intravenous fluids and/or $Rh_o(D)$ immune globulin.
- Check laboratory values, such as hemoglobin, hematocrit, blood type and Rh factor, and clotting factors. Kleihauer-Betke (K-B) testing identifies fetal-maternal hemorrhage.
- Keep the woman as comfortable as possible.
- Consider the psychologic needs of the family members, who usually experience an acute sense of loss and grief when the fetus does not survive.
    - Acknowledge the parents' emotions.
    - Allow time to listen and to reflect family feelings.
    - Provide reassurance to lessen feelings of self-blame.

— Help woman express her feelings to partner and other trusted family members.
- Keep the family informed of preoperative procedures that are often performed quickly.
- Reinforce necessary follow-up care.
- Teach the family how to prevent and recognize signs of infection that may occur as a result of blood loss. Some specific measures include:
  — Instructing her to check her temperature every 8 hours for the first 3 days at home. Validating that the woman knows how to use a thermometer.
  — Emphasizing the importance of careful handwashing before and after changing pads.
  — Suggesting that she consult with health care provider before resuming use of tampons or sexual intercourse.
  — Advising her to consume foods high in iron to increase hemoglobin and hematocrit values.

DISSEMINATED INTRAVASCULAR COAGULATION

Disseminated intravascular coagulation (DIC) is a life-threatening complication in which anticoagulation and procoagulation factors are activated at the same time. The result is a simultaneous decrease in clotting factors and an increase in anticoagulant factors that leave the circulating blood unable to clot.

ETIOLOGY AND PREDISPOSING FACTORS

Major predisposing factors include:

- Missed abortion.
- Abruptio placentae.
- Preeclampsia or eclampsia.

Signs and Symptoms
- Profuse bleeding from any vulnerable area, such as intravenous sites, incisions, the gums, or nose
- Profuse bleeding from the site of placental attachment

Management

- Delivery of the fetus and placenta to stop the production of thromboplastin, which is fueling the process
- Blood replacement with whole blood, packed red blood cells, plasma, and cryoprecipitate
- Continuous monitoring of maternal vital signs to detect hypovolemia
- Documentation of location and severity of bleeding

DIABETES MELLITUS
TYPES OF DIABETES MELLITUS

- Diabetes mellitus that exists prior to pregnancy may be type 1 (insulin dependent, also known as insulin deficient) or type 2 (non–insulin dependent, also known as insulin resistant with a relative deficiency of insulin to metabolize carbohydrate). *Oral hypoglycemic medications are not presently advised for use during pregnancy.*
- Diabetes that develops during pregnancy is termed gestational diabetes mellitus (GDM).

EFFECTS OF PREGNANCY ON INSULIN PRODUCTION

Significant changes in insulin production affect all women during pregnancy. Women without diabetes adapt easily to the changes, but those with diabetes of all types must adjust their insulin dose, diet, and exercise regimen. Changes include:

- A decrease in the amount of insulin needed during the first trimester, when the expectant woman experiences anorexia, nausea, and vomiting.
- An increase in the amount of insulin needed during the second and third trimesters, when placental hormones create resistance to insulin.
- Either an increase or a decrease in insulin during the intrapartum, depending on the exertion of labor, food and fluid intake, and blood glucose levels. Insulin is often administered by insulin infusion ("insulin drip"), with the dose adjusted based on frequent blood glucose levels.

- A decrease in the amount of insulin needed during the postpartum period, when the hormones of pregnancy decline after the delivery of the placenta.

EFFECTS OF DIABETES ON PREGNANCY

Women with diabetes mellitus are at increased risk for complications that may include:

- Chronic hypertension or preeclampsia, possibly related to maternal vascular damage secondary to diabetes.
- Urinary tract infections that may be due to glycosuria, which provides a nutrient-rich medium for bacterial growth.
- Hydramnios (excessive amniotic fluid) as a result of fetal hyperglycemia and consequent fetal polyuria.
- Premature rupture of membranes and preterm labor that may be related to overdistention of the uterus by hydramnios or a large fetus.
- Difficult labor, injury to birth canal, cesarean birth, and postpartum hemorrhage that are associated with fetal macrosomia.
- Ketoacidosis due to increase in ketones when fats and proteins are metabolized for energy instead of glucose.

INCREASED FETAL AND NEONATAL RISKS

- Congenital anomalies, such as neural tube defects, caudal regression syndrome, and cardiac defects that are related to maternal hyperglycemia during the first trimester while fetal organs are being formed
- Perinatal death due to maternal vascular damage, maternal hypertension, or early deterioration of the placenta
- Large infant (>4000 g) due to fetal hyperglycemia and consequent high levels of fetal insulin (a powerful growth hormone)
- Birth injury related to macrosomia, difficult labor, and shoulder dystocia
- Intrauterine growth restriction if there is damage to maternal arterioles, resulting in poor perfusion of the placenta; inadequate fetal oxygenation may result in

oligohydramnios as the fetus conserves oxygenated blood for circulation to the brain
- Polycythemia in response to frequent episodes of hypoxia
- Neonatal hyperbilirubinemia when excessive red blood cells are broken down, leaving large quantities of unconjugated bilirubin
- Neonatal respiratory distress syndrome due to hyperinsulinemia that retards cortisol, which is necessary for surfactant production
- Neonatal hypoglycemia following birth when serum glucose declines but neonatal insulin production remains high

DIAGNOSIS OF GESTATIONAL DIABETES MELLITUS (GDM)

All women are screened for GDM during pregnancy, usually at 24 to 28 weeks of gestation. Women at high risk to develop GDM may be screened earlier. Screening tests include:

- Glucose challenge test (GCT) 1 hour following ingestion of 50 g of glucose solution. If serum glucose level is 140 mg/dL or greater, a GTT should be performed.
- Three-hour oral glucose tolerance test (OGTT); this test is positive if two or more of the following serum glucose levels are met or exceeded after drinking 100 g of glucose solution:

Fasting	>95 mg/dL
1 hour	>180 mg/dL
2 hour	>155 mg/dL
3 hour	>140 mg/dL

PREDISPOSING FACTORS FOR GESTATIONAL DIABETES MELLITUS

- Overweight (body mass index [BMI] ≥26-29 or obesity [BMI>29])
- Chronic hypertension
- Maternal age older than 25 years
- Family history of diabetes in close relatives
- Previous birth of a large infant (≥4000 g)
- Previous birth of an infant with unexplained congenital anomalies

- Previous unexplained fetal death
- Gestational diabetes in previous pregnancy
- Multifetal pregnancy
- Fasting serum glucose ≥140 mg/dL or random serum glucose ≥200 mg/dL

MANAGEMENT OF GESTATIONAL DIABETES MELLITUS

- Dietary counseling that should emphasize:
  — Adequate calories (average of 30 kcal/kg/day for nonobese woman).
  — Adequate complex carbohydrates to prevent ketosis.
  — Distribution of calories among three meals and three or more snacks.
  — Restriction or elimination of sugars and concentrated sweets.
  — Teaching use of exchange lists or carbohydrate counts to maintain normal glucose levels.
  — Treatment of hypoglycemia with limited amounts of simple carbohydrates (glucose tablets, fruit juice or regular soft drink, saltine crackers, fruit, or small quantities of sugar or honey). Teaching the woman to avoid large amounts of simple carbohydrates reduces the possibility that her blood sugar will abruptly rise and then fall again.
- Exercise regimen
- Instruction in self-evaluation of glucose levels and times when each level (often fasting and 2-hour postprandial) should be done
- Fetal surveillance that may include:
  — Maternal assessment of fetal activity ("kick counts").
  — Nonstress tests.
  — Amniotic fluid index.
  — Biophysical profile.
- Administration of insulin if diet and exercise do not maintain normal blood glucose
- Routine prenatal care
- Opportunities for maternal decision making and control whenever possible

ASSESSMENT AND MANAGEMENT OF PREEXISTING DIABETES MELLITUS

A team, composed of a perinatologist, obstetrician, dietitian, nurse-educator, and diabetologist, help the mother:

- Maintain normal blood glucose levels.
- Give birth to a healthy baby.
- Avoid accelerated impairment of blood vessels and other organs.

Prior to pregnancy, every effort is made to achieve and maintain normal blood glucose levels. This helps prevent congenital anomalies that are strongly associated with hyperglycemia in the first trimester.

In addition, specific evaluation may be done to determine the effects of diabetes on maternal body systems. These tests include:

- Baseline electrocardiogram.
- Evaluation for retinopathy.
- Renal function tests.
- Glycosylated hemoglobin (HbA_{1C}) for average glucose concentration during the preceding 2 to 3 months.
- Maternal serum screen for neural tube or other defects (triple-marker or multiple-marker screening).
- Ultrasound evaluation of fetus, including fetal cardiac structures.
- Fetal surveillance (kick counts, nonstress tests, contraction stress tests, biophysical profiles, amniotic fluid index) to monitor the well-being of the fetus.
- Self-monitoring of blood glucose several times each day to determine amounts of insulin needed to maintain euglycemia.
- Diet of adequate caloric intake that should be distributed among three meals and two to four snacks daily.
- Insulin therapy as necessary to maintain normal blood glucose.

- Recognition and management of hyperglycemia; signs include:
  — Fatigue.
  — Flushed, hot skin.
  — Dry mouth; excessive thirst.
  — Frequent urination.
  — Rapid, deep respirations; odor of acetone on the breath.
  — Drowsiness; headache.
  — Depressed reflexes.
- Instruction to notify the physician when signs or symptoms of hyperglycemia are noted.
- Recognition and management of hypoglycemia; signs include:
  — Shakiness (tremors).
  — Sweating.
  — Pallor; cold, clammy skin.
  — Disorientation, irritability.
  — Headache.
  — Hunger.
  — Blurred vision.
- Timing of delivery as close to term as possible.

NURSING CONSIDERATIONS

Women respond differently to the intense medical supervision that is necessary to maintain normal blood glucose. Some fear they will be unable to control the diabetes to the degree expected. Other women may feel that they are only an "incubator" and that their feelings are unimportant as long as the fetus thrives. Nurses can facilitate communications and provide support by:

- Asking broad, open-ended questions such as, "What are your major concerns?" "How do you feel about the plan of care?"
- Actively listening to concerns of the woman and her family.
- Conveying acceptance of feelings that are expressed, whether they are negative or positive.

- Identifying opportunities for control in exercise and diet whenever possible.
- Teaching and evaluating a woman's understanding of insulin administration: type or types of insulins given, mixing insulins, and length of time to delay meal after insulin injection.
- Recognizing signs of hypoglycemia, treatment, and reevaluation of glucose levels.
- Providing normal pregnancy care, which is sometimes ignored because the focus is on controlling diabetes and preventing complications.
- Providing and reinforcing information about required tests and procedures, such as nonstress tests, biophysical profile, and self-monitoring of blood glucose.
- Giving praise and encouragement for maintaining normal blood glucose and for keeping recommended appointments.

HYPERTENSIVE DISORDERS OF PREGNANCY

In addition to its contribution to disease and mortality among all ages and both genders, hypertension is an important cause of perinatal morbidity and mortality. Hypertension may precede pregnancy or it may first occur during pregnancy. Hypertension that persists well after pregnancy signifies a chronic disease that may have many causes and complications. Pregnancy-related hypertension is a multiorgan disease process that is related to vasospasm and a consequent rise in blood pressure, a decrease in cardiac output, and reduced perfusion of vital organs such as the kidneys, brain, and placenta. Figure 1-11 traces the pathologic processes throughout the body.

Terminology used to describe pregnancy related hypertension was developed within the National Institutes of Health to clarify use of terms among health care providers.

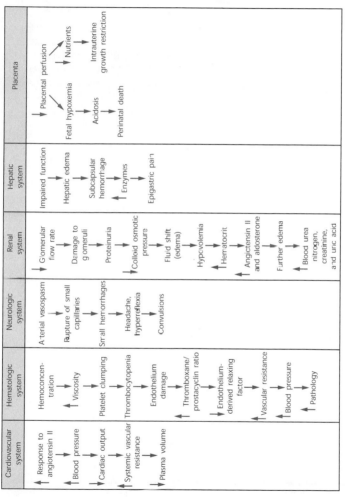

Figure 1-11   The pathologic process of preeclampsia.

Table 1-7	**Classification of Hypertensive Disorders of Pregnancy**

Classification	Comments
Preeclampsia	Systolic blood pressure ≥140 mm Hg or diastolic blood pressure ≥90 mm Hg that develops after 20 weeks of pregnancy and is accompanied by proteinuria >0.3 g in a 24-hr urine collection (random urine dipstick is usually ≥1+).
Eclampsia	Progression of preeclampsia to generalized seizures that cannot be attributed to other causes.
Gestational hypertension	Systolic blood pressure ≥140 mm Hg or diastolic blood pressure ≥90 mm Hg that develops after 20 weeks of pregnancy, but without significant proteinuria (negative or trace on a random urine dipstick).
Chronic hypertension	Systolic blood pressure ≥140 mm Hg or diastolic blood pressure ≥90 mm Hg that was known to exist before pregnancy or develops before 20 weeks of gestation. Also diagnosed if the hypertension does not resolve during the postpartum period.
Preeclampsia superimposed on chronic hypertension	Development of new-onset proteinuria >0.3 g in a 24-hr collection in a woman who has chronic hypertension. In women who had proteinuria before 20 weeks, preeclampsia should be suspected if the woman has a sudden increase in proteinuria from her baseline levels, a sudden increase in blood pressure when it had been previously well controlled, development of thrombocytopenia (platelets <100,000/mm^3), or abnormal elevations of liver enzymes (AST or ALT).

ALT, Alanine aminotransferase (formerly SGPT); *AST,* aspartate aminotransferase (formerly SGOT).

RISK FACTORS

Risk Factors for Pregnancy-Related Hypertension (PRH)*

First pregnancy
Age >40 years
Anemia
Family history of PIH
Chronic hypertension or preexisting vascular disease
Chronic renal disease
Obesity
Diabetes mellitus
Antiphospholipid syndrome
Multifetal pregnancy
Angiotensin gene T235
Mother or sister who had preeclampsia

SIGNS AND SYMPTOMS

The classic signs of preeclampsia are: (1) hypertension, (2) proteinuria, and (3) generalized edema. Edema is currently considered a nonspecific sign of pregnany related hypertension because it may occur in the woman who is not hypertensive and may be absent if the woman does have preeclampsia. See Table 1-8 for a description of mild versus severe preeclampsia. Because of potential errors, the procedure for determining blood pressure should be standardized in each facility. The woman should be sitting with the arm supported in a horizontal position at heart level. The diastolic pressure should be recorded at Korotkoff phase V, disappearance of sound (National High Blood Pressure Education Program Working Group on High Blood Pressure in

---

*From Poole, J.H., Sosa, M.E., Freda, M.C., Kendrick, J.M., Luppi, C.J., Krening, C.F., & Dauphinee, J.D. (2001). High-risk pregnancy. In K.R. Simpson & P.A. Creehan (Eds.), *AWHONN perinatal nursing* (2nd ed., pp. 173-296). Philadelphia: Lippincott; Martin, J.A., Hamilton, B.E., Sutton, P.D., Ventura, S.J., Menacker, F., & Munson, M.L. (2003). Births: Final data for 2002. *National Vital Statistics Reports,* 52(10). Hyattsville, MD: National Center for Health Statistics, 2003; Roberts, J.M. (2004). Pregnancy-related hypertension. In R.K. Creasy, R. Resnik, & J.D. Iams (Eds.), *Maternal-fetal medicine: Principles and practice* (5th ed., pp. 859-899). Philadelphia: Saunders.

Table 1-8	Mild versus Severe Preeclampsia	
Parameter Evaluated	**Mild**	**Severe**
Systolic blood pressure	≥140 but <160 mm Hg	≥160 mm Hg (2 readings, 6 hours apart, while on bed rest)
Diastolic blood pressure	≥90 but <110 mm Hg	≥110 mm Hg
Proteinuria (24-hr specimen is preferred to eliminate hour-to-hour variations)	≥0.3 g but <2 g in 24-hr specimen (1+ on random dipstick)	≥5 g in 24-hr specimen (3+ or higher on random dipstick sample)
Creatinine, serum (renal function)	Normal	Elevated (>1.2 mg/dL)
Platelets	Normal	Decreased (<100,000 cells/mm^3)
Liver enzymes (alanine aminotransferase [ALT] or aspartate aminotransferase [AST])	Normal or minimal increase in levels	Elevated levels
Urine output	Normal	Oliguria common, often <500 mL/day
Severe, unrelenting headache not attributable to other cause; mental confusion (cerebral edema)	Absent	Often present

Persistent right upper quadrant or epigastric pain or pain penetrating to the back (distention of the liver capsule); nausea and vomiting	Absent	May be present and often precedes seizure
Visual disturbances (spots or "sparkles"; temporary blindness; photophobia)	Absent to minimal	Common
Pulmonary edema; heart failure; cyanosis	Absent	May be present
Fetal growth restriction	Normal growth	Growth restriction; reduced amniotic fluid volume

From American Academy of Pediatrics & American College of Obstetricians and Gynecologists. (2002). *Guidelines for perinatal care* (5th ed.). Elk Grove Village, IL: Author; National High Blood Pressure Education Program Working Group on High Blood Pressure in Pregnancy. (2000). Report on the national high blood pressure education program working group on high blood pressure in pregnancy. *American Journal of Obstetrics and Gynecology,* 183(1), S1-S22.

Pregnancy, 2000). Hospitalizing the woman for serial observations of her blood pressure may identify true elevations from those induced by anxiety.

MANAGEMENT OF MILD PREECLAMPSIA

Management in the home may be possible if the woman is in stable condition with no evidence of worsening maternal or fetal status. The woman and her family must be able to adhere to a prescribed treatment plan that often includes:

- Bed rest or reduced activity—a lateral position for at least 1½ hours per day.
- Fetal movement monitoring (kick counts).
- Home blood pressure monitoring, often two to four times per day, using a cuff of the correct size, the same arm, and the same maternal position each time the blood pressure is checked.
- Daily weights, usually each morning and wearing clothing of similar weight.
- Daily urine dipstick for protein using first voided specimen. Normal is negative or trace.
- Uterine activity monitoring for signs of preterm labor.
- Documentation for home health care nurse.
- Additional fetal surveillance such as serial sonography, weekly nonstress testing, contraction stress testing, or biophysical profiles as necessary.
- Reporting nonreassuring signs such as reduced fetal movement, persistent or severe headache, visual disturbance, or epigastric pain.

MANAGEMENT OF SEVERE PREECLAMPSIA

Goals of management are to prevent generalized seizures and to maintain the pregnancy until it is safe to deliver the fetus. Home care is not appropriate for severe preeclampsia. The woman will be hospitalized for constant assessment and management that includes:

- Bed rest with reduced environmental stimuli. Include seizure precautions.

- Intravenous administration of magnesium sulfate (the drug of choice in the United States to prevent convulsions). See Drug Guide for Magnesium Sulfate in Section Seven, p. 462.
- Administration of antihypertensive medications. See Drug Guide for Hydralazine in Section Seven, p. 461.
- Delivery by induction or ccsarean, depending on gestation and added complications.
- Continuing magnesium sulfate infusion for 24 hours after birth.

NURSING CONSIDERATIONS

Careful nursing assessment is the only way to determine whether the disease is responding to medical management or is worsening. Nursing assessments include:

- Daily weights (rapid increase indicates fluid retention). Significant edema of upper body often accompanies a rapid weight increase.
- Blood pressure to determine response to treatment.
- Respiratory rate (magnesium sulfate causes respiratory depression; rate <12 per minute should be reported at once).
- Breath sounds (moist breath sounds suggest pulmonary edema).
- Hourly urinary output via indwelling catheter (≥30 mL/hr indicates adequate perfusion of kidneys).
- Urine dipstick for protein level.
- Electronic monitoring for changes in fetal heart rate or variability.
- Periodic monitoring for signs of labor or uterine irritability.
- Deep tendon reflexes (biceps, triceps, radial, patellar, Achilles), especially if associated with clonus. Hyperreflexia suggests increasing cerebral irritability; hyporeflexia suggests magnesium excess. See Procedure Guide in Section Six, Assessing Deep Tendon Reflexes, p. 420.
- Level of consciousness (drowsiness, dulled sensorium indicate therapeutic effects of magnesium; nonresponsive behavior or muscle weakness suggest magnesium toxicity).
- Pulse oximetry; oxygen administration at 8 to 10 L/minute.

- Symptoms such as headache, visual disturbances, epigastric pain (indicate increasing severity of the condition and the development of eclampsia).
- Laboratory data (elevated creatinine, elevated liver enzymes, or decreased platelets signify increasing severity of the disease, possibly HELLP syndrome. Serum magnesium levels should be in therapeutic range (4-8 mg/dL).

SPECIFIC NURSING INTERVENTIONS

- Respond to signs of magnesium toxicity.
  - Discontinue magnesium and notify physician if respiratory rate is <12 per minute, if deep tendon reflexes are absent, or if urinary output falls below 30 mL per hour (magnesium is excreted by the kidneys).
  - Have calcium gluconate (an antidote for magnesium sulfate) available. Magnesium toxicity can be reversed by intravenous administration of calcium gluconate 1 g (10 mL of 10%) given at 1 mL/minute.
- Initiate measures to prevent eclamptic seizures.
  - Admit to private room where environmental stimuli (lights, noise, activity) can be controlled; keep the door closed.
  - Pad the door if needed to reduce noise when it must be opened and closed.
  - Collaborate with family to reduce visitors and incoming telephone calls.
  - Group nursing assessments and care to allow long periods of quiet.
  - Move carefully and calmly around the room.
- Intervene to prevent seizure-related injury.
  - Keep the bed in the lowest position with wheels locked and side rails raised at all times.
  - Pad the side rails to prevent trauma should the woman hit them during a seizure.
  - Assemble suction and oxygen equipment in the room. Check the equipment each shift.
  - Keep a preeclampsia tray or supply box in the room. Equipment should include an airway, Ambu bag with

mask, ophthalmoscope, syringes, needles, tourniquet, and reflex hammer. Medications that should be readily available to the woman's location include magnesium sulfate, sodium bicarbonate, heparin sodium, epinephrine, phenytoin, and calcium gluconate.

- Protect the woman and fetus during a convulsion.
  - Remain with the woman and press the emergency call for assistance.
  - Turn the woman onto her side when the tonic phase begins if there is time.
  - Note the time and sequence of the convulsive activity.
  - Insert an airway after the seizure and suction the nose and mouth to prevent aspiration.
  - Administer oxygen by mask.
  - Notify the physician as soon as possible because eclampsia is an obstetric emergency associated with cerebral hemorrhage, premature separation of the placenta, fetal hypoxia, and death of mother or infant.
  - Administer medications and prepare for additional medical intervention as directed by the physician.
- Provide information and support for the family.
  - Explain to the family what has happened after the convulsion has ended.
  - Acknowledge that a convulsion is frightening and that it indicates worsening of the condition.
  - Respond to questions and prepare the family for future medical management that may include delivery of the infant as soon as possible.

HEART DISEASE

A healthy heart can adapt to the increased work of pregnancy and birth without difficulty. If there is preexisting or underlying heart disease, however, the changes can impose a burden on an already compromised heart, resulting in cardiac decompensation and congestive heart failure. The two major categories are rheumatic heart disease and congenital heart disease. The severity of heart disease is determined by the woman's ability to endure physical activity (Table 1-9).

Table 1-9	Functional Classification of Heart Disease

Class I
Uncompromised. No limitation of physical activity. Asymptomatic with ordinary activity.
Class II
Slightly compromised, requiring slight limitation of physical activity. Comfortable at rest, but ordinary physical activity causes fatigue, dyspnea, palpitations, or anginal pain.
Class III
Marked limitation of physical activity. Comfortable at rest, but less than ordinary activity causes excessive fatigue, palpitation, dyspnea, or anginal pain. Markedly compromised.
Class IV
Inability to perform any physical activity without discomfort. Symptoms of cardiac insufficiency even at rest.
 In general, maternal and fetal risks for class I and II disease are small but are greatly increased with classes III and IV.

Additional cardiac complications may affect pregnancy or postpartum women and include mitral valve prolapse and cardiomyopathy.

SIGNS AND SYMPTOMS
- Dyspnea, paroxysmal nocturnal dyspnea, and hemoptysis
- Syncope (fainting) with exertion
- Cyanosis or clubbing of the fingers
- Chest pain with exertion
- Heart murmurs
- Cardiac enlargement
- Serious dysrhythmias
- Diagnostic studies that often include imaging of the chest, electrocardiography, or echocardiography

ANTEPARTUM MANAGEMENT
The goal of treatment is to ensure that cardiac demand does not exceed the functional capacity of the heart.

To accomplish this goal, all pregnant women with heart disease should:

- Limit physical activity to remain free of symptoms of cardiac stress such as dyspnea, chest pain, or tachycardia.
- Avoid excessive weight gain that places greater demands on the heart.
- Prevent anemia, which decreases the oxygen-carrying capacity of the blood and results in a compensatory increase in heart rate.
- Prevent infection that may include immunizations for influenza or pneumonia, administration of prophylactic antibiotics, and rapid treatment of infections. Avoiding those who are ill should be emphasized.
- Undergo careful assessment for the development of congestive heart failure, pulmonary edema, or cardiac arrhythmias.
- Anticoagulant therapy with enoxaparin (Lovenox) or heparin.
- Antidysrhythmic therapy may be necessary for those with arrhythmias (digoxin, adenosine and calcium channel blockers appear to be safe). Beta blockers may be required but have been associated with neonatal respiratory depression, sustained bradycardia, and hypoglycemia if given late in pregnancy. Atenolol and metoprolol may be preferred beta blockers.
- Diuretics such as furosemide or thiazides are rarely used in pregnancy and require careful monitoring of fluid and electrolyte balance if they are required.

INTRAPARTUM MANAGEMENT

Every effort is made to minimize the effects of labor on the cardiovascular system. Because of surgical risks to the cardiovascular system, vaginal birth is ideal unless there are specific indications for cesarean birth. Care includes:

- Careful management of fluid administration to prevent fluid overload.
- Side-lying position with head and shoulders elevated.
- Pulse oximetry with oxygen supplementation as required.

- Cardiac monitoring as required.
- Sedation and epidural anesthesia to reduce discomfort.
- Quiet, calm environment to decrease anxiety.
- Keeping the legs level with the body during birth or lowering the legs during the third stage to minimize the risks of fluid overload when blood from the uteroplacental unit is added to central circulation.
- Using vacuum extraction or outlet forceps to limit the pushing and duration of second stage.
- Carefully assessing signs of circulatory overload (bounding pulse, distended neck and peripheral veins, moist rales in the lungs) during the fourth stage.

POSTPARTUM MANAGEMENT

Women who have shown no evidence of distress during pregnancy, labor, or childbirth may decompensate during the postpartum period. They must be observed closely for signs of:

- Cardiac decompensation, possibly manifested by:
  — Cough (frequent, productive, hemoptysis).
  — Moist rales in lower lobes.
  — Progressive dyspnea with exertion; low pulse oximetry or arterial line oxygen levels.
  — Orthopnea.
  — Pitting edema of legs and feet or generalized edema of face, hands, or sacral area.
  — Palpitations of the heart.
  — Progressive fatigue or syncope.
- Fluid overload; inadequate urine output to excrete high volume of postdelivery fluid.
- Infection.
- Hemorrhage.
- Signs of superficial or deep vein thrombosis.

NURSING CONSIDERATIONS

Nursing care focuses on teaching the woman and her family about measures that reduce the workload of the heart during pregnancy and postpartum recovery. Measures are individualized to the patient but may include:

- Avoiding excessive weight gain while achieving necessary nutrients.
- Modifying activities that require energy.
  - Rest for an hour after meals.
  - Sit rather than stand whenever possible.
  - Rest whenever an activity increases heart rate.
  - Stop any activity that produces dyspnea, tachycardia, or chest pain.
- Avoiding unnecessary exposure to extreme temperatures.
- Identifying and reducing emotional stress.
- Maintaining contact between the mother and newborn in the most effective way.

HYPEREMESIS GRAVIDARUM

Hyperemesis gravidarum (HEG) is persistent, uncontrollable vomiting that begins in the early weeks and may continue throughout pregnancy. Consequences may include:

- Severe weight loss.
- Ketosis, acid-base imbalance, and electrolyte imbalance.
- Metabolic alkalosis (due to loss of large amounts of hydrochloric acid from the stomach).
- Vitamin K deficiency and clotting disorders.

ETIOLOGY AND PREDISPOSING FACTORS

The cause is unknown; however, some demographic factors have been studied. The condition is more prevalent in unmarried white women, first pregnancies, and multifetal pregnancies. Other risks may include elevated pregnancy-related hormone levels, thyroid dysfunction, or psychologic factors. Additional causes may include maternal allergy to fetal proteins or *Helicobacter pylori,* an organism that causes peptic ulcer disease.

MANAGEMENT

- Exclusion of other possible causes for extreme nausea and vomiting, such as cholecystitis or a peptic ulcer
- Lab studies: hemoglobin and hematocrit to identify hemoconcentration; electrolyte studies to identify deficient sodium, potassium, and chloride; metabolic studies to identify elevated creatinine that may indicate renal dysfunction
- Administration of pyridoxine (vitamin B_6); prenatal vitamins taken at the best time
- Medications that may include promethazine, diphenhydramine, histamine-receptor antagonists (famotidine, ranitidine); gastric acid inhibitors (esomeprazole, omeprazole); metoclopramide; ondansetron
- Possibly minimal steroids to control
- Intravenous fluids to replace electrolytes and total parenteral nutrition
- Periodic brief rehospitalizations if needed to correct hydration, electrolyte imbalances, and reestablish food intake

NURSING CONSIDERATIONS

Care usually takes place in the home, and nurses are responsible for assessing and providing care if they work in the home care setting. Nursing assessments include:

- Daily weights at home or when hospitalized.
- Intake (oral and intravenous).
- Output (emesis, urine, bowel; 1 mL/kg/hr of urinary output suggests adequate perfusion of the kidneys).
- Urine dipsticks to identify elevated ketone levels or other abnormalities.
- Measures to reduce nausea and vomiting.

Nursing interventions focus on reducing nausea and vomiting and maintaining nutrition and fluid balance. Specific interventions include:

- Offering small, frequent feedings, approximately every 2 to 3 hours.

- Describing potassium- and magnesium-rich foods such as fruits, vegetables, meat, seeds or nuts, legumes. Salting foods may replace some that is lost with vomiting.
- Suggesting low-fat foods and easily digested carbohydrates (fruit, bread, rice, cereal, pasta).
- Recommending that soups and other liquids be taken between meals to reduce nausea after eating.
- Instructing that sitting upright after meals reduces gastric reflux.
- Providing emotional support as needed.

Rh INCOMPATIBILITY
ETIOLOGY
If blood from the Rh-positive fetus enters the bloodstream of the Rh-negative mother, her body reacts by developing antibodies to the foreign antigen. Fetal Rh-positive blood may leak across the placenta in very small amounts during pregnancy. During labor or childbirth, small placental tears may allow fetal blood to mix with maternal blood in small quantities. The antibodies that develop as a consequence may cause problems for a subsequent pregnancy with an Rh-positive fetus (Figure 1-12).

FETAL-NEONATAL IMPLICATIONS
Red blood cells of an Rh-positive fetus are destroyed by maternal antibodies that cross the placenta, producing:

- Anemia.
- Hyperbilirubinemia.
- Hypoxemia.
- Generalized fetal edema.
- Fetal death.

MANAGEMENT
- Prenatal screening for Rh factor for all women
- Antibody titer for all Rh-negative women
- Administration of $Rh_o(D)$ immune globulin (see Drug Guide, $Rh_o(D)$ Immune Globulin, Section Seven, p. 471 to:

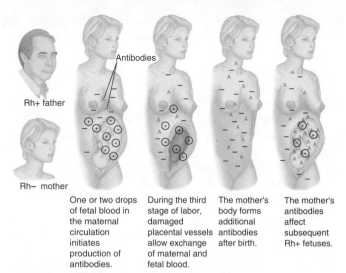

One or two drops of fetal blood in the maternal circulation initiates production of antibodies.

During the third stage of labor, damaged placental vessels allow exchange of maternal and fetal blood.

The mother's body forms additional antibodies after birth.

The mother's antibodies affect subsequent Rh+ fetuses.

Figure 1-12 The process of maternal sensitization to the Rh factor.

— Unsensitized, Rh-negative woman at 28 weeks
— After amniocentesis or chorionic villus sampling
— With bleeding episodes or after trauma if needed
— Following the birth of an Rh-positive infant

• Evaluation of fetal bilirubin (by amniocentesis for optical density of the fluid or DNA analysis of fetal cells to determine Rh factor) if antibody titer indicates maternal sensitization

• Ultrasound examination to identify fetal edema, presence of ascites, heart enlargement, or hydramnios

• Cordocentesis for severe fetal anemia and transfusion of blood in the preterm fetus

INFECTIONS

Infections can be mild or even asymptomatic in adults, but they are of great concern during pregnancy because they can cause catastrophic consequences for the fetus or neonate. See Table 1-10 for the most common viral and nonviral infections. The most common sexually transmitted diseases and their effects on pregnancy are described in Table 1-11.

Table 1-10	Common Viral and Nonviral Infections	
Maternal Effects	**Fetal-Neonatal Effects**	**Treatment**
	Viral Infections	
	Cytomegalovirus Infection	
Mild, flulike symptoms after exposure to body fluids such as saliva, semen, cervical mucus, breast milk, stool, and urine.	2% of all live neonates are infected with virus; 5%-13% may be symptomatic at birth. Most serious complications are deafness, mental retardation, seizures, IUGR, blindness.	No effective therapy; antiviral agents are toxic and only temporarily suppress shedding of the virus.
	Rubelia	
Fever, maculopapular rash, general malaise; maternal infection in first trimester results in multiorgan complications for the fetus.	Increase in spontaneous abortion, deafness, cataracts, mental retardation, cardiac defects, and microcephaly. Neonates shed the virus for many months.	Vaccine available for prevention; blood test of rubella titers determines maternal immunity.
	Varicella Infection (Chickenpox)	
Fever, anorexia, progressive rash (macules, papules to vesicles that	If infection occurs during first trimester, fetus is at risk for congenital varicella	Avoid contact with infected people; report symptoms

Continued

Table 1-10	Common Viral and Nonviral Infections—cont'd	
Maternal Effects	**Fetal-Neonatal Effects**	**Treatment**
crust and dry); varicella-zoster immune globulin (VZIG) administered after exposure to lessen fetal effects.	that includes limb hypoplasia, cutaneous scars, cataracts; exposure in later pregnancy may develop life-threatening varicella infection.	immediately; administer VZIG to infants whose mothers have chickenpox.
	Genital Herpes	
Virus shed from active lesions; vertical transmission from mother to infant when virus ascends after rupture of membranes, or when fetus comes into direct contact with infectious genital secretions; antiviral chemotherapy (acyclovir) is pregnancy risk category C and is used with caution during pregnancy.	Neonatal herpes infection is a major perinatal problem; symptoms are usually present within 2 to 3 days; mortality rate is 50% for disseminated herpes infection in newborn.	Cesarean birth if active genital lesion is present; protect infant from direct contact with lesions after birth.
	Hepatitis B	
Vomiting, pain, fever, jaundice, painful joints; hepatitis B vaccine available for	Prematurity, low birth weight, neonatal death.	HBIG is administered to newborns whose mothers

prevention; hepatitis B immune globulin (HBIG) is administered to women who carry surface antigen (HBsAG positive). *Clinical Tip:* Newborn should be bathed carefully before any injections are given to prevent infections from skin surface contamination.

are HBsAg-positive; Hepatitis B vaccine is also given soon after birth; within 12 hours to the newborn whose mother is HBsAg positive.

Acquired Immunodeficiency Syndrome

Vertical transmission from mother to infant is between 20% and 40% if the mother had no antiretroviral therapy during pregnancy.

No evidence of fetal embryopathy. Antiretroviral drug therapy through pregnancy and after birth can limit newborn infection. Breastfeeding not advised.

Encouraging results have been obtained from antiviral medications and protease inhibitors that reduce replication of the virus and reduce vertical transmission.

Nonviral Infections

Toxoplasmosis (Protozoa Toxoplasma gondii)

Often subclinical; fatigue, muscle pains, swollen glands; transmitted through undercooked meat, contact with infected cat feces, or transplacentally.

Spontaneous abortion, low birth weight, jaundice, anemia; neurologic damage may develop years later.

To prevent, cook meat thoroughly, avoid touching mouth or eyes while handling raw meat, wash

Continued

Table 1-10	Common Viral and Nonviral Infections—cont'd	
Maternal Effects	**Fetal-Neonatal Effects**	**Treatment**
		hands often, wash raw fruits and vegetables, avoid uncooked eggs and unpasteurized milk; avoid contact with materials contaminated with cat feces.
Group B Streptococcus Infection (Group B Streptococci)		
Colonizes in the vagina, cervix, urethra, and rectum of women; usually asymptomatic, although intermittent maternal infections can occur.	Sepsis, pneumonia, meningitis of newborn; permanent neurologic sequelae are possible.	Prenatal screening cultures and intrapartum administration of penicillin to prevent neonatal infection.
Tuberculosis (Mycobacterium tuberculosis)		
Transmitted by aerosolized droplets of liquid containing the bacterium that is inhaled by noninfected person; PPD is used to screen for disease during pregnancy.	Perinatal infection is rare; diagnosis made by finding bacilli in gastric aspirate of newborn.	Isoniazid (INH) plus rifampin; pyridoxine may be given with INH to prevent fetal neurotoxicity; skin-test infant and begin preventive INH therapy if necessary.

Table 1-11	Sexually Transmitted Diseases, Vaginal Infections, and Urinary Tract Infections During Pregnancy

Maternal, Fetal, and Neonatal Effects	Nursing Considerations

Sexually Transmitted Diseases

Syphilis (Causative Organism: Spirochete Treponema pallidum)

If untreated, the infection may cross the placenta to the fetus and result in spontaneous abortion, a stillborn infant, premature labor and birth, or congenital syphilis. Major signs of congenital syphilis are enlarged liver and spleen, skin lesions, rashes, osteitis, pneumonia, and hepatitis.	Penicillin is the primary treatment to cure the disease in both the woman and fetus. Women who are allergic are desensitized and then treated.*

Gonorrhea (Causative Organism: Bacterium Neisseria gonorrhoeae)

Not transmitted via the placenta; vertical transmission from mother to newborn during birth may cause ophthalmia neonatorum. Endocervicitis and weakness of the fetal membranes increase the risk for premature rupture of membranes and preterm labor. Chlamydial infection is likely to accompany the gonorrhea infection.	Ceftriaxone or cefixime plus amoxicillin or azithromycin are now recommended for penicillin-resistant organisms because 20%-50% of women with gonorrhea will also have chlamydial infection.*† The partner must also be treated to prevent reinfection. Infants are treated with an ophthalmic antibiotic such as ceftriaxone at birth to prevent ophthalmia neonatorum.

Continued

Table 1-11	Sexually Transmitted Diseases, Vaginal Infections, and Urinary Tract Infections During Pregnancy—cont'd

Maternal, Fetal, and Neonatal Effects	Nursing Considerations
Chlamydial Infection (Causative Organism: Bacterium Chlamydia trachomatis)	
Chlamydial infection is the most common sexually transmitted disease in the United States. The fetus may be infected during birth and suffer neonatal conjunctivitis or pneumonitis. Conjunctivitis is prevented by erythromycin ophthalmic ointment. *Chlamydia* may also be responsible for premature rupture of membranes, premature labor, and chorioamnionitis.	Education is particularly important because *Chlamydia* infection is the most common sexually transmitted disease in the United States and infection is usually asymptomatic. Both partners should be treated to prevent recurrent infection. As with all sexually transmitted diseases, the use of condoms decreases the risk for infection. Erythromycin or amoxicillin is the recommended treatment. Azithromycin is an alternate treatment.[†]

Trichomoniasis (Causative Organism: Protozoan Trichomonas vaginalis)

Common cause of vaginitis in 10%-50% of pregnant women. Associated with preterm rupture of membranes and postpartum endometritis.[†]

Metronidazole (Flagyl) may be given to the pregnant woman as a 2-g single oral dose. Consistent association between fetal abnormalities or injury and metronidazole use has not been upheld.[†]

Condyloma Acuminatum (Causative Organism: Human Papillomavirus)

Transmission of condyloma acuminatum, also called *venereal* or *genital warts*, may occur during vaginal birth and is associated with the development of epithelial tumors of the mucous membranes of the larynx in children. Pregnancy can cause proliferation of lesions, which are associated with cervical dysplasia and cancer.

The common choices for nonpregnant therapy (podophyllin, podofilox, imiquimod) are not recommended during pregnancy. Excision of the maternal lesions by cryotherapy or cautery may be done.[†]

Vaginal Infections

Candidiasis (Causative Organism: Yeast Candida albicans)

Oral candidiasis (thrush) may develop in newborns if infection is present at birth. Thrush is treated with application of nystatin (Mycostatin) over the surfaces of the oral cavity four times a day for several days.

Candidiasis (sometimes called *Monilia vaginitis*) is a persistent problem for many women during pregnancy. Examples of maternal treatment choices include miconazole, clotrimazole, or fluconazole.[†]

Continued

Table 1-11	Sexually Transmitted Diseases, Vaginal Infections, and Urinary Tract Infections During Pregnancy—cont'd
Maternal, Fetal, and Neonatal Effects	**Nursing Considerations**
Bacterial Vaginosis‡ (Causative Organism: Gardnerella vaginalis)	
Characteristic "cottage cheese" vaginal discharge with vulvar pruritus, burning, and dyspareunia. Vulva may be red, tender, and edematous.	
No known fetal effects. May be associated with postpartum endometritis; has been associated with preterm birth. Marked by a major shift in vaginal flora from the normal predominance of lactobacilli to a predominance of anaerobic bacteria. Causes profuse, malodorous, "fishy" vaginal discharge, itching, and burning.	Metronidazole (oral therapy or intravaginal gel) or clindamycin intravaginal cream may be used in the pregnant woman.
Urinary Tract Infections	
Asymptomatic Bacteriuria (Causative Organisms: Escherichia coli, Klebsiella, Proteus)	
Ascending bacterial infection can result in cystitis or pyelonephritis in later pregnancy if condition remains untreated.	Recovery of a urinary pathogen from a midstream, clean-catch urine specimen is defined as 100,000 colony-forming units (CFUs) per mL of urine.

Rapid, less-expensive office tests to identify the infection may also be used. Treatment for asymptomatic bacteriuria may include treatment for pathogens that also cause symptomatic cystitis.

Cystitis (Causative Organisms: *E. coli, Klebsiella, Proteus*)

Signs and symptoms include dysuria, frequency, urgency, and suprapubic tenderness. Ascending infection may lead to pyelonephritis.

Antibiotics used for both asymptomatic bacteriuria and cystitis may include amoxicillin, sulfisoxazole, trimethoprim-sulfamethoxazole, nitrofurantoin, or third-generation cephalosporins such as cefixime or cefpodoxime. Emphasize importance of reporting signs of urinary tract infection. Stress the importance of taking all the medication prescribed even if the symptoms abate. Provide information about hygiene measures.

Acute Pyelonephritis (Causative Organisms: *E. coli, Klebsiella, Proteus*)

Increased risk for preterm labor and premature delivery. Maternal complications include a high fever, septic shock, and adult respiratory distress syndrome.

Inform women with asymptomatic bacteriuria or cystitis of signs and symptoms, such as sudden onset of fever (often higher than 39° C (102.2° F), chills, flank pain or tenderness, nausea, and vomiting, so that treatment

Continued

Table 1-11	Sexually Transmitted Diseases, Vaginal infections, and Urinary Tract Infections During Pregnancy—cont'd
Maternal, Fetal, and Neonatal Effects	**Nursing Considerations**
	can begin promptly. Skin cooling equipment may be used to lower her temperature below 38° C (100.4° F), reducing possible compromise of fetal oxygen level. Woman may be hospitalized for intravenous administration of antibiotics. Common combinations include ampicillin or a cephalosporin plus an aminoglycoside. Serum levels of aminoglycosides are often done to ensure an adequate dose without its reaching a toxic level.

*Centers for Disease Control and Prevention. (2002). Sexually transmitted diseases treatment guidelines, 2002. *Morbidity and Mortality Weekly Report, 51*(RR-6). Retrieved February 20, 2005, from www.cdc.gov/STD/treatment/rr5106.pdf.
†Gibbs, R.S., Sweet, R.L., & Duff, W.P. (2004). Maternal and fetal infectious diseases. In R.K. Creasy, R. Resnik, & J.D. Iams (Eds.), *Maternal-fetal medicine: Principles and practice* (5th ed., pp. 741-801). Philadelphia: Saunders.
‡Formerly called *nonspecific vaginitis* or *Gardnerella vaginitis*.

Section 2

Intrapartum

NURSING CARE DURING LABOR AND BIRTH

The intrapartum period begins with the first true labor contraction and ends with the immediate recovery period after birth.

COMPONENTS OF CHILDBIRTH

The four major components of the birth process, often called the "four Ps" of childbirth, are the powers, the passage, the passenger, and the woman's psyche.

Powers
- Two components
  — Uterine contractions: first and second stages
  — Maternal bearing-down (pushing) efforts: second stage
- Contraction cycle
  — Increment: The period of increasing strength
  — Peak (acme): The period of greatest contraction strength
  — Decrement: The period of decreasing strength
  — Interval: The period of uterine relaxation between contractions

Passage
- Bony pelvis
  — False pelvis: Above linea terminalis
  — True pelvis: Below linea terminalis; the part most important to birth
- Divisions of true pelvis
  — Inlet: The upper portion, bounded by the upper border of the symphysis pubis, the sacral promontory, and the linea terminalis

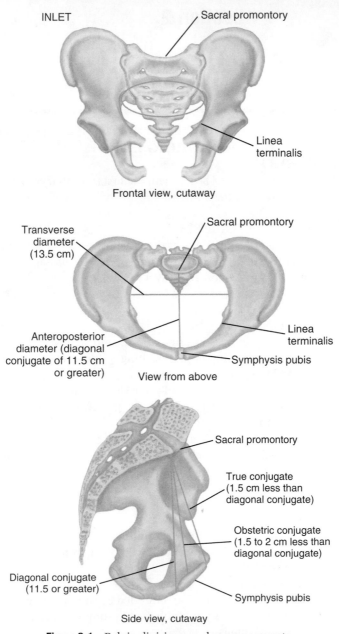

Figure 2-1 Pelvic divisions and measurements.

MIDPELVIS

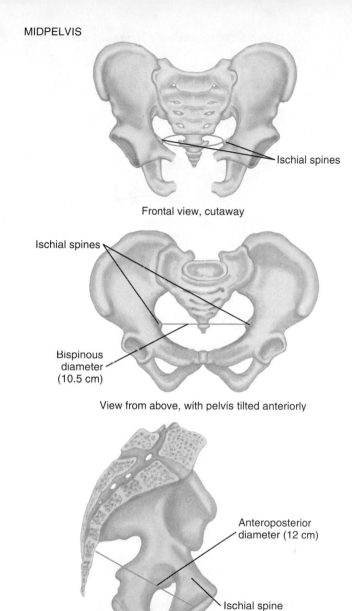

Frontal view, cutaway

Ischial spines

Ischial spines

Bispinous
diameter
(10.5 cm)

View from above, with pelvis tilted anteriorly

Anteroposterior
diameter (12 cm)

Ischial spine

Ischial tuberosity

Side view, cutaway

Figure 2-1, cont'd Pelvic divisions and measurements.

Continued

OUTLET

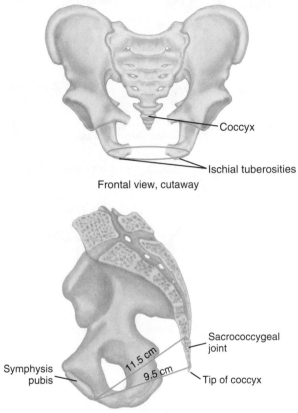

Coccyx

Ischial tuberosities

Frontal view, cutaway

Sacrococcygeal joint

Symphysis pubis

11.5 cm

9.5 cm

Tip of coccyx

Side view, cutaway

Figure 2-1, cont'd Pelvic divisions and measurements.

— Midpelvis (pelvic cavity): Between the boundaries for the pelvic inlet and outlet
— Outlet: The plane of the pelvis that lies at the level of the ischial tuberosities, the lower border of the symphysis pubis, and the coccyx
• Pubic arch: Angle should be 90 degrees or wider to allow the fetus to pass under it easily

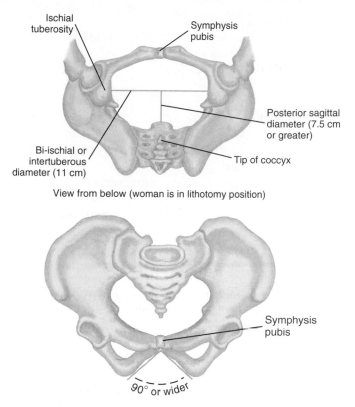

Ischial tuberosity

Symphysis pubis

Posterior sagittal diameter (7.5 cm or greater)

Bi-ischial or intertuberous diameter (11 cm)

Tip of coccyx

View from below (woman is in lithotomy position)

Symphysis pubis

90° or wider

Frontal view, with pelvis tilted anteriorly

Figure 2-1, cont'd Pelvic divisions and measurements.

Passenger. The passenger is the fetus, plus the membranes and placenta.

- Fetal lie: Fetal orientation to the mother's vertebral column, either longitudinal, with the fetal spine parallel to the mother's spine, or transverse, with the fetus at right angles to her spine
- Fetal presentation: The fetal part that enters the pelvis, with cephalic presentations being most common (96%)

— Cephalic presentations
  - Vertex: Most common; fetal head is fully flexed, with the chin on the chest
  - Military: The fetal head is in a neutral position, neither flexed nor extended
  - Brow: The fetal head is partly extended, and may change to a vertex or face presentation as labor progresses
  - Face: The fetal head is fully extended, with the occiput near the fetal spine
— Breech presentations have three variations.
  - Frank breech: The fetal legs extend across the abdomen toward the shoulders, with the buttocks presenting
  - Full (complete) breech: The fetus is flexed, with the buttocks and feet presenting
  - Footling breech: One or both feet presenting
- Fetal position (abbreviations describe the relationship of a fixed fetal part in relationship to one of the four quadrants of the maternal pelvis)
  — Right (R) or left (L) of the maternal pelvis; if the fetal part is directly anterior or posterior, this letter is omitted.
  — Occiput (O), chin (M for *mentum*), or sacrum (S) describes the fetal part used in the abbreviation. Other abbreviations may be used for less common fetal presentations.
  — Anterior (A), posterior (P), or transverse (T) describes whether the fetal point is in the mother's front or rear pelvis, or if it is between the front and back of her pelvis (transverse).

Psyche. Stress hormones called *catecholamines* can inhibit uterine contractions and placental blood flow. Excess muscle tension means that each contraction or maternal bearing-down effort must work against more resistance than if the tension is less. Excess anxiety and fear consume maternal

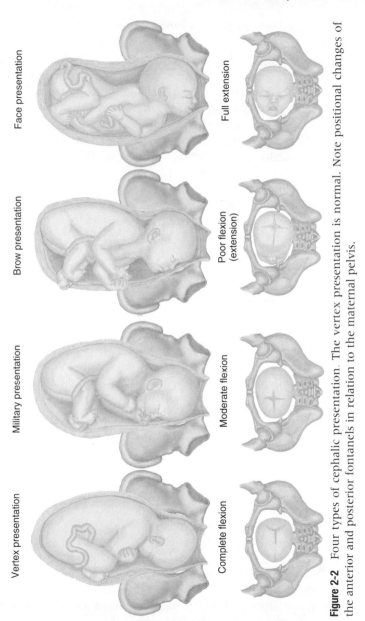

Figure 2-2 Four types of cephalic presentation. The vertex presentation is normal. Note positional changes of the anterior and posterior fontanels in relation to the maternal pelvis.

Face presentation

Full extension

Brow presentation

Poor flexion (extension)

Military presentation

Moderate flexion

Vertex presentation

Complete flexion

energy that she could otherwise use to cope with the demands of labor.

Cultural values affect the family's expectations of birth and satisfaction with it. Cultural values influence who the woman wants to support her during labor, how she expresses pain, and specific practices that are important to her and her family. The nurse must explore with each woman and her family what values are important to them to best determine how to make the experience as satisfying as possible.

CERVICAL CHANGES

- Effacement (thinning): Commonly described as a percentage of its usual length or as length in centimeters; a multigravida's cervix is often thicker than a primigravida's, even during late labor
- Dilation (opening): Described in centimeters

MECHANISMS OF LABOR

The mechanisms (or cardinal movements) of labor occur as the contractions and maternal pushing efforts propel the fetus through the pelvis.

- Descent, engagement, and flexion: The fetal head is pushed downward through the pelvis, causing the head to flex sharply on the chest
  — Engagement occurs when the largest fetal head diameter has passed the pelvic inlet. It is described as *station,* or centimeters above or below the ischial spines, which are a 0 station.
  — Internal rotation occurs when the fetal head rotates from a transverse orientation (side-facing) within the maternal pelvis to an occiput anterior orientation (facing the mother's spine).
  — Extension occurs as the flexed fetal head descends under the symphysis pubis and meets resistance from the perineum.
  — External rotation occurs after the head is born, when it rotates passively to face one of the mother's legs.

The wide diameter of the shoulders is now aligned with the anteroposterior maternal pelvic diameter.
— Expulsion occurs as the anterior, then posterior, fetal shoulders pass beneath the maternal symphysis pubis. The rest of the fetal body follows quickly (Figure 2-3).

STAGES OF LABOR
Labor is divided into four stages.

• First stage is from onset of true labor until full effacement and dilation of the cervix; this stage has three phases
  — Latent phase: 0 to 3 cm of cervical dilation
  — Active phase: 4 to 7 cm of cervical dilation
  — Transition phase: 8 to 10 cm (full) cervical dilation
• Second stage is from full effacement and dilation of the cervix until the birth of the infant
• Third stage is from the birth of the infant until the birth of the placenta
• Fourth stage is 1 to 4 hours after birth for physiologic stabilization and attachment within the new family

TRUE LABOR AND FALSE LABOR
Three categories help the woman and the nurse distinguish contractions that are probably false labor from those that are likely to be true labor.

WHEN TO GO TO THE BIRTH CENTER
When a woman should go to the birth center depends on several factors, such as the number and duration of previous labors, transportation factors, and child care needs. These are typical guidelines:

• Contractions that become progressively more regular, frequent, and have a longer duration and greater intensity
  — Nullipara: Regular contractions, about 5 minutes apart, for 1 hour
  — Multipara: Regular contractions, about 10 minutes apart, for 1 hour

DESCENT, ENGAGEMENT,
AND FLEXION

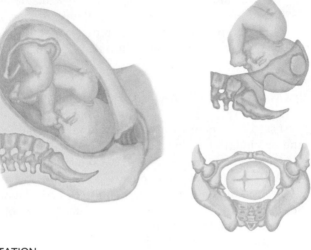

STATION

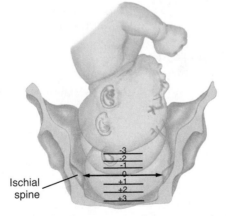

Ischial
spine

Figure 2-3 Mechanisms (cardinal movements) of labor.

- Rupture of the membranes, with or without contractions
- Bright red vaginal bleeding that is not mixed with mucus
- A substantial decrease in fetal movement

Text continued on p. 126

INTERNAL ROTATION

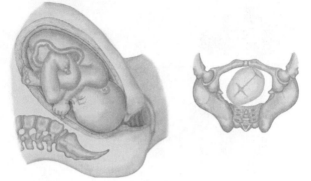

EXTENSION

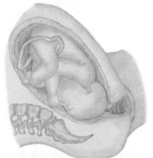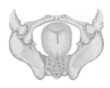

Extension beginning (internal rotation complete)

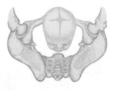

Extension complete

Figure 2-3, cont'd Mechanisms (cardinal movements) of labor.

Continued

EXTERNAL ROTATION

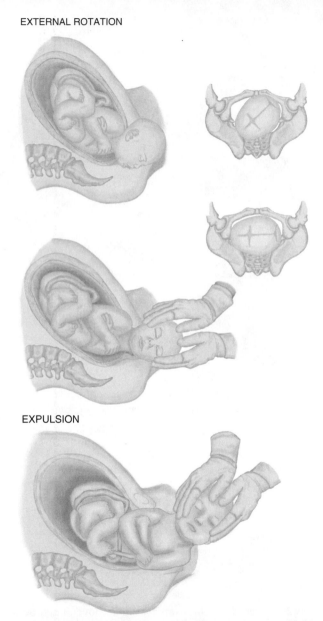

EXPULSION

Figure 2-3, cont'd Mechanisms (cardinal movements) of labor.

Table 2-1	Characteristics of Normal Labor		
First Stage	**Second Stage**	**Third Stage**	**Fourth Stage**
	Duration		
Nullipara: 8-10 hours after reaching active phase (range 6-18 hr); average rate of dilation is 1.2 cm/hr	Nullipara: 50 minutes (range 30 min-3 hr)	5-10 minutes; up to 30 minutes; parity does not affect duration of third stage	First 1-4 hours after birth
Multipara: 6-7 hours after reaching active phase (range 2-10 hr); average rate of dilation is 1.5 cm/hr	Multipara: 20 minutes (range 5-30 min)		

Continued

Table 2-1	Characteristics of Normal Labor—cont'd			
First Stage		**Second Stage**	**Third Stage**	**Fourth Stage**
		Uterine Contractions		
Latent phase: Mild and irregular at first, becoming more regular and longer. Frequency is about 5 minutes and duration is about 30-40 seconds by the end of latent phase		Strong, about 2-3 minutes apart; duration about 40-60 seconds. Maternal bearing-down efforts (pushing) adds to the force of contractions in propelling the fetus through the pelvis	Firmly contracted after the placenta and membranes are expelled	Uterus should be firmly contracted to control bleeding
Active phase: Frequency is 2-5 minutes; duration 40-60 seconds Moderate to strong intensity Transition: Strong contractions, 1½-2 minutes apart; duration 60-90 seconds				

Sensations

Often begins with a low backache or menstrual-like cramping Gradually sweeps to the lower abdomen in a girdle-like fashion	Urge to push or bear down with contractions Distention of vagina and vulva may cause sensation of intense stretching or splitting	Little discomfort; sometimes slight cramping as the placenta is passed	Afterpains may occur, especially in multiparous women, when the uterus alternately contracts and relaxes rather than remaining continuously contracted

Maternal Behaviors

Sociable and relaxed during early labor. Becomes more inwardly focused as labor intensifies. May temporarily lose control during transition	Intense concentration when pushing with contractions. May seem oblivious to surroundings and doze between contractions	Excited and relieved after baby's birth. Anxious to inspect the baby to see if he or she is normal	Tired, but excitement may make rest difficult. Eager to become acquainted with the infant

Table 2-2	How to Know Whether Labor Is "Real"

True labor differs from false labor in three categories

False Labor	True Labor
Contractions	
Inconsistent in frequency, duration, and intensity	A consistent pattern of increasing frequency, duration, and intensity usually develops
A change in activity, such as walking, does not alter contractions, or activity may decrease them	Walking tends to increase contractions
Discomfort	
Felt in the abdomen and groin	Begins in lower back and gradually sweeps around to lower abdomen like a girdle
May be more annoying than truly painful	Back pain may persist in some women
	Early labor often feels like menstrual cramps
Cervix	
No significant change in effacement or dilation of the cervix	Effacement and/or dilation of cervix occurs
	Progressive effacement and dilation of cervix are most important characteristics

Text continued from p. 120.

Text continued from p. 120.

- Other concerns that do not fit these guidelines, because some women will have an atypical labor

ADMISSION TO THE BIRTH CENTER

If focus assessments upon admission are normal and birth is not imminent, additional nursing assessments are done.

Focus Assessments
- Fetal heart rate (FHR) and pattern: An external fetal monitor is usually applied for at least 20 minutes to obtain a baseline.
- Maternal vital signs.
- Impending birth is possible if the woman says her baby is coming, if she makes grunting sounds, or is bearing down. If the woman displays signs similar to these, look at her perineum and/or perform a vaginal examination to determine her actual labor status. A vaginal examination is *not* done if the woman has bleeding other than bloody show.

CONTINUING INTRAPARTUM CARE

Fetal Assessments. Fetal heart rate and pattern: Assess either by intermittent auscultation or with intermittent or continuous electronic fetal monitoring (EFM). Guidelines for FHR assessment vary according to the mother's risk status and with labor events (Table 2-4, p. 146.)

Amniotic fluid: Assess for color, quantity, and odor when the membranes rupture. Prepare for infant respiratory suctioning and support at birth if the fluid is meconium stained.

Maternal Assessments
- Check vital signs every 2 to 4 hours.
- Labor progress: Perform vaginal exams to determine cervical effacement, dilation, and fetal descent; limit as much as possible because of possible introduction of infection.
- Monitor intake and output.
- Response to labor: Observe for the behavioral changes that are associated with labor progress. Signs that the woman may need help dealing with pain (pharmacologic or non-pharmacologic) include:
  — Inability to use learned breathing techniques or ineffectiveness despite varying the ones used.
  — Arching her back or muscle tension that persists between contractions.

Text continued on p. 148

Table 2-3	Intrapartum Assessment Guide		

Women who have had prenatal care have much of this information available on their prenatal record. The nurse need only verify it or update it as needed.

Assessment, Method (Selected Rationales)	Common Findings	Significant Findings, Nursing Action
	Interview	
Purpose: To obtain information about the woman's pregnancy, labor, and conditions that may affect her care. The interview is curtailed if she seems to be in late labor.		
Introduction: Introduce yourself and ask the woman how she wants to be addressed. Ask her if she wants her partner and/or family to remain during the interview and assessment. (Shows respect for the woman and gives her control over those she wants to remain with her.)	Many women prefer to be addressed by their first names during labor.	The surname (family name) precedes the given name in some cultures. Clarify which name is used to properly address the woman and to properly identify both mother and newborn.
Culture/language: If she is from another culture, ask what her preferred language is and what language(s) she speaks, reads, or verbally understands.	Common non-English languages of women in the United States are Spanish or one of the	Try to secure an interpreter fluent in the woman's primary language. Ask her if there are people who are not acceptable to her as interpreters

(Enables the most accurate data collection.)	Asian dialects. The most common non-English language varies with location.	(e.g., males or one from a group in conflict with her culture). Family members may not be the best interpreters because they may interpret selectively, adding or subtracting information as they see fit.
Communication: Ask the woman to tell you when she has a contraction, and pause during the interview and physical assessment. (Shows that the nurse is sensitive to her comfort and allows her to concentrate more fully on the information the nurse requests.)	Women in active labor have difficulty answering questions or cooperating with a physical examination while they are having a contraction.	If contractions are very frequent, assess the woman's labor status promptly rather than continuing the interview. Ask only the most critical questions.
Nonverbal cues: Observe the woman's behaviors and interactions with her family and the nurse. (Permits estimation of her level of anxiety. Identifies behaviors indicating that she should have a vaginal examination to determine whether birth is imminent.)	Latent phase: Sociable and mildly anxious.	The unprepared or extremely anxious woman may breathe deeply and rapidly, displaying a tense facial and body posture during and between contractions.
	Active phase: Concentrating intently with contractions; often uses prepared childbirth techniques.	

Continued

Table 2-3	Intrapartum Assessment Guide—cont'd	
Assessment, Method (Selected Rationales)	**Common Findings**	**Significant Findings, Nursing Action**
		These behaviors suggest that birth is imminent: 1. Her statement that the baby is coming 2. Grunting sounds (low-pitched, guttural sounds) 3. Bearing down with abdominal muscles 4. Sitting on one buttock
Reason for admission: "What brings you to the hospital/birth center today?" (Open-ended question promotes more complete answer.)	Labor contractions at term are the usual reason. Observation for false labor is another common reason for admission.	Euphoria, combativeness, or sedation suggest recent illicit drug ingestion. Bleeding, preterm labor, pain other than labor contractions. Report these findings to the physician or nurse-midwife promptly.
Prenatal care: "Did you see a physician or nurse-midwife during your pregnancy?" "Who is your physician or nurse-midwife?" "How far along were you in your pregnancy when you saw the physician	Early and regular prenatal care promotes maternal and fetal health.	No prenatal care or care that was irregular or begun in late pregnancy means that complications may not have been identified.

or nurse-midwife?" (Enables location of prenatal record.)

Estimated date of delivery (EDD): "When is your baby due?" (Determines if gestation is term.) "When did your last menstrual period begin?" (For estimation of EDD if woman did not have prenatal care.)

Term gestation: 38-42 weeks. The woman's gestation may have been confirmed or adjusted during pregnancy with an ultrasound or other clinical examination.

Gestations earlier than 38 weeks (preterm) or later than the end of 42nd week (postterm) are associated with more fetal or neonatal problems.

Gravidity, parity, abortions: "How many times have you been pregnant?" "How many babies have you had? Were they full-term or premature?" "How many children are living?" "Have you had any miscarriages or abortions?" "Were there any problems with your babies after they were born?" (Helps estimate probable speed of labor and anticipate neonatal problems.)

Labor may be faster for the woman who has given birth before than for the nullipara. Miscarriage is used to describe a spontaneous abortion because many laypeople associate the term "abortion" with only induced abortions.

Parity of 5 or more (grand multiparity) may be associated with placenta previa (see p. 73) or postpartum hemorrhage (see p. 329). Women who have had several spontaneous abortions or who have given birth to infants with abnormalities may face a higher risk for an infant with a birth defect.

Continued

Table 2-3	Intrapartum Assessment Guide—cont'd	
Assessment, Method (Selected Rationales)	**Common Findings**	**Significant Findings, Nursing Action**
Pregnancy History (Identifies Problems That May Affect This Birth)		
Present pregnancy: "Have you had any problems during this pregnancy, such as high blood pressure, diabetes, or bleeding?"	Complications are not expected.	Women having diabetes or hypertension may have poor placental blood flow, possibly resulting in fetal compromise. Some complications of past pregnancies, such as diabetes, may recur in another pregnancy. The woman who plans a vaginal birth after cesarean section (VBAC) may need more support and reassurance to give birth vaginally.
Past pregnancies: "Were there any problems with your other pregnancy(ies)?" "Were your other babies born vaginally or by cesarean birth?"	Women who had previous cesarean birth(s) often have a trial of labor and vaginal birth (VBAC). A woman who previously had a difficult labor may be more anxious than one who had an uncomplicated labor and birth.	
Other: "Is there anything else you think we should know so that we can better care for you?"	This open-ended question gives the woman a chance to share information that	

Labor status: "When did your contractions become regular?" "What time did you begin to think you might really be in labor?" (Facilitates a more accurate estimation of the time labor began.)	may not be elicited by other questions. Varies among women. Many women go to the birth facility when contractions first begin. Others wait until they are reasonably sure that they are really in labor.	Women who say they have been "in labor" for an unusual length of time (for example, "for 2 days") have probably had false labor. These women may be very tired from the annoying contractions that seem nonproductive.
Contractions: "How often are your contractions coming?" "How long do they last?" "Are they getting stronger?" "Tell me if you have a contraction while we are talking." (Obtains the woman's subjective evaluation of her contractions. Alerts the nurse to palpate contractions that occur during the interview.)	Varies according to her stage and phase of labor. Labor contractions are usually regular and show a pattern of increasing frequency, duration, and intensity.	Irregular contractions or those that do not increase in frequency, duration, or intensity are more likely to represent false labor. Contractions with a duration of longer than 90 seconds or intervals of full uterine relaxation shorter than 60 seconds can reduce placental blood flow.
Membrane status: "Has your water broken?" "What time did it break?" "What did the fluid look like?" "About how much fluid did you lose—was it a big gush or a trickle?" (Alerts the nurse of the need to verify whether the membranes have ruptured if it is not obvious. Identifies possible prolonged rupture of membranes.)	Most women go to the birth facility for evaluation soon after their membranes rupture. If a woman is not already in labor, spontaneous contractions usually begin within a few hours after the membranes rupture at term.	If the woman's membranes have ruptured and she is not in labor or if she is not at term, a vaginal examination is often deferred. Labor may be induced if she is at term with ruptured membranes.

Continued

Table 2-3	Intrapartum Assessment Guide—cont'd	
Assessment, Method (Selected Rationales)	**Common Findings**	**Significant Findings, Nursing Action**
Allergies: "Are you allergic to any foods or medicines?" "What kind of reaction do you have?" "Have you ever had a problem with anesthesia when you had dental work?" (Determines possible sensitivity to drugs that may be used.) "Are you allergic to latex?" (most common in healthcare providers or those who wear protective gloves).	Record any known allergies to food and medication. As needed, describe how they affected the woman. Ask about possible allergies to latex.	Allergy to seafood, iodized salt, or x-ray contrast media may indicate iodine allergy. Because iodine is used in many "prep" solutions, alternative ones should be used. Allergy to dental anesthetics may indicate possible allergy to the drugs used for local or regional anesthetics. These drugs usually end in the suffix *-caine*. Allergy to latex is more likely in women who wear gloves in their workplace.
Food intake: "When was the last time you had something to eat or drink?" "What did you have?" (Helps evaluate risk for regurgitation and aspiration of stomach contents during general anesthesia.)	Record the time of the woman's last food intake and what she ate. Include both liquids and solids.	If the woman says she has not had any intake for an unusual length of time, question her more closely: "Is there any food you may have forgotten, such as a snack or a drink of water?"
Recent illness: "Have you been ill recently?" "What was the problem?" "What did you do for it?" "Have you been around anyone with a contagious illness recently?"	Most pregnant women are healthy. An occasional woman may have had a minor illness such as an	Untreated urinary tract infections are associated with preterm labor. The woman who has had contact with someone having a communicable

Medications: "What drugs do you take that your physician or nurse-midwife has prescribed?" "Are there any over-the-counter drugs that you use?" "I know this may be uncomfortable to discuss, but we need to know about any illegal substances that you use to more safely care for you and your baby." (Permits evaluation of the woman's drug intake and encourages her to disclose nonprescribed use.)

Tobacco or alcohol: "Do you smoke or use tobacco in any other form? About how many cigarettes a day? "Do you use alcohol? About how many drinks do you have each day (or week)?" (Evaluates use of these legal substances.) Birth plans (shows respect for the woman and her family as individuals and promotes achievement of their expectations. Enables more culturally appropriate care):

upper respiratory infection.

Prenatal vitamins and iron are commonly prescribed. Record all drugs the woman takes, including time and amount of last ingestion. Women who use illegal substances often conceal or diminish the extent of their use because they fear reprisals.

As in substance abuse, women may underreport the extent of their use of tobacco or alcohol.

disease may become ill and possibly infect others in the facility.

Drugs may interact with other medications given during labor, especially analgesics and anesthetics. Substance abuse is associated with complications for the mother and infant. If the woman discloses that she uses illegal drugs, ask her what kind and the last time she ingested them (often referred to as a "hit"). A nonjudgmental approach is more likely to result in honest information.

Infants of heavy smokers are often smaller and may have reduced placental blood flow during labor. Infants of women who use alcohol may show fetal alcohol effects.

Continued

Table 2-3	Intrapartum Assessment Guide—cont'd	
Assessment, Method (Selected Rationales)	**Common Findings**	**Significant Findings, Nursing Action**
Coach or primary support person: "Who is the main person you want to be with you during labor?" Ask that person how he or she wants to be addressed, such as "Mr. Smith" or "Bob."	This is usually the woman's husband or the baby's father, but it may be her mother, sister, or a friend, especially if she is single.	The woman who has little or no support from significant others probably needs more intense nursing support during labor and after the birth. These clients are more likely to have problems with parent-infant attachment.
Other support: "Is there anyone else you would like to be present during labor?" Preparation for childbirth: "Did you attend prepared childbirth classes?" "Did someone go with you?"	Women often want another support person present. Ideally, the woman and a partner have had some preparation in classes or self-study. Women who attended classes during previous pregnancies do not always repeat the classes during subsequent pregnancies.	The unprepared woman may need more support with simple relaxation and breathing techniques during labor. Her partner may need to learn techniques to assist her.

Preferences: "Are there any special plans you have for this birth?" "Is there anything you want to avoid?" "Did you plan to record the birth with pictures or video?"	Some women or couples have strong feelings regarding certain interventions. Common ones are (1) analgesia or anesthesia; (2) intravenous lines; (3) fetal monitoring; (4) shave prep or enema; or (5) use of episiotomy or forceps.	Conflict may arise if the woman has not previously discussed her preferences with her physician or nurse-midwife or if she is unaware of what services are available where she gives birth.
Cultural needs: "Are there any special cultural practices that you plan when you have your baby?" "How can we best help you to fulfill these practices?"	Women from Asian and Hispanic cultures often subscribe to the "hot/cold" theory of illness and want specific foods after birth, such as soft-boiled eggs. They may not want their water iced.	Try to incorporate all positive or neutral cultural practices. If a practice is harmful, explain why and try to find a way to work around it if the family does not want to give it up.

Continued

Table 2-3	Intrapartum Assessment Guide—cont'd		
Assessment, Method (Selected Rationales)	**Common Findings**	**Significant Findings, Nursing Action**	
	Fetal Evaluation		
Purpose: To determine if the fetus seems to be healthy and tolerating labor well. Fetal heart rate (FHR): Assess by intermittent auscultation, or apply an external fetal monitor if that is the facility's policy (most common in the United States). Document FHR at least this often for the fetus at low risk for complications: 1. Every hour during the latent phase 2. Every 30 minutes during active and transition phases 3. Every 15 minutes during second stage	Average at term is a lower limit of 110-120 bpm and an upper limit of 150-160 bpm. Rate of the term or near-term fetus should increase when the fetus moves.	These signs may indicate fetal stress and should be reported to the physician or nurse-midwife: 1. Rate outside the normal limits 2. Slowing of the rate that persists after the contraction ends 3. No increase in rate when the fetus moves More frequent assessments should be made of the FHR if these occur.	
	Labor Status		
Purpose: To identify whether the woman is in labor and if birth is imminent. If she displays signs of imminent birth, this assessment is done as soon as she is admitted.			

Contractions (Yields objective information about labor status): In addition to asking the woman about her contraction pattern, assess the contractions by palpation with the fingertips of one hand. A guideline is to assess: 1. Hourly during the latent phase 2. Every 30 minutes during the active phase 3. Every 15 minutes during transition and second stage	See interview section earlier in table	See interview section earlier in table. Women who have intense contractions or who are making rapid progress need to be assessed more frequently.
Vaginal examination (Determines cervical dilation and effacement; fetal presentation, position, and station; bloody show; and status of the membranes)	Varies according to the stage and phase of labor. It may not be possible to determine fetal position by vaginal examination when membranes are intact and bulging over the presenting part.	A vaginal examination is not performed if the woman reports or has evidence of active bleeding (not bloody show). Report reasons for omitting a vaginal examination to the physician or nurse-midwife.

Continued

Table 2-3	Intrapartum Assessment Guide—cont'd	
Assessment, Method (Selected Rationales)	**Common Findings**	**Significant Findings, Nursing Action**
Status of membranes: During a vaginal examination a flow of fluid suggests ruptured membranes. A Nitrazine or amniostat test and/or fern test may be done. (Test needed only if it is not obvious that the membranes have ruptured.)	Amniotic fluid should be clear, possibly containing flecks of white vernix. Its odor is distinctive but not offensive. Nitrazine test with a color change to blue-green to dark blue (pH >6.5) suggests true rupture of the membranes but is not conclusive. Fern test is more diagnostic of true rupture of membranes.	A greenish color indicates meconium staining, which may be associated with fetal compromise or postterm gestation. Thick meconium with much particulate matter ("pea soup") is most significant (see Clinical Tip, p. 148). Thick green-black meconium may be passed by the fetus in a breech presentation and is not necessarily associated with fetal compromise. Cloudy, yellowish, strong- or foul-smelling fluid suggests infection. Bloody fluid may indicate partial placental separation (p. 74).
Leopold's maneuvers: Often done before assessing the FHR because they help locate the best place to assess the FHR. (Identifies fetal presentation and position. Most accurate when combined with information from vaginal examination.)	A cephalic presentation with the head well flexed (vertex) is normal. The fetal head is often easily displaced upward ("floating") if the woman	A hard, round, freely movable object in the fundus suggests a fetal head, meaning the fetus is in a breech presentation. Less commonly, the fetus may be crosswise in the uterus: a transverse lie.

Assessment	Normal Findings	Deviations
Pain: Note discomfort during and between contractions. Note tenderness when palpating contractions. (Distinguishes between normal labor pain and abnormal pain that may be associated with a complication.)	is not in labor. When the head is engaged, it cannot be displaced upward with Leopold's maneuvers. There may be verbal or nonverbal evidence of pain with contractions, but the woman should be relatively comfortable between contractions. The skin around the umbilicus is often sensitive.	Constant pain or a tender, rigid uterus suggests a complication, such as abruptio placentae (separated placenta) (see p. 74) or, less commonly, uterine rupture (see p. 200).

Physical Examination

Assessment	Normal Findings	Deviations
Purpose: To evaluate the woman's general health and identify conditions that may affect her intrapartum and postpartum care.		
General appearance: Observe skin color and texture, nutritional state, and appearance of rest or fatigue. Examine the woman's face, fingers, and lower extremities for edema. Ask her if she can take her rings off and on.	Women are often fatigued if their sleep has been interrupted by Braxton Hicks contractions, fetal activity, or frequent urination.	Pallor suggests anemia.

Continued

Table 2-3	Intrapartum Assessment Guide—cont'd	
Assessment, Method (Selected Rationales)	**Common Findings**	**Significant Findings, Nursing Action**
	Mild edema of the lower extremities is common in late pregnancy.	Edema of the face and fingers or extreme (pitting) edema of the lower extremities is associated with pregnancy-related hypertension (see p. 87).
Vital signs: Take the woman's temperature, pulse, respirations, and blood pressure. Reassess the temperature every 4 hours (every 2 hr after membranes rupture or if elevated); repeat blood pressure, pulse, and respirations every hour.	Temperature: 35.8°-37.3° C (96.4°-99.1° F) Pulse: 60-100/min Respirations: 12-20/min, even and unlabored. Blood pressure near baseline levels established during pregnancy. Transient elevations of blood pressure are common when the woman is first admitted, but they return to baseline levels within about ½ hour.	Report abnormalities to physician or nurse-midwife. Temperature of 38° C (100.4° F) or higher suggests infection. Pulse, respirations, and FHR may also be elevated. Pulse and blood pressure may be elevated if the woman is extremely anxious or in pain. A blood pressure of 140/90 or higher is considered hypertensive. For women who did not have prenatal care, there is no baseline to compare.

Heart and lung sounds: Auscultate all areas with a stethoscope.	Heart sounds should be clear with a distinct S_1 and S_2. A physiologic murmur is common because of the increased blood volume and cardiac output. Breath sounds should be clear, with respirations even and unlabored.	The woman who is breathing rapidly and deeply may have symptoms of hyperventilation: tingling and spasm of the fingers, numbness around the lips.
Breasts: Palpate for a dominant mass.	Breasts are full and nodular. Areola is darker, especially in dark-skinned women. Breasts may leak colostrum (clear, sticky, straw-colored fluid) during labor.	Report a dominant mass to the physician or nurse-midwife.
Abdomen: Observe for scars at the same time Leopold's maneuvers and the FHR are assessed. It is usually sufficient to assess the fundal height by observing its relation to the xiphoid process.	Striae (stretch marks) are common. If scars are noted, ask the woman what surgery she had. The fundus at term is usually slightly below the xiphoid process.	Report a previous cesarean birth to the physician or nurse-midwife. Transverse uterine scars are least likely to rupture if the woman is in labor (see p. 200). Measure the fundal height (see Fig. 1-10 on p. 32) if the fetus seems small or if the gestation is questionable.

Continued

Table 2-3	Intrapartum Assessment Guide—cont'd		
Assessment, Method (Selected Rationales)	**Common Findings**	**Significant Findings, Nursing Action**	
Deep tendon reflexes: Assess patellar reflex. Upper extremity deep tendon reflexes should be used after epidural block analgesia.	Brisk knee jerk without spasm or sustained muscle contraction is normal. Some women normally have hypoactive reflexes.	Report absent (uncommon unless the woman is receiving magnesium sulfate) or hyperactive reflexes. Hyperactive reflexes and clonus (repeated tapping when the foot is dorsiflexed) are associated with pregnancy-induced hypertension and often precede a seizure (see p. 84).	
Midstream urine specimen: Assess protein and glucose levels with a dipstick. Follow instructions on the package for waiting times. Send for urinalysis if ordered.	Negative or trace of protein; negative glucose.	Proteinuria is associated with pregnancy-induced hypertension but may also be associated with urinary tract infections or a specimen that is contaminated with vaginal secretions. Glucosuria is associated with diabetes.	
Laboratory tests: Women who have had prenatal care may not need additional tests. Common tests include:			

1. Complete blood count (or hematocrit done on unit)	1. Hemoglobin at least 10.5 g/dL–11 g/dL; hematocrit at least 33%
2. Blood type and Rh factor	2. The woman who is Rh-negative usually has received Rh immune globulin at about 28 weeks of gestation to prevent formation of anti-Rh antibodies
3. Serologic tests for syphilis	3. Negative
4. Rubella immunity	4. Positive immunity

Second column notes:

1. Values lower than these reduce maternal reserve for normal blood loss at birth.
2. Rh-negative mothers need Rh immune globulin if their infant is Rh-positive.
3. A positive test may indicate that the baby is infected and needs treatment after birth. The mother should be treated if she has not been treated already.
4. Negative or equivocal immunity increases a woman's risk for having rubella if she is exposed. Maternal rubella during pregnancy increases the risk for birth defects.

Continued

Table 2-4	**Assessment and Documentation of Fetal Heart Rate**

Low-Risk Patients	**High-Risk Patients**
First stage of labor Every 1 hour in latent phase Every 30 minutes in active phase	First stage of labor Every 30 minutes in latent phase Every 15 minutes in active phase
Second stage of labor Every 15 minutes	Second stage of labor Every 5 minutes

Labor Events

Other Times to Document Fetal Heart Rate

- Before artificial rupture of the membranes; after rupture of the membranes, either artificially or spontaneously
- Before and after ambulation
- If contractions become too frequent or last too long or there is an inadequate interval between them
- Before administration of oxytocin and when evaluating the dose for increase, maintenance, or decrease
- Before administration of sedative medications or central nervous system depressants and at time of peak action
- Before epidural analgesia is started and every 15 minutes 1 hr after it is started

From NAACOG. (1990). *Fetal heart rate auscultation*. Washington, D.C.: Author.

Text continued from p. 127.

— A tense facial expression.
— Statements similar to "I can't take it anymore."
— Request for pain medication or other specific interventions to help her manage pain.

Common Intrapartum Nursing Diagnoses and Collaborative Problems

- Risk for Ineffective Health Maintenance related to Deficient Knowledge regarding characteristics of false and true labor
- Anxiety or Fear related to ability to meet demands of labor and labor's uncertain outcome
- Potential complication: Fetal compromise
- Pain related to uterine contractions and vaginal/perineal distention
- Risk for Injury (maternal and/or fetal) related to unexpected rapid birth

Nursing Interventions

- Promoting fetal oxygenation and observing for compromise
  — Assess the fetus at appropriate intervals and labor events.
  — Encourage the woman to assume positions other than the supine, which can reduce blood flow to the placenta because of aortocaval compression.
  — Observe contractions for:
    – Excessive duration (more than 90 seconds)
    – Inadequate relaxation interval (less than 60 seconds)
  — Observe maternal blood pressure (hypotension and hypertension reduce placental blood flow).
  — Observe maternal temperature (increases fetal body temperature, which increases fetal oxygen demands).
  — Teach the woman to avoid sustained breath-holding during pushing (the Valsalva maneuver). Prolonged breath-holding reduces placental blood flow.
- Promoting comfort
  — Reduce irritants: Dim bright lighting, especially if it shines in the woman's eyes.

Clinical Tip

Conditions associated with fetal compromise include the following:

- FHR outside normal range for a term fetus: lower limit of 110 to 120 bpm and upper limit of 150 to 160 bpm
- Little or no variability in the electronically monitored FHR
- Slowing of the FHR persisting after contraction ends
- Meconium-stained (greenish) amniotic fluid
- Cloudy, yellowish, or foul odor to amniotic fluid (suggesting infection)
- Contractions lasting longer than 90-120 seconds
- Incomplete uterine relaxation or intervals shorter than 30 seconds between contractions
- Maternal hypotension (may divert blood flow away from the placenta to ensure adequate perfusion of the maternal brain and heart)
- Maternal hypertension (may be associated with vasospasm in spinal arteries, which supply the intervillous spaces of the placenta)
- Maternal fever (38° C [100.4° F] or higher)

— Alter the temperature
  - Adjust the thermostat to a comfortable level.
  - Use a fan or blankets as needed.
  - Provide a cool, damp washcloth for the mother's face and neck.
  - Socks provide warmth for cold feet.
— Change the underpad regularly. A folded terry towel absorbs more amniotic fluid than does a disposable underpad.
— Offer hard candy, a Popsicle, or ice chips to reduce mouth dryness if not contraindicated. A moist washcloth on the lips reduces a dry mouth if the woman cannot have oral intake.
— Observe the bladder for filling that may cause discomfort or reduce the effectiveness of pharmacologic pain relief methods. The woman will usually need to void

every 2 hours, or more often if she has large quantities of IV fluids.
— Have the woman change positions regularly to reduce pressure and help the fetus adapt to pelvic contours. Any position of comfort (other than supine) is usually permissible. Vertical positions work with gravity. "Back labor" may be eased by having the woman assume a position in which the back of the fetal head falls away from the maternal sacral promontory, such as leaning forward or assuming a hands and knees position. During second stage, squatting enlarges the pelvic outlet slightly.
— Water therapy in the form of a shower, tub, or whirlpool is relaxing and improves the tolerance of contractions. Nipple stimulation by the water currents promotes natural oxytocin release from the posterior pituitary, which then stimulates contractions.
• Teaching
— Breathing techniques.
— Usual course of labor.
— Avoiding pushing before full cervical dilation, or pushing most effectively after full dilation.
— Avoiding prolonged breath-holding (the Valsalva maneuver) during second stage.
• Providing encouragement
— Provide nursing presence with the laboring woman, which conveys respect and support.
— Reinforce techniques the woman uses that are effective, and help her find others that may be more effective if needed.
— Care for the woman's support person. Involve the birth partner as the couple desires. Do not expect more support of the partner than he or she can provide. Do not interfere with the woman and partner who are coping well. Encourage the partner to take a break. Food and drink can mean the difference between an effective birth partner and one who faints at birth.

Nursing Responsibilities during Birth

- Transferring the woman to a delivery room if a birthing room is not being used
- Preparing a sterile delivery table, which includes gowns, gloves, drapes, solutions, and instruments
- Performing a perineal cleansing prep
- Performing initial care and assessment of the newborn; using personal protective equipment when caring for the infant before the first bath
- Administering maternal medications, such as oxytocin, as ordered

Nursing Responsibilities Immediately after Birth

- Care of the infant
  — Observe and support respiratory function.
    – Perform an Apgar at 1 and 5 minutes (Table 2-5).
    – Suction excess secretions with a bulb syringe or suction catheter; teach parents the use of the bulb syringe at the first opportunity.
  — Support temperature regulation.
    – Dry the infant thoroughly, including the hair, and wrap in warm blankets.
    – A hat reduces heat loss from the large surface area of the head.

Clinical Tip

If a woman will give birth before her birth attendant arrives, get the emergency delivery tray ("precip tray"), calling for another person to bring it if it is not in the room. Put on gloves, preferably sterile, to catch the baby as it emerges. Suction the infant's mouth and nose with a bulb syringe. Dry the infant and place skin-to-skin with the mother or wrap in warmed blankets. Infant suckling at the breast stimulates maternal oxytocin release to promote placental expulsion and control of bleeding.

Text continued on p. 153.

Table 2-5	Apgar Score*		
	Points		
Assessment	**0**	**1**	**2**
Heart rate	Absent	Less than 100/min	100/min or more
Respiratory effort	No spontaneous respirations	Slow respirations or weak cry	Spontaneous respirations with a strong, lusty cry
Muscle tone	Limp	Minimal flexion of extremities; sluggish movement	Flexed body posture; spontaneous and vigorous movement
Reflex response	No response to suction or gentle slap on soles	Minimal response (grimace) to suction or gentle slap on soles	Responds promptly to suction or a gentle slap to the sole with cry or active movement
Color	Pallor or cyanosis	Bluish hands and feet	Pink (light skinned) or absence of cyanosis (dark skinned)

Continued

Table 2-5										Apgar Score*—cont'd	
0	1	2	3	4	5	6	7	8	9	10	
	Infant needs resuscitation.				Gently stimulate by rubbing the infant's back while administering oxygen. Determine whether mother received narcotics, which may have depressed infant's respirations. Have naloxone (Narcan) available for administration.			Provide no action other than support of the infant's spontaneous efforts and continued observation.			

Points

*The Apgar score is a method of rapid evaluation of the infant's cardiorespiratory adaptation after birth. The nurse scores the infant at 1 minute and 5 minutes in each of five areas. The assessments are arranged from most important (heart rate) to least important (color). The infant is assigned a score of 0 to 2 in each of the five areas and the scores are totaled.

General guidelines for the infant's care are based on three ranges of 1-minute scores.

Text continued from p. 150.

Clinical Tip

A rising pulse is the first sign of hypovolemic shock; the blood pressure usually falls later.

— Methods to add heat
  - Place the infant in skin-to-skin contact with a parent.
  - Place the infant in a radiant warmer without hat and blankets; a skin probe allows the warmer heat to rise and fall according to the infant's needs.
• Care of the mother
  — Observe for hemorrhage
    - Check vital signs every 15 minutes during the first hour, every 30 minutes during the second hour, and hourly until discharge from the recovery area.
    - Observe uterine fundus for firmness, height, and position. The uterus should be firm, midline, and about halfway between the symphysis and umbilicus. Actual height varies with the woman's parity and the size of her infant. If the uterus is soft, it should be massaged until firm.
    - Observe bladder with fundal checks. A high uterine fundus that may be displaced to one side suggests a full bladder, which interferes with uterine contraction. Measure the first two voidings; each should be about 300 to 400 mL. Expect more rapid bladder filling and possible difficulty voiding if the woman received epidural anesthesia for birth.
    - Observe lochia with each vital sign and fundal check.

  — Watch for excess lochia pooling under the woman's buttocks and back.
  — More than one saturated standard pad (not those having cold packs in them) per hour is excessive.

- Report large clots (small ones are common) or a continuous bright red trickle of blood when the fundus remains firm (suggests a bleeding laceration in the birth canal).

— Promote comfort
  - Provide warmth in the form of a warm blanket and/or a portable radiant warmer. Warm drinks may be comforting.
  - Apply cold packs to the perineal area in the form of a glove filled with shaved ice or a chemical cold pack. Wrap the glove in a washcloth or similar wrap to avoid placing the latex next to the woman's perineal skin.
  - Provide analgesia: Oral analgesic drugs such as hydrocodone with acetaminophen are common.
- Early care of the new family
  — Provide time for the parents and newborn to get acquainted, with as little interruption as possible. Do infant assessments and care while parents hold the baby, if possible.
  — Initiate breastfeeding. The infant is often alert at this time, and stimulating the woman's nipples causes oxytocin secretion from her pituitary, aiding in control of bleeding.
  — Observe for expected behaviors in early parent-infant interactions.
    - Use of high-pitched, affectionate tones
    - Seeking eye contact with the infant
    - Gradually progressing from tentative fingertip touching of the infant, to palm touch, to enfolding the infant

INTRAPARTUM FETAL ASSESSMENT
FACTORS THAT AFFECT FETAL OXYGENATION
- Maternal blood flow to the placenta
- Maternal blood oxygen saturation
- Exchange of oxygen and carbon dioxide in the placenta
- Blood flow from the placenta, through the umbilical vessels, to the fetus
- Fetal circulatory and oxygen-carrying functions

Table 2-6	**Conditions Associated with Decreased Fetal Oxygenation**

Antepartum Period

Maternal history
  Prior stillbirth
  Prior cesarean birth
  Chronic diseases, such as cardiac disease, hypertension, and
    diabetes
  Drug abuse
Problems identified during pregnancy
  Fetal growth restriction
  Gestation >42 weeks
  Marked decrease in fetal movement
  Multifetal gestation
  Pregnancy-related hypertension
  Gestational diabetes
  Placenta previa
  Maternal severe anemia
  Maternal infection

Intrapartum Period

Maternal problems
  Hypotension
  Hypertonic uterine contractions
  Abnormal labor: preterm or dysfunctional
  Prolonged ruptured membranes
  Chorioamnionitis
  Fever
Fetal or placental problems
  Abnormal fetal heart rate
  Meconium-stained amniotic fluid
  Abnormal presentation or position
  Prolapsed cord
  Abruptio placentae

TYPES OF INTRAPARTUM FETAL ASSESSMENT

Intrapartal fetal assessment primarily involves observation of the fetal heart rate and uterine contractions. Other factors that relate to fetal well-being include maternal vital signs and character of amniotic fluid.

Low-Tech Approach

- Involves intermittent auscultation of fetal heart rate with Doppler or fetoscope (see Procedure: Auscultating the Fetal Heart Rate, p. 428). plus intermittent palpation of uterine contractions for frequency, duration, intensity, and resting interval. See Procedure: Palpating Contractions, p. 418.
- Provides a more natural birthing environment.
- Assesses the fetus and uterine activity for a small percentage of the total labor.

Electronic Fetal Monitoring (EFM)

- Variations
  - Continuous, with only occasional interruptions (such as toileting)
  - Intermittent, assessed at regular intervals during labor
- EFM provides more total information and allows identification of subtle trends in the fetal response to labor.
- EFM lends a more technical atmosphere to the birthing room.

ELECTRONIC FETAL MONITORING EQUIPMENT

- External equipment is noninvasive, but less accurate than internal. See Procedure: External Fetal Heart Rate and Contraction Monitoring, p. 425.
- Internal equipment has greater accuracy, but is invasive and requires ruptured membranes and some cervical dilation. See Procedure: Internal Fetal Heart Rate and Contraction Monitoring, p. 427.

EVALUATING ELECTRONIC FETAL MONITORING STRIPS

- The fetal heart rate is recorded in the upper grid of the paper strip on computer screen; uterine activity is recorded in the lower grid.
- Fetal heart rate and uterine activity patterns must be evaluated together.

Fetal Heart Rate

- Baseline rate
  - Normal: For the term fetus, a lower limit of 110 to 120 bpm, and an upper limit of 150 to 160 bpm (some sources say that 120 bpm is the lower limit of normal); preterm fetus generally has a higher rate
  - Bradycardia: Less than 110 to 120 bpm, persisting at least 10 minutes
  - Tachycardia: Greater than 150 to 160 bpm, persisting at least 10 minutes
- Variability: fluctuations in the baseline FHR. Two types are:
  - Short-term variability (STV): Changes in the fetal heart rate from one beat to the next (beat to beat); most accurately assessed with an internal spiral electrode
  - Long-term variability (LTV): Broader fluctuations that are apparent over 1-minute intervals (about 3-6 cycles/min)
- Presence of periodic changes
  - Accelerations: Increase in the FHR of at least 15 bpm above the baseline, lasting at least 15 seconds in a term or near term fetus (10 bpm above baseline lasting 10 seconds in the preterm fetus); reassuring pattern
  - Decelerations
    - Early: Usually caused by fetal head compression
      Begin after the contraction begins
      End before contraction ends
      Reassuring pattern
    - Late: Associated with uteroplacental insufficiency
      Begin after the contraction begins (often after it peaks)
      End after the contraction is over
      Nonreassuring pattern
    - Variable: Associated with umbilical cord compression
      Variable in appearance
      Often have no consistent relation to contractions
      Sharp in onset and sharp in offset

No uniform agreement about classification; ACOG guideline (1995) states that variable decelerations are significant
Text continued on p. 160

Table 2-7	**Reassuring and Nonreassuring Fetal Heart Rate Patterns**

Reassuring Patterns

Baseline rate: Stable, with a lower limit of 110-120 bpm and an upper limit of 150-160 bpm at term
Variability of 6-25 bpm
Accelerations with fetal movement: At least 15 bpm above the baseline for at least 15 seconds for a term or near-term fetus
Uterine activity:
  Contraction frequency: no more frequent than every 2 min
  Contraction duration: no longer than 90 seconds
  Interval between contractions at least 60 seconds
  Uterine resting tone: uterus relaxed between contractions (with external monitor); uterine resting tone <20 mm Hg (with intrauterine pressure catheter)

Nonreassuring Patterns
Tachycardia

Baseline FHR >160 bpm for at least 10 minutes Mild: 161-180 bpm Severe >181 bpm	Maternal fever (fetal tachycardia may be the first sign of an intrauterine infection) Maternal dehydration Maternal or fetal hypoxia Fetal acidosis Maternal or fetal hypovolemia Fetal cardiac arrhythmias Maternal severe anemia Maternal hyperthyroidism Drugs administered to mother (such as terbutaline)

Bradycardia

Baseline FHR <110 bpm for at least 10 minutes Baseline rates between 100 and 110 bpm are usually not associated with fetal compromise if there are no nonreassuring patterns	Fetal head compression Fetal hypoxia Fetal acidosis Fetal heart block Umbilical cord compression Second-stage labor with maternal pushing

Table 2-7	**Reassuring and Nonreassuring Fetal Heart Rate Patterns—cont'd**

Decreased or Absent Variability

FHR baseline has a smooth, flat appearance	Fetal sleep (usually lasts no longer than 30 min at a time) Fetal hypoxia with acidosis Drug effects: CNS depressants Local anesthetic agents

Late Decelerations

Recurrent decelerations with a uniform appearance and a consistent relation to the contraction; begin after the contraction starts (usually at the peak) and do not return to baseline until after the contraction ends	Uteroplacental insufficiency, which may be secondary to: Maternal hypotension Excess uterine activity Placental interruption, such as abruptio placentae or placenta previa Pregnancy-related or chronic hypertension Maternal diabetes Maternal severe anemia Maternal cardiac disease

Variable Decelerations

Sharp in onset and offset	Umbilical cord compression, which may be secondary to:
Appearance and relationship to contractions is not consistent, may occur as a nonperiodic pattern (randomly)	Prolapsed cord Nuchal cord (around fetal neck) Oligohydramnios (abnormally small amount of amniotic fluid) Cord between fetus and mother's uterus or pelvis, without obvious prolapse Cord between fetal body parts Knot in cord

bpm, Beats per minute; *FHR*, fetal heart rate.

when the FHR repeatedly decreases to less than 70 bpm and persists at that level for at least 60 seconds before returning to the baseline.

Clarifying Questionable EFM Data

- Fetal scalp stimulation
  - Apply pressure to the fetal scalp with the gloved finger and sweep the fingers in a circular motion.
  - Acceleration of the FHR (which may not be immediate) of at least 15 bpm for at least 15 seconds is reassuring.
  - Stimulation should not be done if a vaginal examination is contraindicated.
- Vibroacoustic stimulation
  - Apply an artificial larynx to the mother's lower abdomen and turn it on for up to 3 seconds.
  - Acceleration as in fetal scalp stimulation is reassuring.
- Fetal scalp blood sampling: The physician obtains a sample of fetal blood to determine the fetal blood pH
  - Normal fetal scalp pH: 7.25 to 7.35
  - Acidosis: less than 7.20 (birth may be hastened by forceps or cesarean delivery)
  - Borderline: 7.20 to 7.24 (sample may be repeated)
  - Oximetry: Fetal pulse oximetry 30%-70%
- Umbilical cord blood analysis: Sampling after birth to determine pH, P_{CO_2}, P_{O_2}, bicarbonate, and base deficit. Analysis helps identify whether acidosis exists and whether it is respiratory (short-term), metabolic (prolonged), or mixed.
  - Draw blood into heparinized syringes from an umbilical cord artery or a fetal artery on the placental surface.
  - Cap syringes promptly to prevent altering values.
  - Samples are reliable for 30 to 60 minutes at room temperature. Ice the samples if testing will be later than this time.

INTERVENING FOR NONREASSURING EFM PATTERNS
Identifying the Cause

- Assess maternal vital signs to identify hypotension, hypertension, or elevated temperature.

- Review maternal medications.
- Perform vaginal examination to identify palpable prolapsed cord.

Interventions for Nonreassuring Patterns. The specific intervention(s) chosen depend on the probable cause that was identified. Common interventions are listed here.

- Increase placental perfusion.
  — Position on side, or other than the supine, to avoid aortocaval compression.
  — Observe for excess uterine activity.
    – Stop oxytocin if it is causing excess activity.
    – A tocolytic drug, such as terbutaline (0.125-0.25 mg intravenously or 0.25 mg subcutaneously), may be given.
  — Increase nonadditive IV solution to expand maternal blood volume.
- Increase maternal blood oxygen saturation by giving oxygen at 8 to 10 L/min with a snug face mask.
- Reduce cord compression.
  — Reposition woman.
    – Turn side to side
    – Elevate hips
  — Perform amnioinfusion if ordered.
- Initiate internal EFM if no contraindication.
- Notify birth attendant of:
  — Pattern that was identified.
  — Nursing interventions to correct the problem.
  — Fetal response.

PAIN MANAGEMENT DURING CHILDBIRTH
The intrapartum nurse usually employs both nonpharmacologic and pharmacologic pain management to assist women during labor. Examples of possible techniques are described next, but a woman may develop personal techniques that best meet her needs.

NONPHARMACOLOGIC TECHNIQUES FOR LABOR

Assist Relaxation

- Control the environment.
  — Reduce bright lights.
  — Mask outside noise with music or television.
- Increase personal comfort.
  — Keep reasonably clean and dry.
  — Offer ice chips to reduce dry mouth.
- Reduce anxiety and fear.
  — Provide explanations.
  — Call her by her name, a "mother" or a "woman," not "patient."

Cutaneous Stimulation

- Self-massage
  — Effleurage
  — Tracing circles or figure-8s on the bed
- Massage by others
  — Palm or sole stimulation
  — Temples or shoulders
  — Sacral pressure
    – Pressure should be continuous and firm.
    – A hand over the woman's hip helps steady her during sacral pressure.
    – Slight movement of the hand may increase effectiveness.
    – Two tennis balls in a sock may be used.

Thermal Stimulation

- Cool cloths to the face
- Ice in a glove (covered with washcloth) applied to lower back
- Warm whirlpool or shower
- Alternating heat with cold to reduce habituation

Mental Stimulation. Teach woman to use:

- A focal point.
- Imagery, usually of a pleasant scene or experience. The woman imagines herself in that setting. As she breathes,

she can picture oxygen entering her body to nourish her baby and tension leaving as she exhales.
• Music or peaceful sounds. Headphones help mask outside noise. The music's rhythm can help her pace her breathing.

Breathing Techniques
• First stage: Cleansing breath (like a sigh) at beginning and end of contraction
  — Slow paced breathing: Use of slow, deep breathing to promote relaxation and sufficient oxygenation
  — Modified paced breathing: More rapid rate, but more shallow and rapid breathing during the peak of a contraction
  — Patterned paced breathing: Pant-blow in various types of patterns
  — Avoiding pushing: Blowing repeatedly using short puffs when the urge to push occurs before complete cervical dilation
• Second stage
  — Cleansing breaths as usual
  — Pushing: Using either as near continuous pushing as possible, or pushing for 5- to 6-second intervals

PHARMACOLOGIC TECHNIQUES FOR LABOR
Systemic Drugs

Table 2-8	Drugs Commonly Used for Intrapartum Pain Management
Drug/Dose	**Comments**
Opioid Analgesics	
Meperidine (Demerol) 12.5-50 mg every 2-4 hours IV; may be given by PCA	Respiratory depression (primarily in the neonate) is the main side effect

Continued

Table 2-8	**Drugs Commonly Used for Intrapartum Pain Management—cont'd**

Drug/Dose	Comments
Fentanyl (Sublimaze) 50-100 mcg; may be repeated every hour; may be given by PCA Adjunct to epidural analgesia during labor (dose individualized)	Onset is quick (5 min for administration IV), but duration of action is short. Less nausea vomiting, and respiratory depression occurs than with meperidine. Epidural use may cause pruritus.
Butorphanol (Stadol) 1 mg every 3-4 hours; range 0.5-2 mg IV; may be given by PCA	Has some narcotic antagonist effects; should not be given to the opiate-dependent woman (may precipitate withdrawal) or after other narcotics such as meperidine (may reverse their analgesic effects); also a respiratory depressant
Nalbuphine (Nubain) 10 mg every 3-6 hours IV; may be given by PCA	Same as butorphanol 5-10 mg may be given to relieve pruritus associated with epidural narcotics.

Adjunctive Drugs

Promethazine (Phenergan) 12.5-25 mg every 4-6 hours IV	Given for nausea and vomiting in labor Duration of action is longer than most narcotics; enhances respiratory depressant effects of narcotics
Diphenhydramine (Benadryl) 10-50 mg every 4-6 hours IV	Given to relieve pruritus from epidural narcotics
Hydroxyzine (Atarax, Vistaril) 25-100 mg IM Z-track only	See promethazine

Narcotic Antagonists

Naloxone (Narcan) Adult: To reduce respiratory depression induced by opioids; 0.4-2 mg IV	Action shorter than most narcotics it reverses; must observe for recurrent respiratory depression and be prepared to give additional doses

Table 2-8	Drugs Commonly Used for Intrapartum Pain Management—cont'd

Drug/Dose	Comments
To reverse pruritus from epidural opioids: 0.04-0.2 mg IV or IV infusion 5-10 mcg/kg/hr	Small doses (0.04-0.08 mg) may be given to reduce pruritus from epidural opioids.
Neonatal resuscitation: 0.1 mg/kg IV (umbilical vein) or intratracheal	For neonatal resuscitation
Naltrexone (Trexan): 3-6 mg PO × 1 dose	Long-acting drug to relieve pruritus from epidural narcotics (investigational when used for this purpose) May reduce some analgesic effect when given for pruritus.

IM, Intramuscularly; *IV,* intravenously; *PO,* orally.

Regional Techniques for Labor Pain Management
Epidural Block
- Injection of anesthetic into the epidural space, between the dura and the spinal canal
- Local anesthetic (often with a small dose of an opioid analgesic) injected intermittently or continuously during labor
- A small (3 mL) test dose is injected before giving the full dose to distinguish the epidural space from the subarachnoid space; 3 mL does not provide anesthetic effect if catheter is in the epidural space

Clinical Tip

All drugs injected into the epidural or subarachnoid spaces are preservative-free.

- Adverse effects or complications
  - Maternal hypotension
    - Rapid infusion of warmed intravenous solution offsets the vasodilation effects of the epidural.
    - Ephedrine 10-15 mg IV (in 5-mg increments) may be given to raise the blood pressure.
  - Bladder distention
  - Prolonged second stage because of a reduced maternal urge to push
  - Epidural catheter migration, possibly resulting in an intense, absent, too-high, or unilateral block
  - Nausea and vomiting, primarily when opioids are given
  - Pruritus, or itching of the face and neck, with epidural narcotic use
  - Delayed maternal respiratory depression for up to 24 hours, depending on the epidural opioid used (usually postcesarean birth)
  - Dural puncture, leading to cerebrospinal fluid leakage and spinal headache
  - Contraindicated if woman has allergy to anesthetic, coagulation defects, hypovolemia, or infection in area of insertion

Intrathecal Opioid Analgesics

- Injection of a preservative-free opioid analgesic into the subarachnoid space; reinjection may be required
- Advantages
  - Allows smaller dose of opioid for pain relief
  - Reduces pain without sedation
  - No motor block
  - No hypotensive effects
- Disadvantages
  - Limited duration of action
  - Inadequate relief for late labor and birth
- Adverse effects or complications
  - Nausea and vomiting
  - Pruritus

Local Infiltration

- Infiltration of the perineal area just before performing an episiotomy or suturing a laceration
- Few adverse effects

Pudendal Block

- Injection of local anesthetic in the area of the pudendal nerves, near the ischial spines; the perineum is also infiltrated.
- Few adverse effects

Subarachnoid (Spinal) Block

- Injection of a single dose of local anesthetic into the subarachnoid space
- Can be done quicker than epidural, if emergency cesarean birth is required
- Contraindications, adverse effects, and precautions similar to those for epidural block
- May be combined with an epidural for a combined spinal-epidural block (CSE)

Management of Postspinal Headache

- Headache may occur after either epidural or subarachnoid block
- Medical treatment and nursing care
  - Bed rest, with flat head of bed
  - Oral or intravenous hydration
  - Blood patch: Injection of 10 to 15 mL of the woman's blood (obtained by sterile technique) into the epidural space to form a patch over the leaking area

General Anesthesia

- Infrequently used, but may be required for some women having cesarean birth
  - Refusal or a poor candidate for epidural or subarachnoid block
  - When rapid cesarean birth is required and there is not time to establish either epidural or subarachnoid block

- Primary risks and prevention measures
  — Maternal aspiration of acidic gastric contents
    – Restrict intake to clear fluids or nothing by mouth if surgery is anticipated
    – Drugs to reduce gastric acidity, such as:
      Sodium citrate and citric acid (Bicitra)
      Ranitidine (Zantac)
      Cimetidine (Tagamet)
      Famotidine (Pepcid)
    – Drugs to reduce secretions, such as glycopyrrolate (Robinul)
    – Drugs to speed gastric emptying, such as metoclopramide (Reglan)
    – Use cricoid pressure (Sellick maneuver) to block the esophagus by pressing the trachea downward toward the cervical spine
  — Newborn respiratory depression
    – Reduce the time from induction of anesthesia to cord clamping
    – Keep anesthesia level light until cord is clamped.
  — Uterine relaxation: Observe the uterine fundus for firmness, quantity of lochia, and urine output during recovery.

OBSTETRIC PROCEDURES
AMNIOTOMY
Amniotomy is the artificial rupture of the membranes, typically abbreviated AROM.

Indications
- Induce or stimulate labor
- Allow internal electronic fetal monitoring and fetal scalp blood sampling

Contraindications or Precautions
- High fetal presenting part
- Fetal presentation other than cephalic
- Placenta previa
- Any contraindication to labor or vaginal examination

Risks
- Prolapse of the umbilical cord
- Infection
- Abruptio placentae (premature separation of the placenta)

Technique
- Sterile technique is used
- Physician or nurse-midwife does vaginal examination
- Membrane perforator is passed through the cervix, and the membranes are snagged with the hook to create a hole

Nursing Considerations
- Document baseline FHR for 20 to 30 minutes.
- Assist with the procedure.
  - Place several underpads under the woman's buttocks.
  - Open the package containing the hook using sterile technique.
  - Drop sterile lubricant on the birth attendant's sterile gloved fingers.
- Document quantity, color, odor of amniotic fluid; FHR.
- Promote comfort by changing underpads regularly.
- Observe for complications.
  - Assess the fetal heart rate for at least 1 minute after amniotomy. Prolapse of the umbilical cord usually causes slowing of the FHR, with variable decelerations.
  - Check the woman's temperature every 2 hours (or according to facility policy). Report a temperature greater than 38° C (100.4° F). Monitor FHR for a baseline of more than 160 bpm, which may precede maternal temperature elevation. Observe for foul-smelling or yellowish fluid.

INDUCTION AND AUGMENTATION OF LABOR
Induction is the initiation of labor. *Augmentation* is stimulation of labor contractions that have already begun. Techniques are similar for both.

Indications

- Pregnancy-related hypertension
- Premature rupture of the membranes without onset of labor
- Chorioamnionitis
- Maternal conditions, such as diabetes or renal or pulmonary disease
- Conditions suggesting fetal compromise, such as intrauterine growth restriction, postterm gestation, maternal-fetal blood incompatibility
- Fetal death
- Mother having a history of rapid labors who lives a long distance from the birth center
- Arranging the birth of a baby expected to have problems at a specialized center
- Labor that began spontaneously slows or stops because of poor contractions

Contraindications or Precautions

- Placenta previa
- Umbilical cord prolapse
- Abnormal fetal presentation
- High fetal presenting part
- Active genital herpes infection
- Maternal pelvic structural abnormalities
- Previous classic (vertical) uterine incision

Risks

- Hypertonic uterine activity, manifested by contractions that:
  — Are too close (less than 2 min apart).
  — Are too long (more than 90 to 120 sec).
  — Are too strong (higher than 90 mm Hg with intrauterine pressure catheter).
  — Have too short a resting interval (less than 30 sec relaxation) or incomplete relaxation (resting tone higher than 20 mm Hg with intrauterine pressure catheter).
- Uterine rupture

- Maternal water intoxication (more likely if a dextrose and water IV solution is used or if infusion rate is higher than 20 mcg/min)

Technique
- Cervical ripening may be done to soften the cervix before the induction.
  — Prostaglandin E_2
  — Hydrophilic inserts such as Dilapan, Lamicel, or laminaria tents
- Oxytocin
  — Administer intravenously.
  — Oxytocin line is inserted into the primary line as close as possible to the venipuncture site.
  — Start slowly, increase gradually, and regulate with an infusion pump.
  — Infusion rate may be reduced when the woman is in the active phase of labor.
  — May be used for serial induction, with oxytocin solution given over a 2- to 3-day period for 8 to 10 hours each day.
  — A lower rate of oxytocin infusion is usually required for augmentation than for induction of labor.

Nursing Considerations
- Observe for hypertonic contractions as described earlier.
- Observe fetal heart rate and patterns that suggest reduced placental exchange
  — Bradycardia
  — Tachycardia
  — Late decelerations
- Nursing actions for excessive contractions or nonreassuring FHR patterns
  — Reduce or stop the oxytocin infusion.
  — Increase the rate of the primary (nonadditive) IV solution.
  — Do not allow the woman to assume a supine position.
  — Give 100% oxygen by snug face mask at 8 to 10 L/min.

— Give ordered tocolytic drug, such as terbutaline or magnesium sulfate.
— Notify birth attendant.
- Check blood pressure and pulse every 30 to 60 minutes or with each oxytocin rate increase. Check temperature every 2 to 4 hours, depending on previous readings and membrane status.
- Record intake and output to identify fluid retention.
- After birth, observe for uterine atony, especially if the woman receives oxytocin for a long time.

EXTERNAL CEPHALIC VERSION
Version involves changing the fetal presentation, usually from breech to cephalic. External version is the more common, although an internal version is sometimes done in a twin birth.

Contraindications or Precautions
- Vaginal birth is unlikely
- Maternal uterine malformations
- Previous cesarean birth with a vertical uterine incision
- Fetopelvic disproportion
- Placenta previa
- Multifetal gestation
- Oligohydramnios
- Ruptured membranes
- Cord around the fetal body or neck
- Uteroplacental insufficiency
- Engagement of the fetal presenting part into the pelvis

Risks
- Entanglement and compression of the umbilical cord
- Abruptio placentae

Technique
- Perform nonstress test to evaluate fetal health and placental function.
- Perform ultrasound examination to determine fetal gestational age and fetal presentation and to identify the

adequacy of amniotic fluid; ultrasound also guides the fetal manipulations.

- Administer a tocolytic drug to relax the uterus during the version.
- Physician pushes the fetal breech out of the pelvis in a forward or backward roll, guiding the fetal head downward into the pelvis.

Nursing Considerations
- Maintain NPO until after procedure and return of maternal and fetal status to baseline levels.
- Assess maternal vital signs before and every 5 minutes during the procedure.
- Perform nonstress test.
- Explain side effects of the planned tocolytic drug, emphasizing that these abate soon after the drug is stopped.
- Administer the drug as ordered.
- Monitor FHR with Doppler or real-time ultrasound during procedure. Fetal bradycardia may occur during the procedure, but the rate usually returns to normal when manipulations stop.
- Monitor maternal vital signs and FHR; monitor for regular contractions or ruptured membranes after the procedure.
- Give Rh immune globulin (RhoGAM) to the Rh-negative woman, as indicated.
- Review signs and symptoms of true labor and teach guidelines for returning to the birth center.

FORCEPS AND VACUUM EXTRACTION
These procedures assist fetal expulsion by allowing the physician to apply traction to the fetal head. Forceps may assist fetal head rotation as well as descent.

Indications
- Maternal
  — Exhaustion
  — Poor pushing effectiveness

— Cardiac or pulmonary disease
— Intrapartum infection demanding prompt birth
- Fetal
    — Prolapsed umbilical cord (if birth can be accomplished quickly with the procedure; otherwise cesarean delivery is done)
    — Premature separation of the placenta
    — Nonreassuring FHR patterns

Contraindications or Precautions
- Severe fetal compromise
- High fetal station
- Acute maternal conditions, such as congestive heart failure or pulmonary edema
- Fetopelvic disproportion

Risks
- Maternal: laceration or hematoma of the vagina
- Fetal/neonatal
    — Ecchymoses
    — Facial or scalp lacerations or abrasions
    — Facial nerve injury
    — Cephalhematoma
    — Subgaleal or intracranial hemorrhage

Technique
- Complete cervical dilation is required.
- Catheterization provides more room in the pelvis.
- Anesthesia is a regional block such as pudendal or epidural.
- Episiotomy is common.
- Classification of forceps is based on station of the fetal head when forceps are applied.
    — Outlet: The fetal head is on the perineum, with the scalp visible at the vaginal opening without separating the labia.
    — Low: The leading edge of the fetal skull is at station +2 (about 2 cm below the level of the mother's ischial spines) or lower.

— Midforceps: The leading edge of the fetal skull is between a 0 (at the level of the ischial spines) and a +2 station.

Nursing Considerations
- Add a catheter to the delivery instrument set.
- Continue FHR observations and notify the physician if the rate is lower than 100 bpm.
- Observe mother and infant for forceps-related trauma.
- Apply cold to the woman's perineum for 12 hours.
- Reassure parents that the reddening and bruising of the infant's skin where forceps were applied is temporary. Cold is not applied to the infant's skin because it would cause hypothermia.
- Observe infant for infection that may gain entry via skin breaks and for facial asymmetry that suggests facial nerve injury.

EPISIOTOMY
Indications
- Fetal
  - Similar to those for forceps or vacuum extraction
  - Reduction of pressure on the head of a small preterm fetus
- Maternal
  - Control of the direction and extent to which the vaginal opening is enlarged (controversial)
  - A straight, clean-edged incision that can be simpler to repair than a large perineal laceration

Contraindications or Precautions. There are no real contraindications, although routine performance of an episiotomy remains controversial. The physician or nurse-midwife must make the decision just before birth.

Risks
- Infection
- Perineal pain that may last longer than pain associated with spontaneous tears

Technique
- Done when fetal presenting part has crowned to a diameter of about 3 to 4 cm
- Two types
  - Median: Cut along a line from the vaginal fourchette toward the anus
    - Less blood loss, scarring, and postpartum pain
    - More likely to extend into the anal sphincter because of limited room to enlarge vaginal opening
  - Mediolateral: Cut at an angle from the vaginal fourchette toward the left or right
    - More enlargement of vaginal opening and less risk of tearing into the anal sphincter
    - More blood loss, pain, and scarring; longer painful intercourse

Nursing Considerations
- Actions to reduce need for episiotomy
  - Help woman push in an upright position.
  - Apply warm perineal compresses.
  - Perform perineal massage.
- Postdelivery
  - Observe the perineum for hematoma and edema.
  - Apply cold compresses for first 12 hours; apply perineal heat after 12 hours.

CESAREAN BIRTH
Indications
- Maternal or fetal compromise
- Dystocia
- Fetopelvic disproportion
- Pregnancy-related hypertension, if prompt delivery is needed
- Maternal diseases such as diabetes, heart disease, or cervical cancer, if labor is not advisable
  - Active genital herpes
  - Some previous uterine surgical procedures, such as a classic cesarean incision

— Persistent nonreassuring fetal heart rate patterns
— Prolapsed umbilical cord
— Fetal malpresentations, such as breech or transverse lie
— Hemorrhagic conditions, such as abruptio placentae or placenta previa

Contraindications or Precautions
• Fetal death
• Fetus that is not expected to survive
• Maternal coagulation defects

Risks
• Maternal
  — Infection
  — Hemorrhage
  — Urinary tract trauma
  — Thrombophlebitis
  — Paralytic ileus
  — Atelectasis
  — Anesthesia complications
• Neonatal
  — Inadvertent preterm birth
  — Transient tachypnea of the newborn
  — Persistent fetal circulation
  — Injury, such as laceration, bruising, or other trauma

Technique
• The reason for the cesarean (planned or unplanned) and time pressure will modify some of these steps.
• Test for fetal lung maturity before planned cesarean birth (lecithin/sphingomyelin [L/S] ratio and assessment for presence of phosphatidylglycerol [PG] and phosphatidyl-inositol [PI]).
• Initiate fetal monitoring for 20 to 30 minutes before a scheduled cesarean birth.
• Administer drugs to reduce gastric acidity or control respiratory secretions. Other than ordered oral medications, the woman remains NPO.

- Laboratory tests vary with the maternal and fetal conditions.
  — Complete blood count
  — Clotting studies
  — Blood typing and screening; crossmatching may be done if the woman is anemic or if she has an increased risk for hemorrhage.
- Anesthesia
  — Epidural or subarachnoid block is preferred
  — General may be required if regional is not possible or refused
- Incisions
  — Skin
    – Pfannenstiel (transverse, or "bikini")
    – Vertical
  — Uterine
    – Low transverse (preferred)
    – Low vertical
    – Classic (high vertical)

Nursing Considerations
- Provide emotional support; need varies according to the reason for the cesarean birth.
  — Identify concerns and misunderstandings about the current or prior cesarean births. Teach the woman and her support person to reduce their fear of the unknown.
  — Use a calm and confident manner, even if the cesarean is done in an emergency situation.
  — Visit the woman and her partner after birth to answer questions they may have or fill in gaps in their understanding.

Clinical Tip

A woman's support person may be anxious and physically exhausted after hours of supporting her in labor. Do not expect more support from this person than he or she can provide.

Preoperative
- Teach the woman and her partner about cesarean birth.
  — Preoperative procedures and their purposes
  — Intravenous line and catheter, which are usually removed within 24 hours after birth
  — Reassurance that pressure and pulling sensations are normal and that the anesthesia clinician will regularly assess her pain management needs.
  — If general anesthesia is planned, reassure her that she will be asleep before the incision is made even though all preparations are done before anesthesia is begun.
  — Appearance of the operating room and explanations of who will be present
    - Cool room
    - Narrow surgery table
    - When her partner can come in (preoperative preparations may take 30-45 minutes in a nonemergency cesarean birth)
  — Recovery room
    - Equipment, such as a pulse oximeter and automatic blood pressure cuff
    - Routine assessments and interventions
      Vital signs
      Fundus and lochia checks
      Coughing and deep breathing
    - Exercises to promote circulation in her legs
    - Comfort interventions, such as medication and positioning
  — Maintaining NPO status, other than for ordered drugs to control gastric secretions.
- Preoperative preparation
  — Abdominal shave depends on the expected skin incision. Guidelines are:
    - For Pfannenstiel skin incision, shave from about 3 inches above the pubic hairline to the mons pubis (about where her legs come together).

- For vertical skin incision, shave from just above the umbilicus to the mons pubis.
— An indwelling catheter, often inserted after a regional anesthetic takes effect, reduces the chance for bladder injury during the procedure. If a general anesthetic is planned, the catheter is inserted before induction of anesthesia to reduce fetal exposure to the anesthetic.
— Intravenous infusion
- Prophylactic intravenous antibiotic

Intraoperative
- Transfer and position to prevent injury
  — Pad bony prominences.
  — Secure the woman's position with a safety strap across her thighs.
  — Place a wedge under one hip or tilt the operating table to reduce aortocaval compression.
  — Route the indwelling catheter drain tube under her leg and place bag near the head of the table so the anesthesia clinician can monitor urine output.
- Verify instrument, suture, and equipment counts before, during, and after surgery.
- Verify proper function of machines such as suction, monitors, electrocautery.
- Apply leads for cardiac monitoring and pulse oximetry readings.
- Apply a grounding pad for electrocautery use.
- Cleanse the incision with sterile water or saline and apply a sterile dressing.
- Clean blood and amniotic fluid from the woman's abdomen, buttocks, and back before transferring her to a bed after surgery.
- Transfer the woman smoothly to reduce pain and prevent hypotension.
- Care for the infant, as in vaginal birth.

Postoperative
- Assessments are typically done every 15 minutes during the first 1 to 2 hours, then every 30 to 60 minutes until transfer to her postpartum room.
  - Check blood pressure, pulse, and respirations at the intervals noted; check temperature at recovery room admission and according to protocol thereafter.
  - Monitor pulse oximetry (continuous). Have the woman take several deep breaths if oxygen saturation falls below 95%. The anesthesia provider specifies additional assessments based on techniques uses for anesthesia.
  - Assess for return of motion and sensation (if a regional block was given).
  - Assess level of consciousness (particularly if general anesthesia or sedating drugs were given).
  - Check abdominal dressing, including character and amount of drainage.
  - Assess uterine firmness and position (midline or deviated).
  - Note lochia quantity and presence of any clots.
  - Assess urine output (quantity, color, other characteristics).
  - Monitor intravenous infusion (solution, rate of flow, condition of site, secondary infusions).
  - Pain relief needs
    - PCA (patient-controlled analgesia) pump
    - Intermittent injections
    - Epidural narcotics provide long-lasting analgesia.

Clinical Tip

To relax her abdominal muscles during fundal checks, have the woman flex her knees and take slow deep breaths. Gently "walk" the fingers toward her fundus to determine uterine firmness, fundal height, and if deviated from the midline.

INTRAPARTUM COMPLICATIONS
DYSFUNCTIONAL LABOR
Dysfunctional labor has many causes. Maternal and fetal risks vary with the specific labor dysfunction, but often include:

• Infection.
• Fetal hypoxia.
• Maternal or fetal injury.

Problems of the Powers
Ineffective Contractions
• Causes
  — Maternal fatigue
  — Maternal inactivity
  — Fluid and electrolyte imbalance
  — Hypoglycemia
  — Excessive analgesia or anesthesia
  — Maternal catecholamines secreted in response to stress or pain
  — Disproportion between the maternal pelvis and the fetal presenting part
  — Uterine overdistention, such as with multiple gestation or hydramnios
• Characteristics
  — Ineffective contraction patterns are classified as hypotonic or hypertonic.
  — The characteristics and therapeutic management differ.
• Nursing considerations
  — Hypotonic dysfunction
    – Encourage position changes.
    – An abdominal binder may help if the woman's abdominal wall is very lax (usually multiparas).
  — Hypertonic dysfunction
    – Promote uterine blood flow by avoiding the supine position.
    – Provide pain relief.
    – Promote general comfort.

— Provide emotional support and reassurance to the woman and her family.

Ineffective Maternal Pushing

- Causes
  - Use of incorrect pushing techniques or inappropriate pushing positions
  - Fear of injury because of pain and tearing sensations felt by the mother when she pushes
  - Decreased or absent urge to push
  - Maternal exhaustion
  - Analgesia or anesthesia that suppresses the woman's urge to push
  - Psychologic unreadiness to "let go" of her baby
- Therapeutic management: Forceps or cesarean birth may be required if the woman continues to be unable to push her baby out.
- Nursing considerations
  - Observe maternal and fetal vital signs for signs that either is not tolerating the prolonged second stage.
    Maternal fever (more than 38° C [100.4° F])
    - Fetal tachycardia (often the first sign of infection)
    - Any other nonreassuring fetal heart rate pattern
    - Amniotic fluid having a foul or strong odor or a cloudy or yellow appearance
  - Encourage upright positions while pushing, such as squatting, semisitting, side-lying, or pushing while sitting on the toilet.
  - Teach the woman how her tissues gradually stretch to accommodate the baby. Warm perineal compresses or perineal massage may increase perineal distensibility.
  - Coach the woman to push if she cannot feel the urge because of regional block analgesia.
  - Have the exhausted woman push only when she feels the urge, or with every other contraction.
  - Provide oral and/or intravenous fluids, as ordered.
  - Reassure the woman that there is no arbitrary time limit for the duration of second stage labor.

Problems with the Passenger
Fetal Size
Macrosomia. Birth weight is greater than 4000 g (8.8 lb). Size is relative, however, and a woman with a large pelvis may easily give birth to an infant larger than this, whereas a woman with a small or abnormally shaped pelvis may be unable to deliver a smaller infant. Also, a woman with a small pelvis may be able to deliver a large infant if all other factors (fetal position, uterine contractions, etc.) are favorable.

Shoulder Dystocia. The fetal shoulders are trapped behind the woman's symphysis after the fetal head is born. The "turtle sign" is characteristic of shoulder dystocia: the fetal head retracts against the perineum as soon as it emerges. Shoulder dystocia is more likely to occur if the fetus is large.

- Therapeutic management involves the birth attendant and the nurse.
  - McRobert's maneuver: The woman flexes her thighs sharply against her abdomen to straighten the pelvic curve.
  - A supported squat has an effect similar to that of McRobert's maneuver and adds gravity to the forces of maternal pushing.
  - Suprapubic pressure toward the maternal sacrum displaces the fetal shoulder from above the maternal symphysis.
  - *Fundal pressure should not be used* because it can further impact the fetal shoulders above the maternal symphysis.

Clinical Tip

A shoulder dystocia is an urgent situation because the umbilical cord is deep in the pelvis, subject to compression. Yet the infant cannot breathe because the thorax is compressed.

- Nursing considerations
  - Assist the birth attendant in the listed methods to relieve shoulder dystocia.
  - Check the newborn's clavicles for crepitus, deformity, or bruising that suggests fracture.

Abnormal Fetal Presentation or Position

Rotation Abnormalities. The fetus in a vertex presentation does not complete rotation into the occiput anterior position. The fetal head may remain in an occiput posterior or occiput transverse position. Some women may be able to deliver their infants in an occiput posterior position, but most cannot.

- Causes
  - Large fetus
  - Poor fetal head flexion, which increases the diameters presented to the maternal pelvis
  - Small or abnormally shaped maternal pelvis
  - Inadequate contractions or maternal pushing to assist fetal rotation
- Characteristics
  - Prolonged labor
  - The woman usually feels intense back and/or leg pain ("back labor") that is poorly relieved with analgesia.
- Therapeutic management
  - Forceps to assist rotation and descent of the fetal head
  - Cesarean birth if the rotation abnormality persists
- Nursing considerations
  - Encourage position changes to favor fetal head rotation
    - Hands and knees; rocking the pelvis back and forth while on hands and knees encourages rotation.
    - Side-lying (on her left side if the fetus is in a right occiput posterior [ROP] position and on her right side for a left occiput posterior [LOP] position)
    - The lunge, in which the mother places one foot on a chair with her foot and knee pointed to that side.

She lunges sideways repeatedly during a contraction for 5 seconds at a time. It can also be done in a kneeling position. The nurse or her partner must secure the chair and help her balance.
   – Squatting (for second-stage labor)
   – Sitting, kneeling, or standing while leaning forward.
— Pain management techniques
— Check for maternal and newborn injuries after birth
   – Vaginal hematoma
   – Newborn cephalhematoma or forceps marks

Breech Presentation. External version may be attempted if the fetus remains in a breech presentation near term. If the fetus remains breech, cesarean birth is common. Vaginal breech birth may be offered if:

• The maternal pelvis is of normal size and shape.
• The estimated fetal weight is under 3600 g (8 lb).
• Other complications, such as placenta previa or prolapsed cord, are not present.

Multifetal Gestation
• Intrapartum risks include:
   — Dysfunctional labor caused by uterine overdistention (hypotonic dysfunction).
   — Abnormal presentation of one or both fetuses.
   — Greater risk for fetal hypoxia.
   — Maternal postpartum hemorrhage caused by uterine atony.
• Vaginal birth considerations include:
   — Fetal presentations.
   — Maternal pelvic size.
   — Presence of other complications.
   — Number of fetuses.
• Nursing considerations
   — Monitor each fetus's FHR separately. Continue monitoring the second twin after the first twin's birth.

— Observe for hypotonic labor dysfunction.
— Duplicate equipment and staff to care for each infant.
— One nurse remains free to care for the woman.
— Observe fundal height and firmness, lochia, and maternal vital signs after birth to detect uterine atony.

Problems of the Passage

Pelvis. Women may have any of four types of pelvis, and most women have characteristics of more than one type. The different pelvic types have different prognoses for vaginal birth. Those other than the gynecoid are likely to cause dysfunctional labor. Therapeutic management and nursing considerations are similar to those listed for dysfunctional labor.

- Gynecoid (50% of women)
  — Round, cylindrical with a wide pubic arch
  — Good prognosis for vaginal birth
- Anthropoid (25% of white women, 50% of nonwhite women)
  — Long, narrow oval with a narrow pubic arch
  — Fetus is more likely to be born in an occiput posterior (face up) position
- Android (30% of women)
  — Heart shaped or triangular with narrow diameters and a narrow pubic arch
  — Poor prognosis for vaginal birth
- Platypelloid (3% of women)
  — Flat with a wide, short oval and a wide pubic arch
  — Poor prognosis for vaginal birth

Maternal Soft Tissue. The most common soft tissue obstruction of labor is a full bladder. The woman often has pain that remains after epidural analgesia. Assess for bladder filling and encourage the woman to void every 1 to 2 hours, or more often if she has received large amounts of intravenous fluids. Catheterize her if she cannot void.

Problems of the Psyche. Nursing care of the woman's psyche is directed toward helping her relax and work with the forces of labor.

- Establish a trusting relationship with the woman and her family.
- Make the environment comfortable by adjusting temperature and light.
- Promote physical comfort, such as cleanliness.
- Provide accurate information.
- Implement nonpharmacologic and pharmacologic pain management.
- Implement appropriate nursing care for any other type of labor dysfunction.

Abnormal Labor Duration
Prolonged Labor
- Parameters for normal labor progress
  — Cervical dilation rate of at least 1.2 cm/hr in the nullipara and 1.5 cm/hr in the parous woman
  — Fetal descent rate of at least 1 cm/hr in the nullipara and 2 cm/hr in the parous woman
- Causes and characteristics: Any of the previously discussed problems of the powers, passenger, passage, or psyche usually cause a prolonged labor. If the cause can be identified, specific therapeutic management and nursing care is directed toward that cause.
- Risks
  — Maternal infection, intrapartum or postpartum, particularly with prolonged membrane rupture
  — Neonatal infection, which may be severe or fatal
  — Maternal exhaustion
  — Higher levels of anxiety and fear during a subsequent labor
- Nursing considerations
  — Limit vaginal examinations as much as possible. Use behavioral cues to help determine when a vaginal examination is truly necessary.

— Observe maternal vital signs every 2 to 4 hours and FHR with fetal monitoring. Note particularly fetal or maternal tachycardia, or elevated maternal temperature. Report a temperature of 38° C (100.4° F) or higher.

— Observe amniotic fluid for a cloudy or yellow color and a strong or foul odor. Change underpads regularly to keep the woman relatively dry.

— Observe for signs associated with fetal hypoxia, such as bradycardia, tachycardia, loss of variability, and/or late decelerations (see Table 2-7 on pp. 159-161).

— Use appropriate position changes to foster labor progress.

— Promote comfort and conservation of maternal energy.

— Observe intake and output. Provide ordered IV fluids. If oral fluids are allowed, juice, lollipops, Popsicles, or other clear liquids help moisten the woman's mouth and maintain her hydration and energy stores.

— Provide emotional support. Encourage and praise her use of coping skills. Tell her when she makes progress. Reassure her of fetal well-being, if true.

— Observe the newborn for signs of sepsis (see p. 292, 298).

— Obtain cultures of maternal (uterine cavity or placenta) and newborn (multiple cultures) secretions as ordered. Use correct specimen containers for aerobic and anaerobic organisms. Transport to the lab promptly.

— Administer prophylactic antibiotics to mother and infant as ordered.

Precipitate Labor
• Causes
  — Unusually strong labor contractions (natural or oxytocin stimulated)
  — Large maternal pelvis relative to the fetal size
• Characteristics: Birth occurs within 3 hours of labor onset.
• Risks
  — Maternal trauma: Uterine rupture, cervical lacerations, or vaginal or vulvar hematoma.
  — Fetal trauma: Fetal hypoxia, intracranial hemorrhage, or nerve damage

- Therapeutic management
  - No specific interventions if contractions are not so strong that they impair fetal oxygenation
  - Tocolytic drugs to reduce contractions that are too intense
  - Supplemental oxygen
- Nursing considerations
  - Promote fetal oxygenation.
    - Maintain a side-lying position.
    - Administer oxygen at 8 to 10 L/min by face mask.
    - Maintain adequate blood volume by titrating the nonadditive IV flow rate.
  - Stop any oxytocin infusion.
  - Give ordered tocolytic drugs.
  - Help woman use nonpharmacologic pain management measures because progress may be too fast to allow medications such as opioid analgesia or regional block. Focus on helping the woman cope with one contraction at a time.
  - Be prepared to assist with birth if it occurs before the birth attendant arrives.

PREMATURE RUPTURE OF THE MEMBRANES
- Definitions
  - Premature rupture of the membranes (PROM): Rupture of the amniotic sac before true labor, regardless of gestational age.
  - Preterm premature rupture of the membranes (PPROM): Rupture of the amniotic sac earlier than the end of the 37th week of gestation, with or without contractions.
- Causes
  - Infections of the vagina or cervix, such as gonorrhea, group B streptococci, and *Gardnerella vaginalis*
  - Chorioamnionitis
  - Incompetent cervix
  - Fetal abnormalities or malpresentation
  - Hydramnios
  - Amniotic sac with a weak structure

— Recent sexual intercourse
— Nutritional deficiencies
- Risks
  — Infection, maternal and newborn, either before or after birth; infection can be both a cause and a result of prematurely ruptured membranes.
  — Newborn complications of prematurity, particularly if birth occurs before 34 weeks of gestation
  — Umbilical cord compression
  — Fetal/neonatal complications of reduced amniotic fluid volume: reduced lung volume with respiratory distress, deformities secondary to compression.
- Therapeutic management
  — Determining if membranes are truly ruptured with a Nitrazine, Amniostat, and/or fern test
  — Assessment of fetal lung maturity
  — Culture of secretions to identify infection
- If gestation is at or near term, management may include:
  — Walking to stimulate contractions.
  — Oxytocin induction of labor.
- If gestation is preterm, management may include observation in the hospital for a few days to rule out infection.
- Nursing considerations
  — Specific care depends on whether the gestation is term or preterm, whether labor will be induced, or whether the woman will be discharged to await labor.
  — Client teaching before discharge (undelivered)
    – Avoid sexual intercourse, orgasm, or insertion of anything into vagina, which increases the risk for infection caused by ascending organisms and can stimulate contractions.
    – Avoid breast stimulation if the gestation is preterm; breast stimulation can cause release of oxytocin from the posterior pituitary and thus stimulate contractions.
    – Check temperature at least four times a day, reporting any temperature greater than 37.8° C (100° F).

– Maintain any activity restrictions recommended.
– Note uterine contractions.

PRETERM LABOR

Labor is preterm if it begins after the 20th week but before the end of the 37th week of gestation.

- Risks (see Table 2-9)
- Characteristics
  — Uterine contractions that may or may not be painful; the woman may not feel contractions at all
  — A sensation that the baby is frequently "balling up"
  — Cramps similar to menstrual cramps
  — Constant low backache
  — Sensation of pelvic pressure or a feeling that the baby is pushing down
  — Pain, discomfort, or pressure in the vulva or thighs
  — Change or increase in vaginal discharge (increased, watery, bloody)
  — Abdominal cramps with or without diarrhea
  — A sense of "just feeling bad" or "coming down with something"
- Therapeutic management
  — More frequent prenatal visits for women at increased risk for preterm labor
  — Fetal fibronectin determination to help the health care provider decide on the best course of action: watchful observation, or more aggressive treatment with tocolytic drugs and drugs to accelerate fetal lung maturity
  — Identifying conditions that contraindicate continuing the pregnancy, such as pregnancy-related hypertension, maternal hypovolemia, chorioamnionitis, or fetal compromise
  — Treating conditions associated with preterm labor, such as urinary tract infection
  — Transport of a woman who is likely to deliver preterm to a facility with neonatal intensive care facilities

Table 2-9	Maternal Risk Factors for Preterm Labor		
Medical History	**Obstetric History**	**Present Pregnancy**	**Lifestyle and Demographics**
Low weight for height	Previous preterm birth	Uterine distention (such as	Little or no prenatal care
Obesity	Previous preterm labor	multifetal pregnancy	Poor nutrition
Uterine or cervical	Previous first trimester	or hydramnios)	Age <18 or >40 yr
anomalies, uterine fibroids	abortions (>2)	Abdominal surgery	Low educational level
History of cone biopsy	Previous second trimester	during pregnancy	Low socioeconomic
Diethylstilbestrol (DES)	abortion	Uterine irritability	status
exposure as a fetus	History of previous pregnancy	Uterine bleeding	Smoking >10 cigarettes
Chronic illness (e.g., cardiac,	losses (2 or more)	Dehydration	daily
renal, diabetes, clotting	Incompetent cervix	Infection	Nonwhite
disorders, anemia,	Cervical length 25 mm	Anemia	Employment with
hypertension)	(2.5 cm) or less at	Incompetent cervix	long hours and/or
Periodontal disease	midtrimester of pregnancy	Pre-eclampsia	long standing
	Number of embryos implanted	Preterm premature rupture	Chronic physical or
	(assisted reproductive	of membranes (PPROM)	psychological stress
	techniques ART)	Fetal or placental	Intimate partner
		abnormalities	violence
			Substance abuse

— Home uterine activity monitoring, which includes transmission of uterine activity data over the phone and 24-hour availability of perinatal nurses
— Measures to stop preterm labor before it reaches the point of no return, usually after 3 cm of cervical dilation; measures chosen depend on the probable cause of preterm labor, but may include the following:
  – Restricting activity, although the usefulness of this measure has been questioned
  – Hydration with oral and/or intravenous fluids
  – Tocolytic drugs
  – Corticosteroids to accelerate fetal lung maturation
- Nursing considerations
  — Teach pregnant women the signs of early preterm labor. Reinforce these and inquire about them at each office visit, particularly for women at increased risk.
  — Help the woman change risk factors that can be changed, such as nutritional deficiencies or smoking.
  — Refer for assistance, such as to food supplement programs (WIC).
  — Teach woman and her partner to promptly report signs or symptoms associated with preterm birth. Teach her how to be assertive in seeking prompt care so measures to prevent preterm birth are likely to be more effective.
  — Observe for conditions that may contraindicate continuing the pregnancy.
    – Assess the blood pressure to identify hypotension or hypertension.
    – Assess temperature and pulse to detect elevations associated with infection.
    – Monitor the FHR for patterns associated with compromise, such as abnormal rates, loss of variability, and late or severe variable decelerations. Significant reduction of fetal movement also suggests compromise.
  — Observe for treatable conditions that increase the likelihood of preterm birth, such as urinary or reproductive tract infections.

Text continued on p. 198.

Table 2-10	Drugs Used in Preterm Labor	
Drug/Purpose	**Common Dose Regiments***	**Side or Adverse Effects**
Terbutaline (beta-adrenergic for tocolysis)	See Drug Guide: Terbutaline (p. 473). *Intravenous (IV):* Begin at 0.01-0.05 mg/min. Increase by 0.01 mg/min increments every 10-30 min until contraction frequency is 6 or fewer per hr or significant side effects develop. Maximum dose guideline 0.08 mg/min. When contraction frequency is no higher than 4-6 per hr, maintain the infusion for 1 hr; then reduce rate at 20-min intervals to reach the minimum maintenance dose, which may be continued for 12 hr after contractions stop or stabilize at acceptable maximum levels. *Subcutaneous (SC):* 0.28 mg q3-4h (maximum dose interval may be q6h, depending on client response).	Cardiovascular: Maternal and fetal tachycardia, palpitations, cardiac dysrhythmias, chest pain, wide pulse pressure. Respiratory: Dyspnea, chest discomfort, pulmonary edema. Central nervous system: Tremors, restlessness, weakness, dizziness, headache. Metabolic: Hyperglycemia, hypokalemia. Gastrointestinal: Nausea, vomiting, reduced bowel motility. Skin: Flushing, diaphoresis. Infection at injection site for subcutaneous infusion pump.

Continued

Table 2-10	Drugs Used in Preterm Labor—cont'd	
Drug/Purpose	**Common Dose Regiments***	**Side or Adverse Effects**
	By SC infusion pump: continuous low dose baseline infusion plus intermittent bolus doses of 0.25 mg at times of greatest uterine activity. *Oral (PO):* 2.5 to 5 mg q2-4h. Hold for maternal pulse>120/min.	
Magnesium sulfate (use as tocolytic)	*IV:* Loading dose, 4-6 g in 15-20 min. Maintenance dose for tocolysis, 1-4 g/hr. When contraction frequency is no higher than 4-6 per hr, maintain infusion rate for 12-24 hr; then reduce rate. An oral drug may be ordered to continue tocolysis after magnesium sulfate is stopped for this purpose.	Side and adverse effects are dose-related, occurring at higher maternal serum levels. Depression of deep tendon reflexes, which should be present, although less active. Respiratory of cardiac depression if serum levels are high; greatest risk is in woman with poor urine elimination of drug. Less serious side effects: Lethargy, weakness, visual blurring, headache, sensation of heat, nausea, vomiting, constipation. Fetal-neonatal effects: Reduced fetal heart rate (FHR) variability hypotonia

Drug	Administration	Adverse Effects
Indomethacin (Indocin); sulindac (Clinoril) (prostaglandin synthesis inhibitors)	Loading dose: up to 100 mg (rectal) or 50 mg (oral). Rectal preparation usually prepared by birth facility's pharmacy. Maintenance dose: 25-50 mg orally q6h. Ideal duration of treatment has not been established. Ultrasound examinations and fetal echocardiography help determine if maternal indomethacin has adverse effects on the fetus.	Epigastric pain, nausea, gastrointestinal bleeding. Asthma in aspirin-sensitive woman. Increased blood pressure in hypertensive women. **Fetus: Adverse fetal effects may include constriction of the ductus arteriosus, particularly if the mother receives indomethacin for more than 48-72 hr and the gestation is earlier than 32 weeks. Impairs fetal renal function, which may reduce the volume of amniotic fluid and result in cord compression.**
Nifedipine (Procardia); nicardipine (Cardene) (calcium channel blockers for tocolysis)	Oral loading dose of 10-20 mg. Continued oral therapy: 10-20 mg q4-6h. Duration of calcium channel blocking drug for tocolysis has not been established.	Maternal flushing, dizziness, headache, nausea. Transient maternal tachycardia. Mild hypotension. Modest increases in blood glucose levels.

*Doses and frequency of administration are examples; actual protocols vary.
Data from American Academy of Pediatrics (AAP), & American College of Obstetricians and Gynecologists (ACOG). (2002). *Guidelines for perinatal care* (5th ed.). Elk Grove Village, IL, and Washington, DC: Author; Blackburn, S.T. (2003). *Maternal, fetal, & neonatal physiology: A clinical perspective*. Philadelphia: Saunders; Goldenberg, R.L. (2002). The management of preterm labor. *Obstetrics & Gynecology, 100*(5 Pt. 1), 1020-1037; Iams, J.D., & Creasy, R.K. (2004). Preterm labor and delivery. In R.K. Creasy & R.Resink (Eds.), *Maternal-fetal medicine: Principles and practice* (5th ed., pp. 498-531). Philadelphia: Saunders.

— Observe for preterm premature ruptured membranes.
— Help woman cope with activity restrictions.
— Provide oral and/or intravenous hydration as ordered. Observe for signs of dehydration if the woman has had a febrile illness or has vomiting and/or diarrhea (dry skin and mucous membranes, elevated temperature, scant and concentrated urine).
— Administer ordered tocolytic drugs and steroids to speed fetal lung maturation. Teach the woman correct use and precautions if she will be self-administering these drugs.

INTRAPARTUM EMERGENCIES

Medical and nursing management often overlap when caring for a woman and her fetus during an intrapartum emergency. Written standard protocols often provide direction for nursing actions in an emergency.

Prolapsed Umbilical Cord

- Characteristics
  — Umbilical cord slips into a position to be compressed between the maternal pelvis and the fetal body.
  — Cord compression is more severe during contractions.
- Risks
  — A fetus that remains at a high station
  — A very small fetus
  — Breech presentations, especially a footling breech
  — Transverse lie
  — Hydramnios
- Signs
  — Complete: Cord is visible at vaginal opening
  — Partial: Cord is not visible externally, but is palpated during vaginal examination
  — Occult: Cord is neither visible nor palpable, but FHR patterns, such as severe variable decelerations or bradycardia, suggest cord compression
- Management
  — Relieve pressure on the cord.

- – Position the woman's hips higher than her head
    Knee-chest position
    Trendelenburg position
    Elevate hips with pillows while maintaining a side-
    lying position
- – With a gloved hand, push the fetal presenting part
    upward. Maintain this position until the physician
    orders it stopped, which may not be until a
    cesarean incision is made.
— Give oxygen at 8 to 10 L/min by face mask.
— Give a tocolytic drug, such as terbutaline, to inhibit
    contractions.
— If cord protrudes, do not attempt to replace it. Towels
    moistened with warm saline retard cooling and drying
    if there will be any delay in delivery.
— Delivery will be as rapid as possible, usually by
    cesarean.
— Provide emotional support. Explain what is happen-
    ing simply and calmly. Encourage the woman and her
    partner to ventilate their feelings after birth.

Uterine Rupture
- Characteristics
    — The uterine wall is torn to a varying degree.
        Classifications of uterine rupture
        - – Complete: Having a direct communication between
            the uterine and peritoneal cavities
        - – Incomplete: Rupture into the peritoneum covering
            the uterus or into the broad ligament but not into
            the peritoneal cavity
        - – Dehiscence: A partial separation of an old uterine scar
    — Signs and symptoms vary with the degree of rupture.
        Dehiscence may have no signs or symptoms.
        - – Abdominal pain and tenderness, which may or may
            not be severe
        - – Chest pain, pain between the scapulae, or pain on
            inspiration
        - – Hypovolemic shock

- FHR patterns associated with impaired fetal oxygenation, such as late decelerations, reduced variability, tachycardia, or bradycardia
- Absent fetal heart tones
- Cessation of uterine contractions
- Palpation of the fetus outside the uterus

- Causes and risks
  — Previous uterine incision; the woman who has had a classic cesarean incision has a greater risk than does the woman who has had a low transverse incision.
  — High parity, with a thin uterine wall
  — Blunt trauma
  — Intense labor contractions, particularly if there is fetopelvic disproportion

- Management
  — Identify women who have increased risk for rupture and remain alert for its signs and symptoms.
  — Give ordered tocolytic drugs for hypertonic contractions.
  — Give oxygen at 8 to 10 L/min.
  — Expedite birth, usually by cesarean.
  — Provide blood and fluid replacement.
  — Observe for excessive postpartum bleeding and hypovolemic shock that may occur if a rupture was not detected earlier.

Uterine Inversion

- Characteristics
  — The uterus turns inside out, either partially or completely.
  — Signs and symptoms
    - Absence of the uterus from the lower abdomen
    - Depression in the fundus of the uterus, felt with palpation
    - Interior of the uterus visible through the cervix or protruding into the vagina
    - Hemorrhage, shock
    - Severe pelvic pain

- Causes and risks
  - Pulling on the umbilical cord before the placenta detaches from the uterine wall
  - Fundal pressure during birth
  - Increased intraabdominal pressure
  - An abnormally adherent placenta
  - Congenital weakness of the uterine wall
  - Fundal placenta implantation
  - Fundal pressure on an incompletely contracted uterus after birth
- Management
  - Establish two IV lines for fluid and blood replacement.
  - Give tocolytic drugs to stop uterine contractions. General anesthesia may be needed.
  - Give oxytocin after the uterus is replaced. Oxytocin is not given until the uterus is repositioned to avoid trapping the inverted fundus in the cervix.
  - Observe for signs of hypovolemia after birth (tachycardia, falling blood pressure, inadequate [less than 30 mL/hr] or absent urine output with an indwelling catheter in place). Cardiac monitoring to identify dysrhythmias and invasive hemodynamic monitoring may be ordered.
  - Observe the uterus for firmness, height, and deviation from the midline.

Amniotic Fluid Embolism. Amniotic fluid embolism occurs when amniotic fluid is drawn into the maternal circulation and carried to the woman's lungs. It is most likely to occur if labor contractions are very intense. Embolism of meconium-stained amniotic fluid is often fatal.

- Characteristics: Amniotic fluid embolism usually becomes apparent after birth.
  - Abrupt respiratory distress
  - Heart failure
  - Circulatory collapse
  - Disseminated intravascular coagulation (see p. 77)

- Management
  - Cardiopulmonary resuscitation
  - Oxygen with mechanical ventilation
  - Blood transfusion
  - Correction of coagulation deficits with platelets or fibrinogen

Trauma
- Causes
  - Accidents
  - Assault
  - Suicide
- Types of trauma
  - Blunt (automobile accidents, battering)
  - Penetrating (knife or gunshot wounds)
  - Burns
  - Electrical injuries
- Fetal/neonatal complications
  - Direct injury due to skull fracture, intracranial hemorrhage
  - Indirect injury due to abruptio placentae, maternal hypovolemia, or uterine rupture
  - Death of the mother (most common cause of fetal death)
  - Neurologic deficits sometimes found in survivors
- Management
  - Stabilization and care of maternal life-threatening injuries, then stabilization of the fetus
  - Delivery if the maternal condition warrants and the fetus is likely to survive
  - Delivery of the dead or extremely immature fetus if that will improve the maternal outcome
- Nursing considerations
  - Place a wedge under one hip to prevent supine hypotension and improve placental blood flow.
  - Observe vital signs (frequency depends on maternal condition). Monitor FHR if the fetus has reached a viable gestational age.

Clinical Tip

Although the nurse is usually anxious in an emergency situation, it is important to keep a calm attitude. The woman and her family quickly pick up on the staff's anxiety, and theirs will escalate. Remain with the woman to reduce fears of abandonment. If possible, hold her hand. Speak in a low, calm voice.

— Observe urine output for quantity (at least 30 mL/hr), and for presence of blood.
— Observe for and report signs of abruptio placentae (vaginal bleeding with uterine pain and tenderness; increase in uterine height).
— Palpate for contractions because pain from injury or impairment of consciousness may mask labor symptoms. Contractions may not be evident on a fetal monitoring strip.
— Prepare for birth of an infant who may be immature and/or need resuscitation.
— Provide emotional support. Explain what is occurring simply and honestly. Support the partner. Give the woman and her family an opportunity to ventilate their feelings after the emergency has passed.

Section 3

The Newborn

THE PROCESSES OF ADAPTATION
RESPIRATORY SYSTEM

- Initiation of respirations occurs by stimulation of the respiratory center in the brain.
  - Chemical factors: Decreased blood oxygen (Po_2) and pH and increased blood carbon dioxide (Pco_2) levels
  - Mechanical factors: Compression and release of the chest during birth
  - Thermal factors: Change in temperature from the uterus to the colder air environment
  - Sensory factors: Stimuli from handling, sound, light, and pain
- Surfactant production
  - Reduces surface tension within the alveoli and prevents collapse of alveoli with exhalation
  - Produced in adequate amounts by 34 to 36 weeks of gestation
- Fetal lung fluid is absorbed by the pulmonary circulatory and lymphatic systems. Absorption is accelerated by labor and may be delayed by cesarean birth.

CARDIOVASCULAR SYSTEM

- Closure of the ductus arteriosus causes blood to flow to the lungs for oxygenation.
- Closure of the foramen ovale directs blood from the right atrium to the right ventricle.
- Closure of the ductus venosus causes blood to pass through the liver for filtration.
- Dilation of the pulmonary vessels allows blood flow into the lungs.

- Closure of structures is functional at first and not permanent for weeks after birth. It can be reversed in the early days.

NEUROLOGIC SYSTEM
Thermoregulation
- Neonates lose heat by four methods.
  - Evaporation from exposure of wet surfaces to air and from insensible water loss from the skin and respiratory tract; examples include amniotic fluid on the skin at birth, bathing.
  - Conduction from direct contact with objects cooler than the infant's skin (cold hands, scale). Heat can also be gained by conduction (warm blankets, the mother's skin).
  - Convection: heat transfers to air surrounding the infant (air conditioning, people moving).
  - Radiation: heat transfers to cooler objects that are not in direct contact with the infant (cold windows, outside walls, walls of incubators).
- Effects of cold stress
  - Increased metabolism (with increased use of glucose and oxygen)
  - Decreased surfactant production
  - Respiratory distress
  - Hypoglycemia
  - Metabolic acidosis
  - Jaundice
  - Vasoconstriction
- Cold may lead to *nonshivering thermogenesis,* the oxidation of brown fat to produce heat.
  - It begins before there is a change in core (rectal) temperature.
  - It increases the need for oxygen and glucose.
  - It produces fatty acids that interfere with bilirubin transport and increase risk for jaundice.
- A neutral thermal environment is one in which infants maintain a stable body temperature without an increase

in oxygen or metabolic rate. The range of neutral thermal environmental temperatures is 32° to 33.5° C (89.6°-92.3° F) for healthy, full-term newborns.

* Hyperthermia
  — Caused by overheating from poorly regulated heating equipment (radiant warmers, warming lights, or incubators)
  — Increases metabolic rate and need for oxygen and glucose
  — Vasodilation causes insensible fluid losses

HEMATOLOGIC SYSTEM

* Normal breakdown of unneeded erythrocytes may cause physiologic jaundice (see Hyperbilirubinemia, p. 256).
* Polycythemia increases the risk of jaundice and may damage the brain or other organs from stasis.
* High leukocyte levels do not necessarily indicate infection. Increased numbers of immature leukocytes or decreased platelets are signs of infection.
* Newborns cannot synthesize vitamin K, which is necessary for normal clotting, until normal flora are established in the intestines.
* Maternal intake of drugs such as phenytoin, phenobarbital, or aspirin during pregnancy interferes with clotting ability in the newborn.
* See Laboratory Values in the Newborn, Appendix B

GASTROINTESTINAL SYSTEM

* The stomach capacity is about 6 mL/kg at birth but expands to about 90 mL within the first week of life.
* Regurgitation often occurs due to the relaxed cardiac sphincter.
* Normal intestinal flora are established within a few days of birth.
* The stools pass through three stages.
  — Meconium stools are thick, sticky, tarlike, greenish black, and usually passed within 12 hours of birth. Suspect obstruction if meconium is not passed within 48 hours.

— Transitional stools are greenish brown and looser in consistency.
— Milk stools are characteristic of the type of feeding the infant receives.
  – Breast milk stools are seedy, mustard colored, and very soft, with a sweet-sour smell. A newborn should have at least 3 stools a day, but may have 10 or more.
  – Formula stools are pale yellow to light brown, firm, and have the odor of feces. Newborns may have one or several daily.

HEPATIC SYSTEM
- A blood glucose level below 40 to 45 mg/dL in the term infant is often used to indicate hypoglycemia. See Hypoglycemia, p. 262, and Procedure: Blood Glucose Assessment in the Newborn, p. 413.
- The liver conjugates bilirubin by the following steps:
  — Unconjugated bilirubin travels on plasma albumin–binding sites to the liver.
  — It is changed to the conjugated form by glucuronyl transferase and passed into the bile and the duodenum.
  — The conjugated bilirubin is reduced to urobilinogen and stercobilin by normal intestinal flora and is excreted in the stool. Some urobilinogen is excreted by the kidneys.
  — A small percentage of conjugated bilirubin is deconjugated by the intestinal enzyme beta-glucuronidase, reabsorbed into the bloodstream and carried back to the liver, where it must be conjugated again for excretion.

URINARY SYSTEM
- The first voiding is usually within 24 hours of birth. Suspect hypovolemia due to inadequate intake or kidney abnormalities if there is no void within 24 hours. Normal voiding pattern is as few as one or two the first 2 days, and at least six voids daily by the fourth day.
- Normal urine output is 1 to 3 mL/kg/hr.

- Normal specific gravity is 1.001 to 1.020. Large increases in fluids (such as excess intravenous fluid) cause fluid overload.
- Seventy-eight percent of the newborn's body is water, with much of it in the extracellular spaces where it can be easily lost.
- Insensible water loss occurs due to the large body surface area, rapid respiratory rate, and radiant heaters.
- Daily fluid need is 40 to 60 mL/kg (18-27 mL/lb) daily during the first 2 days of life, then 100 to 150 mL/kg (45-68 mL/lb) each day.
- Maintenance of the acid-base and electrolyte balance may be precarious.
- The ability to filter waste products from the blood is decreased.
- Urate crystals may leave a pink or reddish stain on the diaper, but this is normal.

IMMUNE SYSTEM
- The hypothalamus and inflammatory responses are immature. Leukocytes may be slow to respond and inefficient. Fever and leukocytosis are often not present in the newborn with infection.
- Immunoglobulins (serum globulins with antibody activity) help protect newborns from infection.
  - IgG from the mother provides temporary immunity to bacteria, bacterial toxins, and viruses to which the mother has developed immunity. Preterm infants may have much less IgG. Most passive immunity lasts about 6 to 8 months.
  - IgM is produced by the infant and helps protect against gram-negative bacteria. High IgM levels indicate exposure to infection in utero because it does not cross the placenta.
  - IgA does not cross the placenta. It helps protect the gastrointestinal and respiratory systems and may limit absorption of antigenic proteins in the diet. A form of IgA is present in colostrum and breast milk.

PSYCHOSOCIAL ADAPTATION

Periods of Reactivity. In the early hours after birth, the infant goes through changes called the periods of reactivity.

- First period of reactivity
  - Infants are active, alert, and often interested in breast-feeding.
  - Respirations are as high as 80 breaths/min. There may be crackles, retractions, nasal flaring, and increased mucus secretions.
  - The heart rate may be as high as 180 bpm.
  - After 30 minutes to 2 hours, the infant becomes sleepy.
- Period of sleep
  - This period lasts about 2 to 4 hours.
  - The pulse and respirations are normal; the temperature may be low.
- Second period of reactivity
  - This period lasts up to several hours.
  - Infants are alert, interested in feeding, and may pass meconium.
  - Infants may have increased pulse and respirations, cyanosis, or apnea.
  - They may gag or regurgitate and have increased mucus secretions.

Behavioral States. There are six different behavior states in the newborn.

- Quiet sleep state
  - Deep sleep without eye movements
  - Quiet, regular respirations
  - Little or no response to noise or stimuli
- Active sleep state
  - Movement, startles from disturbances, brief fussing
  - Rapid, irregular respirations
  - Rapid eye movement (REM)
  - May return to sleep or awaken

- Drowsy state
  — Eyes closed or glazed and unfocused
  — Startling, slow movement
  — May progress to sleep or awake states
- Quiet alert state
  — Intense gazing at objects or people
  — Excellent time for bonding
- Active alert state
  — Fussy, restless, seems aware of discomfort
  — Respirations faster and irregular
- Crying state
  — Continuous, lusty crying

NURSING ASSESSMENTS
INITIAL ASSESSMENTS

- Examine the infant immediately after birth for cardiorespiratory status, thermoregulation, and presence of anomalies. Intervene appropriately.
- When the infant is stable, perform a more thorough assessment. See Table 3-1, Summary of Newborn Assessments and Table 3-2 Summary of Neonatal Reflexes.
- Assess vital signs every 30 minutes until stable for 2 hours. See Procedure: Vital Sign Assessment in the Newborn, p. 448.

DOCUMENTATION

Document the results of all assessments according to agency policy.

ASSESSMENT OF GESTATIONAL AGE

- This assessment determines the number of weeks from conception to birth based on neurologic and physical characteristics. The New Ballard Score (Figure 3-1 on p. 229) is frequently used.
- Neuromuscular characteristics
  — Posture and degree of flexion: Observe the position of the infant at rest.

Text continued on p. 228

Table 3-1	Summary of Newborn Assessments	
Normal	**Abnormal (Possible Causes)**	**Nursing Considerations**
Initial Assessment		
Assess for obvious problems first. If infant is stable and has no problems that require immediate attention, continue with complete assessment.		
Vital Signs *Temperature*		
36.5°-37.5° C (97.7°-99.5° F) axillary; 36.5°-37.6° C (97.7°-99.7° F) rectal. Axilla is preferred site.	Decreased (cold environment, hypoglycemia, infection, CNS problem). Increased (infection, environment too warm).	Decreased: Institute warming measures and check in 30 minutes. Check blood glucose. Increased: Remove excessive clothing. Check for dehydration. Decreased or increased: Look for signs of infection. Check radiant warmer temperature setting. Check thermometer for accuracy if skin is warm or cool to touch. Report abnormal values to physician.

Continued

Table 3-1	Summary of Newborn Assessments—cont'd	
Normal	Abnormal (Possible Causes)	Nursing Considerations
Pulses		
Heart rate 120-160 bpm (100 sleeping, 180 crying). Rhythm regular. PMI at third to fourth intercostal space, slightly to left of midclavicular line. Brachial, femoral, and pedal pulses present and equal bilaterally.	Tachycardia (respiratory problems, anemia, infection, cardiac conditions). Bradycardia (asphyxia, increased intracranial pressure). PMI to right (dextrocardia, pneumothorax). Murmurs (functional or congenital heart defects). Arrhythmias. Absent or unequal pulses (coarctation of the aorta).	Note location of murmurs. Refer abnormal rates, rhythms and sounds, pulses.
Respirations		
Rate 30-60 (average 40) per minute. Respirations irregular, shallow, unlabored. Chest movements symmetric. Breath sounds present and clear bilaterally.	Tachypnea, especially after the first hour. Slow respirations (maternal medications). Nasal flaring. Grunting (respiratory distress syndrome). Gasping (respiratory depression). Periods of apnea more than 20 seconds or with change in heart rate or color (respiratory depression, sepsis, cold stress).	Mild variations require continued monitoring and usually clear in early hours after birth. If persistent or more than mild, suction, give oxygen, call physician, and initiate more intensive care.

Asymmetry or decreased chest expansion (pneumothorax).
Intercostal, xiphoid, or supraclavicular retractions or seesaw respirations (respiratory distress).
Moist, coarse breath sounds (crackles, rhonchi, fluid in lungs).
Bowel sounds in chest (diaphragmatic hernia).

Blood Pressure

Average BP 65-95 mm Hg systolic, 30-60 mm Hg diastolic. Varies with activity and gestational age and size.

Hypotension (hypovolemia, shock, sepsis). Difference of 15 mm Hg between arms and legs (coarctation of the aorta).

Refer abnormal blood pressures. Prepare for intensive care if very low.

Measurements
Weight

Weight 2500-4000 g (5 lb, 8 oz to 8 lb, 13 oz). Weight loss up to 10% in early days.

High (LGA, maternal diabetes). Low (SGA, preterm, multifetal pregnancy, medical conditions in mother that affect fetal growth). Weight loss greater than 10% (dehydration, feeding problems).

Determine cause. Monitor for complications common to cause.

Continued

bpm, Beats per minute; *PMI,* point of maximum impulse.

Table 3-1	Summary of Newborn Assessments—cont'd	
Normal	**Abnormal (Possible Causes)**	**Nursing Considerations**
Length		
48-53 cm (19-21 inches).	Below normal (SGA, congenital dwarfism). Above normal (LGA, maternal diabetes).	Determine cause. Monitor for complications common to cause.
Head Circumference		
33-35.5 cm (13-14 inches). Head approximately one fourth of infant's length.	Small (SGA, microcephaly, anencephaly). Large (LGA, hydrocephalus, increased intracranial pressure).	Determine cause. Monitor for complications common to cause.
Chest Circumference		
30.5-33 cm (12-13 inches). Is 2-3 cm less than head circumference.	Large (LGA). Small (SGA).	Determine cause. Monitor for complications common to cause.
Posture		
Flexed extremities resist extension, return quickly to flexed state. Hands usually	Limp, flaccid, "floppy," or rigid extremities (preterm, hypoxia, medications, CNS trauma).	Seek cause, refer abnormalities.

clenched. Movements symmetric. Slight tremors on crying. Breech: extended, stiff legs. "Molds" body to caretaker's when held, responds by quieting when needs met.	Hypertonic (neonatal abstinence syndrome, CNS damage). Jitteriness or tremors (low glucose or calcium level). Opisthotonos, seizures, stiff when held (CNS damage).	
Cry		
Lusty, strong.	High-pitched (increased intracranial pressure). Weak, absent, irritable, catlike "mewing" (neurologic problems). Hoarse or crowing (laryngeal irritation).	Observe for changes, report abnormalities.
Skin		
Color pink or tan with acrocyanosis. Vernix caseosa in creases. Small amounts of lanugo over shoulders, sides of face, forehead, upper back. Skin turgor good with quick recoil. Some cracking and peeling of skin. Normal variations: Milia. Erythema	Color: Cyanosis of mouth and central areas (hypoxia). Facial bruising (nuchal cord). Pallor (anemia, hypoxia). Gray (hypoxia, hypotension). Red, sticky, transparent skin (very preterm). Ruddy (polycythemia). Greenish brown discoloration of skin, nails, cord (possible fetal compromise, postterm).	Differentiate facial bruising from cyanosis. Central cyanosis requires suction, oxygen, and further treatment. Refer jaundice in first 24 hours. Watch for respiratory problems in infants with meconium staining. Look for other signs and complications of preterm or postterm birth. Record location, size, shape, color, type of

LGA, large for gestational age; *SGA*, small for gestational age.

Continued

Table 3-1	Summary of Newborn Assessments—cont'd	
Normal	**Abnormal (Possible Causes)**	**Nursing Considerations**
toxicum ("flea bite" rash). Puncture on scalp (from electrode). Mongolian spots. Telangiectatic nevi (nevus simplex, salmon patch, or "stork bites").	Harlequin color (normal or cardiac problems, sepsis.) Mottling (normal or cold stress, hypovolemia, sepsis). Yellow vernix (blood incompatibilities). Jaundice (pathologic if in the first 24 hours). Thick vernix (preterm). Delivery marks: Bruises on body (pressure), scalp (vacuum extractor), or face (cord around neck). Petechiae (pressure, low platelets, infection). Forceps marks. Birthmarks: Mongolian spots. Telangiectatic nevi ("stork bites"). Nevus flammeus (port-wine stain). Nevus vasculosus (strawberry hemangioma). Café-au-lait spots (six or more or >0.5 cm in size, neurofibromatosis). Other: Excessive lanugo (preterm). Excessive peeling, cracking (postterm). Skin tags. Milia. Erythema toxicum. Pustules, or other rashes (infection). "Tenting" of skin (dehydration).	rashes and marks. Differentiate Mongolian spots from bruises. Check for facial movement with forceps marks. Watch for jaundice with bruising. Point out and explain normal skin variations to parents.

Head

Sutures palpable with small separation between each. Anterior fontanel diamond shaped, 2-4 cm, soft and flat. May bulge slightly with crying. Posterior fontanel triangular, 0.5-1 cm. Hair silky and soft with individual hair strands. Normal variations: Overriding sutures (molding). Caput succedaneum or cephalhematoma (pressure during birth).	Head large (hydrocephalus, increased intracranial pressure) or small (microcephaly). Widely separated sutures (hydrocephalus) or hard, ridged area at sutures (craniosynostosis). Anterior fontanel depressed (dehydration, molding), full or bulging at rest (increased intracranial pressure). Woolly, bunchy hair (preterm). Unusual hair growth (genetic abnormalities).	Seek cause of variations. Observe for signs of dehydration with depressed fontanel, increased intracranial pressure with bulging of fontanel and wide separation of sutures. Refer for treatment. Differentiate caput succedaneum from cephalhematoma and reassure parents of normal outcome. Observe for jaundice with cephalhematoma.

Ears

Ears well formed and complete. Area where upper ear meets head even with imaginary line drawn from inner to outer canthus of eye. Startle response to loud noises. Alerts to high-pitched voices.	Low-set ears (chromosomal disorders). Skin tags, preauricular sinuses, dimples (kidney or other anomalies). No response to sound (deafness).	Check voiding if ears abnormal. Look for signs of chromosomal abnormality if position abnormal. Refer for evaluation if no response to sound or if hearing screening is abnormal.

CNS, central nervous system.

Continued

Table 3-1	Summary of Newborn Assessments—cont'd	
Normal	Abnormal (Possible Causes)	Nursing Considerations
Face		
Symmetric in appearance and movement. Parts proportional and appropriately placed.	Asymmetry (pressure and position in utero). Drooping of mouth or one side of face, "one-sided cry" (facial nerve damage). Abnormal appearance (chromosomal abnormalities).	Seek cause of variations. Check delivery history for possible cause of damage to facial nerve.
Eyes		
Symmetric. Eyes clear. Transient strabismus. Scant or absent tears. Pupils equal, react to light. Alerts to interesting sights. Follows objects across midline. Doll's-eye sign, red reflex present. May have subconjunctival hemorrhage or edema of eyelids from pressure during birth.	Inflammation or drainage (chemical or infectious conjunctivitis). Constant tearing (plugged lacrimal duct). Unequal pupils. Failure to follow objects (blindness). White areas over pupils (cataracts). Setting-sun sign (hydrocephalus). Yellow sclera (jaundice). Blue sclera (osteogenesis imperfecta).	Clean and monitor any drainage; seek cause. Reassure parents that subconjunctival hemorrhage and edema will clear. Refer other abnormalities.

Nose

Both nostrils open to air flow. May have slight flattening from pressure during birth.

Blockage of one or both nasal passages (choanal atresia). Malformations (congenital conditions). Flaring, mucus (respiratory distress).

Observe for respiratory distress. Report malformations.

Mouth

Mouth, gums, tongue pink. Tongue normal in size and movement. Lips and palate intact. Sucking pads. Sucking, rooting, swallowing, gag reflexes present. Normal variations: Precocious teeth, Epstein's pearls.

Cyanosis (hypoxia). White patches on cheeks or tongue (candidiasis). Protruding tongue (Down syndrome). Diminished movement of tongue, drooping mouth (facial nerve paralysis). Cleft lip or palate, or both. Absent or weak reflexes (preterm, neurologic problem). Excessive drooling (tracheo-esophageal fistula, esophageal atresia).

Oxygen for cyanosis. Expect loose teeth to be removed. Obtain order for nystatin medication for candidiasis. Check mother for vaginal or breast infection. Refer anomalies.

Feeding

Good suck-swallow coordination. Retains feedings.

Poorly coordinated suck and swallow. Duskiness or cyanosis during feeding (cardiac defects). Choking, gagging, excessive drooling (tracheoesophageal fistula, esophageal atresia).

Feed slowly. Stop frequently if difficulty occurs. Suction and stimulate if necessary. Refer infants with continued difficulty.

Continued

Table 3-1	Summary of Newborn Assessments—cont'd	
Normal	Abnormal (Possible Causes)	Nursing Considerations
Neck and Clavicles		
Short neck turns head easily side to side. Infant raises head when prone. Clavicles intact.	Weakness, contractures, or rigidity (muscle abnormalities). Webbing of neck, large fat pad at back of neck (chromosomal injuries, disorders). Crepitus, lump, or crying when clavicle palpated, diminished or absent arm movement (fractured clavicle).	Fracture of clavicle occurs especially in large infants with shoulder dystocia at birth. Immobilize arm. Look for other injuries. Refer abnormalities.
Chest		
Cylindric. Xiphoid process may be prominent. Nipples present and located properly. May have engorgement, white nipple discharge (maternal hormone withdrawal).	Asymmetry (diaphragmatic hernia, pneumothorax). Supernumerary nipples. Redness (infection).	Report abnormalities.
Abdomen		
Rounded, soft. Bowel sounds present soon after birth. Liver	Sunken abdomen (diaphragmatic hernia). Distended abdomen or	Refer abnormalities. Look for other anomalies if only two vessels in cord.

palpable 1-3 cm below costal margin. Skin intact. Three vessels in cord. Clamp tight and cord drying. Meconium passed within 12-48 hours. Urine passed within 12-24 hours. Normal variation: "Brick dust" staining of diaper (urate crystals).	loops of bowel visible (obstruction, infection, enlarged organs). Absent bowel sounds after first hour (paralytic ileus). Masses palpated (kidney tumors, distended bladder). Enlarged liver (infection heart failure, hemolytic disease). Abdominal wall defects (umbilical or inguinal hernia, omphalocele, gastroschisis, exstrophy of bladder). Two vessels in cord (other anomalies). Bleeding (loose clamp). Redness, drainage from cord (infection). No passage of meconium (imperforate anus, obstruction). Lack of urinary output (kidney anomalies) or inadequate amounts (dehydration).	Tighten or replace loose cord clamp. If stool and urine output abnormal, check to see none was unrecorded, increase feedings, report.
Genitals *Female* Labia majora dark, cover clitoris and labia minora. Small amount	Clitoris and labia minora larger than labia majora (preterm). Large clitoris	Check gestational age if genitalia are immature. Refer anomalies.

Continued

Table 3-1	Summary of Newborn Assessments—cont'd	
Normal	**Abnormal (Possible Causes)**	**Nursing Considerations**
of white mucous vaginal discharge. Urinary meatus and vagina present. Normal variations: Vaginal bleeding (pseudomenstruation). Hymenal tags.	(ambiguous genitalia). Edematous labia (breech birth).	
Male		
Testes within scrotal sac, rugae on scrotum, prepuce nonretractable. Meatus at tip of penis.	Testes in inguinal canal or abdomen (preterm, cryptorchidism). Lack of rugae on scrotum (preterm). Edema of scrotum (pressure in breech birth). Enlarged scrotal sac (hydrocele). Small penis, scrotum (preterm, ambiguous genitalia). Urinary meatus located on upper side of penis (epispadias), underside of penis (hypospadias), or perineum.	Check gestational age for immature genitalia. Refer anomalies. Explain to parents why no circumcision can be performed with abnormal placement of meatus.

Extremities

Upper and Lower Extremities

Equal and bilateral movement of extremities. Correct number and formation of fingers and toes. Nails to ends of digits or slightly beyond. Flexion, good muscle tone.

Crepitus, redness, lumps, swelling (fracture). Diminished or absent movement, especially during Moro reflex (fracture, nerve damage, paralysis). Polydactyly (extra digits). Syndactyly (webbing). Fused or absent digits. Poor muscle tone (preterm, neurologic damage, hypoglycemia, hypoxia).

Refer all anomalies, look for others.

Upper Extremities

Two transverse palm creases.

Simian crease (Down syndrome). Diminished movement of arm with extension and forearm prone (Erb-Duchenne paralysis).

Refer all anomalies, look for others.

Lower Extremities

Legs equal in length, abduct equally, gluteal and thigh creases and knee height equal, no hip "clunk." Normal position of feet.

Ortolani and Barlow tests abnormal, unequal leg length, unequal thigh or gluteal creases (developmental dysplasia of the hip). Malposition of feet (position in utero, talipes equinovarus).

Refer all anomalies, look for others. Check malpositioned feet to see if they can be manipulated back to normal position.

Continued

Table 3-1	Summary of Newborn Assessments—cont'd	
Normal	**Abnormal (Possible Causes)**	**Nursing Considerations**
Back		
No openings observed or felt in vertebral column. Anus patent. Sphincter tightly closed.	Failure of vertebra to close (spina bifida), with or without sac with spinal fluid and meninges (meningocele) or cord (myelomeningocele) enclosed. Tuft of hair over spina bifida occulta. Pilonidal dimple or sinus. Imperforate anus.	Refer abnormalities. Observe for movement below level of defect. If sac, cover with sterile dressing wet with sterile saline. Protect from injury.
Reflexes		
Moro, palmar and plantar grasp, rooting, sucking, swallowing, tonic neck, Babinski, Gallant, and stepping reflexes present (see Table 3-2).	Absent, asymmetric, or weak reflexes.	Observe for signs of fractures, nerve damage, or injury to CNS.

Table 3-2	Summary of Neonatal Reflexes	
Method of Testing	**Expected Response**	**Abnormal Response/Possible Cause**
Babinski		
Stroke the lateral sole of the foot from the heel to across the base of the toes	Toes flare with dorsiflexion of the big toe. Disappears by 12 months.	No response. Bilateral: CNS deficit. Unilateral: Local nerve damage.
Gallant (Trunk Incurvation)		
Lightly stroke the back, lateral to the vertebral column	Entire trunk flexes toward the side stimulated. Disappears by 1 month.	No response. CNS deficit.
Grasp (Palmar and Plantar)		
Press finger against the base of the fingers or toes	Fingers curl tightly, toes curl forward. Palmar: lessens by 3 months. Plantar: lessens by 8 months.	Weak or absent. Neurologic deficit or muscle damage.

Continued

Table 3-2	Summary of Neonatal Reflexes—cont'd	
Method of Testing	Expected Response	Abnormal Response/Possible Cause
Moro		
Let the infant's head drop back approximately 30 degrees	Sharp extension and abduction of the arms with the thumbs and forefingers in a C position. Followed by flexion and adduction to "embrace" position. Legs follow a similar pattern. Disappears by 6 months.	Absent: CNS dysfunction. Asymmetry: brachial plexus injury, paralysis, fractured bone of the extremity. Exaggerated: maternal drug use.
Rooting		
Touch or stroke the side of the mouth toward the cheek	Infant turns to the side touched. Difficult to elicit if infant is sleeping or just fed. Disappears by 3-4 months.	Weak or absent: prematurity, neurologic deficit, depression from maternal drug use.
Startle		
Make a loud noise	Similar to the Moro but the hands remain clenched. Disappears by 4 months.	Weak or absent: Neurologic damage, deafness.

Stepping

Hold the infant so the feet touch a solid surface

Infant lifts alternate feet as if walking. Disappears by 4-7 months.

Asymmetry: Fracture of extremity, neurologic deficit.

Sucking

Place a nipple or finger in the mouth, rub against the palate

Infant begins to suck. Weak if recently fed. Disappears by 1 year.

Weak or absent: prematurity, neurologic deficit, maternal drug use

Swallowing

Place fluid on the back of the tongue

Infant swallows fluid. Should be coordinated with sucking. Present throughout life.

Coughing, gagging, choking, cyanosis: tracheoesophageal fistula, esophageal atresia, neurologic deficit.

Tonic Neck

Gently turn the head to one side while the infant is supine

Extension of the extremities on the side to which head is turned with flexion on the opposite side. May be weak at birth, disappears by 4 months.

Prolonged period of time in position: neurologic deficit.

Text continued from p. 210.

- — Square window sign: Measure the angle between the palm and the forearm when the hand is bent at the wrist as far as possible.
- — Arm recoil: Measure the degree of flexion after the infant's arms are fully flexed at the elbows for 5 seconds, pulled straight down to the sides, and released.
- — Popliteal angle: Measure the angle at the popliteal space when the thigh is flexed against the abdomen and the lower leg is straightened.
- — Scarf sign: Note the position of the elbow when the infant's hand is brought across the body as far as possible without lifting the shoulder.
- — Heel-to-ear: Note how far the leg will extend without resistance when the foot is grasped and pulled toward the ears. Keep the hips flat.
- • Physical characteristics
  Assess each of the following characteristics.
  - — Skin: Color, visibility of veins, peeling and cracking
  - — Lanugo: Amount and placement of lanugo
  - — Plantar surface: Depth of plantar creases and amount of the foot covered by creases
  - — Breasts: Size and development of the nipples, areolae, and breast buds
  - — Eye/ear: Eyelids—fused or open; ear incurving and stiffness; fold ear over and assess how quickly it returns to its original state
  - — Genitals: Female—Size of the clitoris, labia minora, and labia majora. Male—Location of the testes, amount and depth of rugae on the scrotum.
- • Determine gestational age and size
  - — Compare the total score with the corresponding gestational age.
  - — Plot the gestational age, weight, length, and head circumference on intrauterine development graph (Figure 3-2 on p. 231).

NEWBORN MATURITY RATING & CLASSIFICATION

ESTIMATION OF GESTATIONAL AGE BY MATURITY RATING
Symbols: X - 1st Exam   O - 2nd Exam

NEUROMUSCULAR MATURITY

	-1	0	1	2	3	4	5
Posture							
Square Window (wrist)	>90°	90°	60°	45°	30°	0°	
Arm Recoil		180°	140°–180°	110°–140°	90–110°	<90°	
Popliteal Angle	180°	160°	140°	120°	100°	90°	<90°
Scarf Sign							
Heel to Ear							

PHYSICAL MATURITY

Skin	sticky friable transparent	gelatinous red, translucent	smooth pink, visible veins	superficial peeling &/or rash, few veins	cracking pale areas rare veins	parchment deep cracking no vessels	leathery cracked wrinkled
Lanugo	none	sparse	abundant	thinning	bald areas	mostly bald	
Plantar Surface	heel-toe 40–50 mm:–1 <40 mm:–2	>50mm no crease	faint red marks	anterior transverse crease only	creases ant. 2/3	creases over entire sole	
Breast	imperceptible	barely perceptible	flat areola no bud	stippled areola 1–2mm bud	raised areola 3–4mm bud	full areola 5–10mm bud	
Eye/Ear	lids fused loosely:–1 tightly:–2	lids open pinna flat stays folded	sl. curved pinna; soft; slow recoil	well-curved pinna; soft but ready recoil	formed &firm instant recoil	thick cartilage ear stiff	
Genitals male	scrotum flat, smooth	scrotum empty faint rugae	testes in upper canal rare rugae	testes descending few rugae	testes down good rugae	testes pendulous deep rugae	
Genitals female	clitoris prominent labia flat	prominent clitoris small labia minora	prominent clitoris enlarging minora	majora & minora equally prominent	majora large minora small	majora cover clitoris & minora	

Figure 3-1 New Ballard Score. (Courtesy Bristol-Myers Company, Evansville, Indiana. From Ballard, J.L., Khoury, J.C., Wedig, K., Wang, L., Eilers-Walsman, B.L., & Lipp, R. [1991]. New Ballard score, expanded to include extremely premature infants. *Journal of Pediatrics, 19*[3], 417-423.)

Continued

Gestation by Dates_____wks

Birth Date_____ Hour_____am/pm

APGAR_____1 min_____5 min

MATURITY RATING

score	weeks
-10	20
-5	22
0	24
5	26
10	28
15	30
20	32
25	34
30	36
35	38
40	40
45	42
50	44

SCORING SECTION

	1st Exam=X	2nd Exam=O
Estimating Gest Age by Maturity Rating	_____Weeks	_____Weeks
Time of Exam	Date_____ Hour_____am/pm	Date_____ Hour_____am/pm
Age at Exam	_____Hours	_____Hours
Signature of Examiner	_____ M.D.	_____ M.D.

Figure 3-1, cont'd

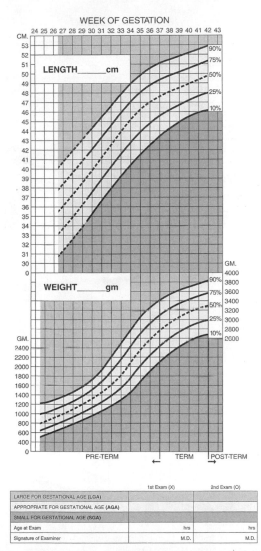

Figure 3-2 Intrauterine growth grids. (Courtesy Bristol-Myers Company, Evansville, Indiana. Adapted from Lubchenko, L.C., Hansman, C., & Boyd, E. [1966]. Intrauterine growth grids, *Pediatrics*, 37, 403; and from Battaglia, F.C. & Lubchenko, L.C. [1967]. Intrauterine growth grids, *Journal of Pediatrics*, 71, 159.)

Continued

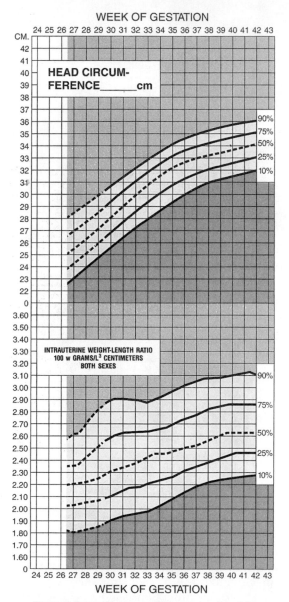

Figure 3-2, cont'd Intrauterine growth grids.

COMMON NURSING DIAGNOSES FOR NORMAL NEWBORNS

- Imbalanced Nutrition: Less Than Body Requirements related to poor infant feeding behaviors
- Health-Seeking Behaviors related to the desire for information about infant care
- Ineffective Airway Clearance related to excessive secretions in the respiratory passages
- Ineffective Thermoregulation related to immature compensation for changes in environmental temperature
- Risk for Ineffective Breastfeeding related to lack of understanding of breastfeeding techniques
- Risk for Ineffective Health Maintenance related to lack of understanding of formula and feeding techniques.
- Risk for Infection related to break in skin integrity at cord or circumcision and immature immune system
- Risk for Impaired Parenting related to stressors involved with new parenting role
- Risk for Injury related to lack of parental knowledge about hyperbilirubinemia

NURSING INTERVENTIONS
PROVIDING EARLY CARE
Early care includes assessment, stabilization, and assignment of an Apgar score (see pp. 151-154).

- Provide resuscitation if necessary (see procedure: Resuscitation in Newborns, p. 439).
- Check and record vital signs.
- Provide for identification: Apply identification bands on the infant, mother, and support person.
- Perform overall assessment (see Table 3-1, Summary of Newborn Assessments).

POSITIONING AND SUCTIONING SECRETIONS
- Position the infant with the head in a neutral position or to the side.
- Use the bulb syringe frequently to suction secretions from the mouth or nose. (See Procedure: Bulb Syringe Use, p. 418.)

- If mechanical suctioning is necessary, choose a small catheter to avoid damaging the tissues. Suction for no more than 5 seconds at a time using minimal negative pressure to avoid trauma, laryngospasm, and bradycardia.

MAINTAINING THERMOREGULATION

- Prevent heat loss
  - Perform initial assessments with the infant under a radiant warmer. Set the servocontrol between 36° and 36.5° C (96.8°-97.7° F).
  - Dry the infant immediately after birth. Cover the infant's head with a cap when the infant is not under a radiant warmer.
  - Warm anything that comes into contact with the infant. Pad cool surfaces such as scales before placing infants on them. Warm stethoscopes and clothing before using them on the infant.
  - Bathe the infant to remove blood and excessive vernix as soon after birth as the temperature is stable. Dry quickly. Keep the infant under a warmer until the temperature is stable.
  - Wrap the infant in two warm blankets and add a hat when moving the infant to a crib.
  - Position the newborn's crib or incubator away from outside walls or windows.
  - Avoid exposing infants to drafts. Reduce traffic near radiant warmers as movement increases air currents.
  - Expose only the parts of the infant's body necessary during assessment or care.
- Restore thermoregulation as necessary with warm blankets or place the infant under a radiant warmer for a short time.
- Perform expanded assessments if the temperature remains low.
  - Assess for signs of respiratory distress from the additional oxygen requirement.
  - Test the blood glucose and feed the infant warm milk to provide glucose.

— Observe for signs of infection, because low temperature may be a sign of infection.

ADMINISTERING PROPHYLACTIC MEDICATIONS

- Vitamin K
  — Given to prevent vitamin K–dependent bleeding (hemorrhagic disease of the newborn).
  — Give only after the infant is bathed if the mother is positive for hepatitis B or HIV.
  — See Procedure: Intramuscular Injection Administration to Newborns, p. 433, and Drug Guide: Vitamin K_1 (Phytonadione), p. 475.
- Eye treatment
  — Prophylactic antibiotic such as erythromycin is applied to the eyes to prevent ophthalmia neonatorum in case the mother is infected with gonorrhea and conjunctivitis if the mother has chlamydial infection.
  — See Drug Guide: Erythromycin Ophthalmic Ointment, p. 457.
  — Mild inflammation occurs in some infants.
  — Purulent discharge from the eyes may indicate infection.

MAINTAINING BLOOD GLUCOSE

- Check blood glucose of infants with signs of hypoglycemia or according to agency policy. See Hypoglycemia, p. 262.
- Feed infants who have low glucose levels according to agency policy (e.g., if the glucose screening test is 40-45 mg/dL or less).
- Retest according to agency policy (e.g., 1 hour after the first test and before feedings several times until results are normal). See Procedure: Blood Glucose Assessment in the Newborn, p. 413.
- Notify the primary caregiver if the glucose level remains low.

GIVING FEEDINGS

- Give (or help mothers give) the first feeding. Watch for cyanosis or choking. If either occurs, stop feeding, suction, and stimulate the infant. Continue feeding when the infant has recovered.

- Determine if the infant is feeding adequately (every 2-3 hours if breastfed, every 3-4 hours if formula fed).
- Record each feeding with the type, amount (or length of the nursing period), regurgitation, and parents' understanding of the feeding method.
- See pp. 241-249 for further information about formula feeding and breastfeeding.

CONTINUING ASSESSMENTS
- Assess the infant at the beginning of each shift or according to agency policy.
- Focus on changes from the original assessment.
- Assess vital signs once a shift according to agency policy or more often if there are abnormalities.
- Observe chest expansion and note signs of respiratory distress.
- Weigh infants every 24 hours at the same time of day.
- Examine all areas of the skin for new marks or changes in existing ones.
- Palpate the fontanels with infants in a slightly upright position. Note changes in molding, caput succedaneum, cephalhematoma.
- Observe the eyes for inflammation or drainage.
- Note the level of alertness, reflexes (see Table 3-2), and changes in behavior.
- Observe the movement of the extremities to see that it is equal.
- Check the cord for bleeding, purulent drainage, or redness at the base.
- Observe the type and number of stools and frequency of voidings.
- Assess the feeding behavior. Note regurgitation or feeding difficulties.

IDENTIFYING INFANTS AND MOTHERS
- Ensure the infant's identification bands remain in place.

• Use the imprinted number to identify the mother and the infant at any time the mother and infant are separated. See Procedure: Infant Identification, p. 433.

CARING FOR THE SKIN
• Remove the cord clamp 24 hours after birth if the end of the cord is dry.
• Teach the parents to care for the cord according to agency policy: apply triple-dye solution, antibiotic ointment, or alcohol; clean with water or a mild soap solution; or allow the cord to dry naturally.
• Explain that the cord will fall off within approximately 10 to 14 days.
• Explain diaper area care to parents. Demonstrate how to fold the diaper below the cord to keep it dry.
• Teach parents of uncircumcised boys that the foreskin may not retract for 3 years or more. It should not be forcibly retracted.

PREVENTING HYPERBILIRUBINEMIA
• Intervene when infants feed poorly to promote stool passage, which aids bilirubin excretion. Explain the relationship of poor feeding and jaundice to parents.
• Notify the primary caregiver of increasing jaundice so treatment may begin early.
• Teach parents how to assess for increasing jaundice after discharge.
• See Hyperbilirubinemia, p. 256.

CARING FOR THE CIRCUMCISED INFANT
• Circumcision is the removal of the prepuce (foreskin) that covers the glans penis. The infant should be at least 12 hours old so that he has recovered from the stress of birth.
• Preparation
   — Obtain informed consent from the parents.
   — Inform the physician of any contraindications to circumcision.

— Check to be sure the infant has received a vitamin K injection.

— Withhold feedings for 2 to 4 hours before the procedure to prevent regurgitation and possible aspiration.

— Gather the equipment and supplies. Place a bulb syringe nearby.

— When the physician and equipment are ready, place the infant on a circumcision board.

— Provide for warmth during the procedure.

— Evaluate the infant's pain and provide pain relief measures such as a pacifier, sucrose, talking to the infant, or local anesthetic.

— Comfort the infant during and after the procedure.

- Aftercare
  — Gomco clamp: Place petroleum jelly or antibiotic ointment over the circumcision site. Plastibell: Do not use petroleum jelly.

  — If excessive bleeding occurs, apply pressure to the penis with sterile gauze and notify the physician.

- Parent teaching
  — Call the physician for signs of complications.
    - Bleeding more than a few drops with the first diaper changes
    - Failure to urinate
    - Signs of infection: fever or low temperature, foul smelling drainage
    - Displacement of the Plastibell

  — Apply petroleum jelly to the penis with each diaper change for the first 24 to 48 hours. If a Plastibell was used, do not apply petroleum jelly.

  — Clean by squeezing warm water over the penis.

  — Fasten the diaper loosely to prevent rubbing or pressure on the incision site.

  — Do not remove the normal yellow crust that forms over the site.

  — The circumcision site should be fully healed in approximately 10 days.

— If a PlastiBell was used, the plastic rim will fall off in 5 to 8 days.

PROVIDING TEACHING

- Assess the parents' interaction with the infant and knowledge of infant care.
- Make a teaching plan.
- Use demonstrations and return demonstrations, videos, and pamphlets in the parents' language.
- Document all teaching performed and the parents' ability to care for the infant.
- Usual topics include handling the infant, use of a bulb syringe, feeding techniques, taking an axillary temperature, elimination norms, and skin care (cord, diaper area, circumcision, bathing).

PREVENTING INFECTION

- Scrub the hands and arms at the beginning of the shift. Wash the hands or use hand disinfectant before and after touching infants. Teach parents and visitors handwashing.
- Keep each infant's supplies separate from those used for other infants to avoid cross-contamination.
- Keep staff or visitors with infections away from infants. If the mother has an infection, consult with the physician as to whether the infant can be with her and can breastfeed. The presence and degree of maternal fever, organisms responsible, and medications will be considered.
- Observe for signs of neonatal infection (temperature instability, poor feeding, lethargy, periods of apnea, unexplained behavior changes). (See Sepsis Neonatorum, p. 292.)

PREVENTING INFANT ABDUCTION

- All personnel must wear appropriate identification at all times.
- Teach parents to allow only a staff person with proper identification to take their infants from them.
- Never give an infant to anyone who does not have an identification bracelet that matches the infant's bracelet or other proper identification.

- Never leave infants unattended in a room or hallway.
- Teach parents to call their nurse if infants cannot be observed at all times.
- Position infants' cribs away from doorways when they are in the mothers' rooms.
- Transport infants only in cribs. Question anyone walking in the hallway carrying an infant.
- Question anyone with a newborn near an exit or in an unusual part of the facility.
- Be suspicious of visitors who move from room to room, ask detailed questions about nursery or discharge routines, or carry large bags or packages that could contain an infant.
- Follow unit policy for security. Keep remote exits locked, codes secret, and respond quickly if an alarm sounds.
- Alert hospital security when any suspicious activity occurs.
- Warn parents that newspaper announcements or signs in their yard may alert abductors about the new baby.

PROVIDING IMMUNIZATION FOR HEPATITIS
- Give hepatitis B vaccine according to agency policy and exposure to mothers with acute or chronic hepatitis. See Drug Guide: Hepatitis B Vaccine, p. 459.
- Give hepatitis B immune globulin (HBIG) within 12 hours of birth to infants exposed to hepatitis during birth. (See Drug Guide: Hepatitis B Immune Globulin [HBIG], p. 458.)

ARRANGING NEWBORN SCREENING TESTS
- All states require that infants receive hearing screening before discharge. Early identification of hearing loss helps prevent developmental delays and enables the child to communicate better.
- Screening tests detect inborn errors of metabolism or other genetic conditions that may cause mental retardation or other serious problems unless treated early.
- Screening for phenylketonuria, hypothyroidism, galactosemia, hemoglobinopathies, and congenital adrenal hyperplasia are most common.

- Tests performed on blood samples obtained before the first 12 to 24 hours of life should be repeated within 1 to 2 weeks of age.

PROVIDING FOLLOW-UP CARE
- Follow-up care should be provided within 48 hours of discharge to all newborns discharged less than 48 hours after birth.
- Care may occur in the home, clinic, or office. Home visits and telephone contact may be made by nurses.

TEACHING ABOUT SUDDEN INFANT DEATH SYNDROME
Teaching parents about reducing the risk of sudden infant death syndrome (SIDS) includes:

- Healthy infants should be placed in a supine position for sleep because there is an increased incidence of SIDS in infants who sleep in a prone position.
- Infants should not sleep on a soft surface or with another person.
- No objects such as pillows, stuffed animals, or loose bedding should be in the infant's bed.
- Infants should not become overheated during sleep.
- Infants should be placed in a prone position with supervision while awake to prevent flattening of the head and to help develop shoulder muscles.

INFANT FEEDING
FORMULA FEEDING
- The most commonly used formulas are made from modified cow's milk, soy, or casein hydrolysate. Other types of formulas are available for specialized needs.
- Available forms include ready-to-use, concentrated, and powdered.
- Correct dilution of concentrated (dilute with equal parts water) or powdered formula (mix one scoop of formula with every 2 oz of water) is essential to prevent serious illness and to promote weight gain and growth.

- Equipment (bottles and nipples) used depends on the mother's preference.
- Preparation may be a single bottle or a 24-hour supply that is capped and refrigerated until needed.
- Wash bottles and nipples with hot sudsy water, rinse well, and air dry. Bottles may be washed in a dishwasher, but nipples tend to deteriorate quickly unless washed by hand
- Sterilization is unnecessary unless the water supply is unsafe. Aseptic method of sterilization: Boil equipment and water for 5 minutes and then assemble and add formula aseptically. Terminal method of sterilization: place formula in bottles, loosely cap, and boil 25 minutes. Refrigerate all prepared formula once cooled.
- Feed approximately every 3 to 4 hours, but avoid a rigid schedule.
- Avoid heating formula in a microwave because the heating is uneven and may result in burning the infant. Test the formula temperature by placing a few drops from the bottle on the inner arm.
- Position the infant in a semiupright position (such as a cradle hold).
- Keep the nipple filled with formula to prevent swallowing of air. Infants typically take 0.5 to 1 ounce per feeding the first day and 2 to 3 ounces per feeding by the third to fifth day.
- Burp the infant after every half ounce at first.
- Do not prop the bottle; doing so increases the risk of aspiration and promotes the growth of bacteria that can lead to ear infections and dental caries when the teeth are in.
- Discard formula not used within an hour because of bacterial growth.

BREASTFEEDING
General Information
- Help the mother assume a comfortable position; use pillows to support her arm and the infant and to protect an abdominal incision.
- Teach the cradle, football, cross-cradle, and side-lying positions to hold the infant (Figures 3-3 to 3-6).

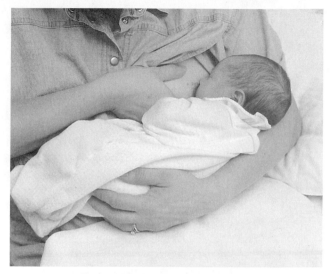

Figure 3-3 Cradle hold position.

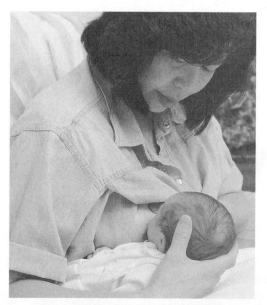

Figure 3-4 Football hold position.

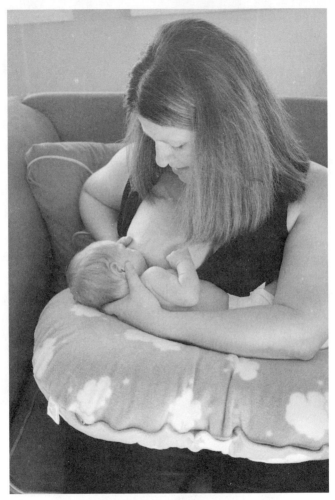

Figure 3-5 Cross-cradle position.

- Position the infant facing the breast and brush the nipple against the infant's lips to elicit latch-on. When the infant's mouth is open wide, insert the nipple with as much of the areola as possible into the infant's mouth.

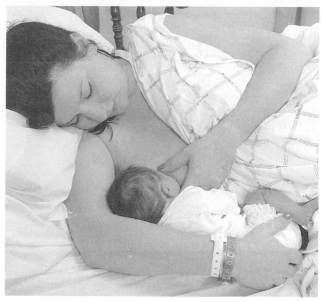

Figure 3-6 Side-lying position.

- Evaluate infant suckling, which should be smooth and continuous with only occasional pauses.
- Take the infant off the breast and start again if suckling is short, choppy, and without audible swallowing sounds.
- Advise the mother to feed the infant when the breasts feel full or when the infant indicates hunger rather than following a rigid schedule but to expect to feed about every 2 to 3 hours with 8 to 12 feedings a day.
- Explain that she should not restrict the duration of breast-feeding, but she should allow adequate time for both breasts to be emptied at each feeding. Feeding time is generally about 10 to 15 minutes on each side.
- Remind her that keeping the breasts dry between feedings helps prevent tissue damage, and wearing a good bra provides necessary support.

Assessing Infant Milk Intake. Signs the infant is getting enough milk:

- Swallowing is audible (a soft "ka" or "ah" sound).
- Nutritive suckling (a smooth series of suckling and swallowing with occasional rest periods) is seen.
- The mother's breast gets softer during the feeding.
- Milk is seen in the baby's mouth or dripping from the mother's breast.
- The infant receives 8 to 12 feedings a day.
- The infant has at least one or two wet diapers a day for the first 2 days and at least six wet diapers by the fourth day. The urine is light yellow in color, not concentrated.
- The infant passes at least three stools daily (after the first few days) and stools are yellow by the fourth day.
- The infant seems satisfied after feedings.
- The infant's checkups show weight gain.

Common Problems of Breastfeeding
Sleepy Infant
- Teach the mother measures to awaken the infant gently (changing the diaper, removing blankets and shirt, rubbing the cheeks or hair, talking, playing, washing the infant's face with a lukewarm washcloth).
- Suggest expressing colostrum onto the nipple to interest the infant in feeding.
- Recommend burping the infant frequently to reduce a feeling of fullness from swallowed air.
- If the infant falls asleep during the feeding, evaluate whether the infant has taken enough. If not, gently reawaken using the above techniques.

Nipple Confusion or Preference. This problem may occur in infants who have received bottles and confuse the tongue movements needed for the two types of feedings. Teaching includes:

- Avoid all bottles unless absolutely necessary.
- Do not give formula during the night or after breastfeeding.

- Avoid pacifiers.
- Nurse more frequently to stimulate milk production and help the infant learn proper suckling.

Suckling Problems. Infants may suck on the end of the nipple, fail to open the mouth widely enough, have dimpling of the cheeks, or make smacking noises. Teaching includes:

- Rub the nipple against the infant's lips to stimulate the infant to open the mouth widely.
- Wait until the infant opens the mouth widely before inserting the nipple. Gently pull down on the infant's chin, if necessary, to open the mouth wider.
- Check the position: Much of the areola should be in the mouth, and the lips should be 1 to 1½ inches from the nipple base.
- Remove the infant and start again if the latch is incorrect.

Engorgement. To prevent engorgement, which may occur when the milk comes in or if feedings are not of sufficient frequency or length, teach the mother to:

- Breastfeed every 2 to 3 hours day and night for approximately 10 to 15 minutes on each side.
- Use a breast pump to empty the breasts if breastfeeding must be interrupted.
- Apply cold packs between feedings to reduce edema and pain. Use commercial packs, a clean glove or plastic bag filled with ice, or a package of frozen vegetables covered with washcloths.
- Apply heat with compresses or a shower prior to feedings.
- Massage the breasts before and during feedings to stimulate the let-down reflex.
- Express milk by hand or use a breast pump before feedings if the areola is too hard for the infant to grasp.
- Take prescribed pain medication before feeding to relieve discomfort.

Sore Nipples. Nursing interventions to prevent sore nipples include:

- Ensure the infant is positioned correctly at the breast.
- Avoid engorgement, which increases the risk of incorrect positioning.
- Avoid using soap or other drying agents on the nipples.
- Change wet nursing pads promptly.
- Avoid creams that must be removed before feedings.
- Check for allergies and irritations caused by use of breast creams.

Teaching includes:

- Begin feeding with the least sore side.
- Vary the position of the infant during feeding (the area of the nipple directly in line with the infant's nose and chin is most stressed during a feeding).
- Avoid nipple shields that decrease milk flow to the infant. Use only with the help of a lactation consultant.
- Apply warm-water compresses, colostrum, or breast milk after feeding.
- Expose the nipples to air between feedings.
- Use hydrogel dressings to relieve pain and promote healing.
- Check the infant's mouth for the white patches of *Candida* infection (thrush). If present, notify the health care provider to obtain medication for the mother and infant.

Flat or Inverted Nipples. Infants may have difficulty grasping flat or inverted nipples. Teaching includes:

- Use breast shells to help the nipples protrude.
- Roll the nipples between the thumb and forefinger to make them more erect just before feedings.
- Use a breast pump just before feedings to draw out inverted nipples.
- Put the baby to breast immediately after pumping makes the nipple become erect.

- Use a nipple shield, but only with the help of a lactation consultant.

Interruption of Breastfeeding. To maintain milk supply when breastfeeding must be interrupted temporarily:

- Teach the mother how to use a breast pump.
- Instruct her to pump for 15 to 20 minutes at least eight times each day.
- Demonstrate breast massage and application of heat before pumping to increase the flow of milk.
- Provide sterile containers for the milk so that the infant can be fed the milk. Instruct the mother about special nursery requirements.

COMPLICATIONS OF NEWBORN
ASPHYXIA
Asphyxia is a lack of oxygen and increase of carbon dioxide in the blood. It can occur before, during, or after birth.

Etiology and Predisposing Factors
- Maternal factors: hypertension, infection, drug use
- Placental conditions: placenta previa, abruptio placentae, postmaturity.
- Other: cord problems, infection, premature birth, multifetal pregnancy

Clinical Signs
- Primary apnea consists of rapid respirations at birth followed by apnea and bradycardia. Stimulation and oxygen may restart respirations.
- Secondary apnea consists of loss of consciousness and metabolic acidosis. Immediate resuscitation is necessary to prevent permanent damage or death.

Therapeutic Management. See Procedure: Resuscitation in Newborns, p. 439.

Nursing Considerations

- Have equipment readily available and functioning properly at all times to prevent delays.
- Begin resuscitation measures quickly, as necessary. Primary asphyxia will progress to secondary asphyxia without immediate intervention.
- Assist the physician with intubation, insertion of umbilical vein catheters, and administration of medications.
- Once the infant is stabilized, assess for further complications.
- Support parents and explain the infant's condition.

BRONCHOPULMONARY DYSPLASIA (BPD)

Bronchopulmonary dysplasia is a serious, chronic lung condition that occurs most often in infants weighing less than 1500 g (3 lb, 7 oz).

Etiology and Predisposing Factors. Treatment with high levels of oxygen, oxygen-free radicals, and high positive-pressure ventilation may damage the lungs, resulting in prolonged oxygen need.

Clinical Signs

- Need for oxygen or mechanical ventilation or both beyond 36 weeks of gestational age.
- Tachycardia, tachypnea, retractions, rales, wheezing, respiratory acidosis, increased secretions, and bronchospasm.
- X-ray: characteristic lung changes.

Therapeutic Management. Treatment is supportive with gradual decrease in the amount of oxygen, bronchodilators, and antibiotics. The infant may go home on long-term oxygen therapy.

Nursing Considerations

- Assess respiratory status frequently.
- Monitor infant's blood oxygen levels and adjust oxygen as indicated.

- Determine infant response to medications.
- Teach parents for home care.

CLEFT LIP AND PALATE
These conditions occur alone or together and affect one or both sides of the mouth. They are among the most common congenital anomalies.

Etiology and Predisposing Factors. Genetic and environmental factors may be involved.

Clinical Signs
- Cleft lip: Minor notching of the lip or extensive cleft through the lip and into the floor of the nose
- Cleft palate: Defect in the soft palate only or extending throughout the hard and soft palates
- Cleft lip and cleft palate: One or both sides involved

Therapeutic Management
- Lip surgery by 3 months with more surgery possible later
- Palate surgery by 1 year usually in stages, depending on degree
- Long term follow-up for orthodontia, speech therapy, hearing problems

Nursing Considerations
- Palpate the hard and the soft palate during the initial assessment to find less obvious clefts.
- Experiment with feeding techniques.
  — Breastfeeding for interested mothers
  — Soft preemie nipples directed away from a cleft palate
  — Nipples with enlarged holes
  — Compressible bottles
  — Special long nipples that extend beyond a cleft palate
  — Nipples with extensions to cover a cleft palate
- Feed in an upright position to prevent aspiration.
- Feed slowly with frequent stops for burping.

- Wash away milk curds after feedings.
- Prevent infections.
- Support the parents.
  — Show "before and after" pictures of plastic surgery.
  — Reinforce explanations of surgery.
  — Teach feeding techniques.
  — Explain the need for long-term follow-up.

CONGENITAL CARDIAC DEFECTS

Common congenital heart defects include:

- Ventricular septal defect is the most common defect. The opening in the septum between the ventricles may be small and close spontaneously. Large defects may cause pulmonary hypertension and heart failure.
- Patent ductus arteriosus is a failure of the vessel to close after birth and is more common in preterm infants. It causes blood to flow into the lungs from the aorta and may result in no symptoms or congestive heart failure.
- Coarctation of the aorta is a narrowing of the aorta near the ductus arteriosus. It causes increased pressure behind the defect and may lead to heart failure.
- In transposition of the great vessels the positions of the aorta and pulmonary artery are reversed. It is fatal without the presence of another defect that allows mixing of oxygenated and unoxygenated blood.

Etiology and Predisposing Factors
- Genetic factors
- Environmental factors such as teratogens or maternal rubella or diabetes
- May occur with other anomalies

Clinical Signs. Signs depend on the type and severity of the defect.

- Cyanosis—may increase with crying or feeding
- Pallor

- Murmurs
- Tachycardia
- Tachypnea
- Dyspnea
- Choking spells
- Poor intake, falling asleep during feedings
- Diaphoresis

Therapeutic Management
- Testing, such as echocardiogram and cardiac catheterization to determine the type of defect
- Oxygen
- Surgery—corrective or palliative, as indicated
- Medications, such as digitalis, diuretics, potassium, sedatives

Nursing Considerations
- Assess for changes in condition.
- Reduce the infant's need for oxygen by providing frequent rest periods.
- Feed by gavage for rapid respirations. Provide oxygen during feedings if necessary.
- Maintain oxygen at the lowest level possible to maintain adequate oxygenation.
- Provide parental support and education about the infant's condition and expected treatment.
- Teach parents home care, including administration of medications, and signs of complications.

DIAPHRAGMATIC HERNIA
Diaphragmatic hernia is a failure of the diaphragm to close during fetal life, allowing intestines to pass through the opening into the chest. It may interfere with lung development.

Etiology and Predisposing Factors
- Exact cause unknown
- Occurs when the diaphragm remains partially open

Clinical Signs. Signs vary according to the size of the herniation and the degree of lung development.

- Mild to severe respiratory distress at birth
- Breath sounds diminished or absent over the affected area
- Barrel chest
- Heartbeat may be displaced to the right
- Scaphoid (concave) abdomen

Therapeutic Management
- May be diagnosed prenatally by ultrasound
- Endotracheal tube for ventilation
- Gastric tube to decompress stomach
- Surgery to replace the intestines and repair the defect when stable
- Extracorporeal membrane oxygenation (ECMO) may be used
- Fetal surgery may be performed

Nursing Considerations
- Position infant on the affected side to allow the unaffected lung to expand.
- Elevate the head.
- Assist with ventilation.
- Monitor the respiratory status.

ERYTHROBLASTOSIS FETALIS
See Hyperbilirubinemia, Complications of Pathologic Jaundice, p. 259.

ESOPHAGEAL ATRESIA AND TRACHEOESOPHAGEAL FISTULA (TEF)
In these conditions, there is most commonly a division of the esophagus into two unconnected segments (atresia) with a blind pouch at the proximal end. The proximal or distal end may be connected to the trachea, resulting in TEF.

Etiology and Predisposing Factors
- Failure of the structures to form normally before birth
- Exact cause unknown

Clinical Signs. Signs vary by the type of anomaly.

- Excessive, frothy mucus
- Drooling
- Regurgitation
- Failure of a catheter to pass into the stomach
- Coughing, choking, cyanosis with feedings
- Distended stomach

Therapeutic Management
- Suspect with polyhydramnios during pregnancy
- Diagnosis by symptoms and x-ray
- Continuous suction to the upper pouch
- Gastrostomy tube
- Surgery to close the fistula and join the esophageal segments
- Long-term follow-up for esophageal reflux and dilation of strictures

Nursing Considerations
- Observe all infants carefully during the first feeding.
- Use a semiupright position to prevent aspiration of gastric fluids.
- Maintain suction equipment.
- Post-surgical care: Maintain ventilator, chest tubes, and parenteral and gastrostomy feedings.

GASTROSCHISIS
See Omphalocele and Gastroschisis, p. 273.

HYDROCEPHALUS
Hydrocephalus is dilation of the cerebral ventricles with cerebrospinal fluid, which may cause compression of the brain and enlargement of the head.

Etiology and Predisposing Factors
- Genetic and environmental factors
- Increased production of cerebrospinal fluid

- Obstruction of flow of cerebrospinal fluid
- Stenosis of the aqueduct
- Neural tube defects
- Hemorrhage that causes obstruction

Clinical Signs of Hydrocephalus
- Full or bulging fontanel
- Separation of sutures
- Head enlargement, especially in the frontal area
- Setting sun sign (sclera visible above the pupils of the eyes)

Therapeutic Management. Surgical correction with insertion of a ventriculoperitoneal shunt.

Nursing Considerations
- Measure the head circumference daily.
- Prevent pressure areas.
- Observe for signs of infection.
- Teach parents how to care for the shunt and how to recognize signs of increased intracranial pressure.

HYPERBILIRUBINEMIA (JAUNDICE)

Hyperbilirubinemia is an elevated level of unconjugated bilirubin, which causes jaundice. Jaundice becomes visible when the serum bilirubin reaches 5 to 7 mg/dL. High levels of bilirubin may stain the brain (kernicterus) and cause bilirubin encephalopathy and severe brain damage. There are three major types of jaundice: physiologic, breast milk, and pathologic jaundice.

Physiologic Jaundice.   Physiologic jaundice is considered normal in newborns.

Etiology
- Normal hemolysis of excessive erythrocytes
- Short red cell life
- Liver immaturity
- Lack of intestinal flora needed to process bilirubin

Predisposing Factors
- Delayed feeding
- Trauma resulting in bruising or cephalhematoma
- Cold stress or asphyxia

Clinical Signs
- Begins after the first 24 hours of life
- Peaks at 5 to 6 mg/dL between the second and fourth days of life
- Falls to 1 mg/dL by 10 to 14 days of age

Breastfeeding Jaundice
Etiology and Predisposing Factors
- Insufficient intake of colostrum and breast milk delays elimination of meconium.
- Conjugated bilirubin may be deconjugated by beta glucuronidase in the intestine and absorbed back into the blood. It must then be conjugated again by the liver.
- The infant may be sleepy, have a poor suck, or nurse infrequently depressing production of breast milk.

Clinical Signs
- Jaundice develops within the first week to more than 12 mg/dL.
- Bilirubin level may become dangerously high if intake is not increased.

Therapeutic Management
- Increase milk intake either by more frequent breastfeeding or temporary supplementation by formula

True Breast Milk Jaundice. Breast milk jaundice is jaundice that occurs in the breastfed infant when physiologic jaundice should be resolving.

Etiology and Predisposing Factors
- The exact cause is unknown.
- Pregnanediol and fatty acids in the milk may interfere with conjugation.

- Beta glucuronidase may be increased.

Clinical Signs
- Late rise in bilirubin (begins after 3-5 days of life)
- Usually peaks at 5 to 10 mg/dL 2 weeks after birth but may reach more than 20 mg/dL
- Bilirubin falls gradually over several months

Therapeutic Management
- Close monitoring of bilirubin levels
- At least 8 to 10 feedings each 24 hours
- Phototherapy if necessary
- Formula supplementation
- Discontinuation of breastfeeding for 24 to 48 hours may be necessary.

Pathologic Jaundice
Etiology and Predisposing Factors
- Blood incompatibilities
  - Rh incompatibility (Rh-negative mother with an Rh-positive infant)
  - ABO incompatibility (type O mother with a type A, B, or AB infant)
- Infection
- Hypothyroidism
- Glucuronyl transferase deficiency
- Polycythemia
- Glucose-6-phosphate dehydrogenase deficiency
- Biliary atresia

Predisposing Factors
- Prematurity
- Cephalhematoma
- Bruising
- Hypoxia
- Cold stress
- Diabetic mother

Clinical Signs
- Appearance of jaundice in the first 24 hours of life
- Laboratory indications of pathologic jaundice
  — Increase of total bilirubin concentration by more than 0.2 mg/dL/hr or 5 mg/dL/day
  — Total serum bilirubin over the 95th percentile for the infant's age in hours
  — Direct bilirubin greater than 1.5 to 2 mg/dL
  — Total bilirubin more than 12 mg/dL in a full-term infant or 10 to 14 mg/dL in a preterm infant
- Jaundice that persists after the second week of life in a full-term infant.

Therapeutic Management
- Phototherapy: Special fluorescent lamps or a fiberoptic phototherapy blanket or both
- Exchange transfusions: When quick reduction of dangerously high bilirubin levels is necessary
  — Removal of small portions of blood and replacement with donor blood, replacing 85% to 90% of the RBCs
  — Complications: Electrolyte imbalances, acidosis, infection, cardiac arrhythmias, necrotizing enterocolitis, thrombosis, and embolism
  — Followed by phototherapy

Complications of Pathologic Jaundice
- Bilirubin encephalopathy
  — This occurs when bilirubin levels are high enough to cause kernicterus (bilirubin staining of the brain).
  — The degree of hyperbilirubinemia necessary to cause bilirubin encephalopathy is unknown.
  — Incidence increases when sepsis, hypoxia, or respiratory acidosis occurs.
  — Bilirubin encephalopathy has a high mortality rate, with possible mental retardation, cerebral palsy, hearing loss, and neurologic and developmental problems in survivors.

- Erythroblastosis fetalis
  - Condition is caused by destruction of fetal red blood cells by maternal antibodies in sensitized Rh-negative women.
  - Severely affected infants may experience hydrops fetalis, a severe anemia that results in heart failure and generalized edema.
  - It is less common now due to use of $Rh_o(D)$ immunoglobulin to prevent maternal antibody formation after exposure to Rh-positive blood.

Nursing Considerations for All Types of Jaundice

- Check for jaundice at each assessment in the birth agency and during follow-up visits. Note areas of the body involved. Jaundice of the midabdomen occurs when the bilirubin is about 15 mg/dL and of the soles of the feet at 20 mg/dL.
- Teach parents the importance of adequate feedings to stimulate passage of stools and excretion of bilirubin. Intervene when infants are feeding poorly. Instruct breastfeeding mothers to nurse every 2 to 3 hours.
- Prevent factors that increase the risk of hyperbilirubinemia: cold stress, hypoglycemia, inadequate intake.
- Note changes in laboratory results and correlate them with the infant's age.
- Teach parents how to check for jaundice at home and to contact their care provider if it occurs.
- Avoid giving water to jaundiced infants because milk stimulates stool excretion better.
- Measure transcutaneous bilirubin or end-tidal carbon monoxide concentration according to agency policy.
- Phototherapy
  - Position the lights or blanket according to the manufacturer's guidelines to prevent overheating or burning the skin. Check the level of irradiance with a light meter once a shift.

— Protect the eyes from retinal damage with eyepatches. Check the position of patches at least every hour. Remove the patches from the eyes during feedings out of the lights. Assess the eyes for infection and provide visual stimulation.

— Dress the infant in only a diaper to increase exposure of the skin to the lights.

— Use a light meter to check the level of irradiance to ensure the equipment is functioning properly.

• Observe for side effects

— Frequent loose, green stools and resulting skin breakdown and fluid loss

— Erythematous macular skin rash or bronzing of the skin

— Temporary lactose intolerance during therapy

• Teach parents care if home phototherapy will be used. Arrange for home visits by nurses and other follow-up care.

HYPOCALCEMIA

Hypocalcemia is a total serum calcium of less than 7 mg/dL.

Etiology and Predisposing Factors

• Preterm birth
• Asphyxia at birth
• Diabetic mother
• Prematurity or low birthweight
• Maternal hyperparathyroidism or infant hypoparathyroidism
• Vitamin D deficiency
• Low magnesium levels

Clinical Signs

• Irritability
• Tremors
• Poor feeding
• High-pitched cry
• Tachycardia, apnea

- Muscle twitching, seizures
- Electrocardiogram changes
- May be asymptomatic

Therapeutic Management
- Laboratory analysis of calcium level
- Intravenous or oral calcium

Nursing Considerations
Consider in infants with tremors who have normal blood glucose levels.
Administer IV calcium slowly and watch for bradycardia or arrhythmia; give oral calcium with feedings.

HYPOGLYCEMIA
Hypoglycemia is a blood glucose level less than 40 to 45 mg/dL on screening tests in the full-term infant.

Etiology and Predisposing Factors
- Prematurity
- Postmaturity
- Intrauterine growth restriction
- Asphyxia
- Cold stress
- Large or small for gestational age
- Maternal diabetes
- Maternal intake of terbutaline or ritodrine

Clinical Signs
- Jitteriness
- Poor muscle tone
- Diaphoresis
- Poor suck
- Tachypnea
- Respiratory distress, cyanosis, apnea
- Low temperature
- High-pitched cry
- Irritability or lethargy

- Seizures, coma
- Some infants may be asymptomatic

Therapeutic Management. Feeding usually alleviates hypoglycemia in the normal newborn. Intravenous glucose may be necessary for repeated episodes of hypoglycemia.

Nursing Considerations
- Screen infants in risk categories and those who show signs of hypoglycemia. See Procedure: Blood Glucose Assessment in the Newborn, p. 413.
- Obtain a laboratory analysis to verify low readings on screening tests because they are less accurate.
- Check the mother's history for diabctcs.
- Assess for sepsis if episodes reoccur.
- Assess for other complications, such as hypocalcemia, if signs continue after feeding.

INFANT OF A DIABETIC MOTHER
The infant of a diabetic mother (IDM) may be normal or have a number of complications.

- Macrosomia from the large supply of glucose from mother
- Trauma due to large size
- Congenital anomalies such as caudal regression syndrome or neural tube, heart, gastrointestinal, and urinary tract anomalies
- Respiratory distress syndrome (RDS) because high levels of insulin interfere with production of surfactant
- Hypoglycemia after birth from sudden loss of maternal glucose at birth and infant's continued insulin production
- Hypocalcemia from decreased production of parathyroid hormone
- Polycythemia
- Prematurity
- Low magnesium levels
- Intrauterine growth restriction from poor placental blood flow

Etiology and Predisposing Factors. Gestational or preexisting maternal diabetes; the level and frequency of maternal hyperglycemia and the functioning of the placenta determine severity of neonatal effects.

Clinical Signs
- Large-for-gestational-age infant with a normal length and head circumference but obese body due to enlargement of organs and fat
- Round, red face
- Poor muscle tone
- See Hypoglycemia, Clinical Signs, p. 262.
- Small for gestational age infant similar to other SGA infants

Therapeutic Management
- Control the mother's diabetes during pregnancy to decrease complications of the fetus
- Cesarean birth if necessary due to the infant's size
- Care of complications as needed
- Intravenous glucose if feeding does not correct hypoglycemia to prevent damage to the brain

Nursing Considerations
- Check the mother's records to determine the severity of her diabetes and how well it was controlled.
- Assess the blood glucose level according to hospital policy or hourly for 4 hours after birth, and every 4 hours twice or until the results are normal.
- Assess for signs of hypoglycemia.
- Observe for signs of respiratory distress, trauma, anomalies, and other complications.
- Feed early and more often if hypoglycemia is a problem. Gavage-feed if sucking is poor or respirations are high.
- Keep hydrated, especially if polycythemia is present.
- Prevent cold stress, which increases the need for glucose and oxygen.
- Explain to parents the need for frequent blood tests.

INTRAUTERINE GROWTH RESTRICTION (IUGR)
See Small-for-Gestational-Age Infants, p. 299.

INTRAVENTRICULAR HEMORRHAGE
See Periventricular-Intraventricular Hemorrhage, p. 274.

JAUNDICE
See Hyperbilirubinemia (Jaundice), p. 256.

KERNICTERUS
See Hyperbilirubinemia, Complications of Pathologic Jaundice, p. 259.

LARGE-FOR-GESTATIONAL AGE INFANTS
Large-for-gestational-age infants are above the 90th percentile in size. Infants are usually full term but may be preterm or postterm.

Etiology and Predisposing Factors
- Multipara mother
- Large parents
- Ethnic groups that have large infants
- Maternal diabetes
- Erythroblastosis fetalis

Clinical Signs
Large size, often more than 4000 g (8 lb, 13 oz)

Therapeutic Management
- Identification of macrosomia during pregnancy
- Delivery by use of vacuum extraction, forceps, or cesarean, if necessary
- Treat complications such as shoulder dystocia, fractures of the clavicle or skull, damage to the brachial plexus or facial or phrenic nerves, cephalhematoma, and bruising.

Nursing Considerations
- Assess for hypoglycemia.
- Feed frequently to provide extra calories.

- Assess temperature regulation.
- Assess for complications.
- Other care depends on complications.

MECONIUM ASPIRATION SYNDROME (MAS)

Meconium aspiration syndrome develops when meconium enters the lungs during fetal life or at birth. It may cause obstruction of the airways, pneumonitis, air trapping, or atelectasis, and may lead to persistent pulmonary hypertension of the newborn.

Etiology and Predisposing Factors

- Meconium may be passed by a normal or hypoxic fetus.
- It enters the lungs in utero if gasping movements occur with asphyxia and acidosis.
- It may be aspirated when the infant takes the first breaths at birth.
- Postmaturity increases the risk.

Clinical Signs

- Mild to severe respiratory distress (tachypnea, cyanosis, retractions, nasal flaring, grunting)
- Rales, rhonchi
- X-rays: atelectasis, hyperexpansion from air trapping
- May have yellow-green nails, skin, and umbilical cord

Therapeutic Management

- If thick meconium is present in the amniotic fluid during labor, amnioinfusion may be performed.
- The infant's mouth and pharynx are suctioned as soon as the head is delivered and before delivery of the rest of the body.
- An endotracheal tube is inserted for deep suction before the first breath to prevent meconium from being drawn into the lower airways.
- If the infant is vigorous with a heart rate greater than 100, spontaneous respirations, and good muscle tone, intubation is unnecessary.

- Warmed, humidified oxygen or a ventilator may be used as necessary.
- Extracorporeal membrane oxygenation (ECMO), a method to oxygenate the blood while bypassing the lungs, may be necessary in some infants.

Nursing Considerations
- Notify the primary caregiver when meconium is noted in the amniotic fluid during labor.
- Ensure that equipment is available and functioning.
- Assist with care at delivery.
- Adapt nursing care to the problems presented and watch for complications.

MENINGOCELE
See Neural Tube Defects, p. 272.

MYELOMENINGOCELE
See Neural Tube Defects, p. 272.

NECROTIZING ENTEROCOLITIS (NEC)
Necrotizing enterocolitis is a serious condition of the intestinal tract that may lead to necrosis, perforation, and peritonitis.

Etiology and Predisposing Factors
- Exact cause unknown
- Hypoxia to the intestines; caused by asphyxia, sepsis, polycythemia, umbilical vessel catheterization, or maternal cocaine use
- Preterm birth and immature intestines

Clinical Signs
- Increased abdominal girth
- Increased gastric residuals
- Decreased or absent bowel sounds
- Loops of bowel seen through the abdominal wall
- Vomiting

- Bile-stained residuals or emesis
- Abdominal tenderness
- Blood in the stools
- Signs of infection—apnea, bradycardia, lethargy, temperature instability, hypotension, shock
- X-ray: Loops of bowel dilated with air and air within the intestinal wall

Therapeutic Management
- Preventive measures
  — Breast milk feedings
  — Slow advancement of feedings
- Treatment
  — Antibiotics
  — Gastric suction
  — Parenteral nutrition
  — Surgery to remove necrotic areas and perform an ostomy

Nursing Considerations
- Early recognition of signs is essential to decrease mortality.
- Withhold the next feeding and notify the physician if one or more signs are present.
- Measure abdominal girth
- Postsurgical care

NEONATAL ABSTINENCE SYNDROME
Neonatal abstinence syndrome is a cluster of physical withdrawal signs in a newborn exposed in utero to maternal use of substances such as heroin or methadone.

Etiology and Predisposing Factors. Maternal use of substances such as cocaine or heroin.

Clinical Signs. Signs usually begin within 48 to 72 hours after birth but may not occur until after 1 week. Signs vary according to the drug or combination of drugs used and the time of the last dose. Some infants show no abnormal signs.

- Behavioral signs
  — Irritability
  — Jitteriness, tremors
  — Muscular rigidity, increased muscle tone
  — Restlessness, excessive activity
  — Exaggerated Moro reflex
  — Prolonged, high-pitched cry
- Difficult to console
  — Poor sleeping patterns
  — Yawning
- Signs related to feeding
  — Uncoordinated sucking and swallowing
  — Frequent regurgitation or vomiting
  — Diarrhea
- Respiratory signs
  — Nasal stuffiness, sneezing
  — Tachypnea
- Other signs
  — Hypertension
  — Fever
  — Diaphoresis
  — Seizures
  — Excoriation
  — Mottling

Therapeutic Management
- Obtain a urine specimen, preferably the first urine output (See Procedure: Pediatric Urine Collection Bag Application, p. 438.) Meconium may also be tested for drugs.
- Treat other complications that occur (respiratory, prematurity, anomalies)
- Administer sedatives for severe irritability. Oral morphine, tincture of opium, methadone, phenobarbital, and benzodiazepines are common.

- Initiate gavage or intravenous feeding as necessary for uncoordinated suck and swallow. See Procedure: Gavage Feeding Administration, p. 430.
- Provide increased calories for excessive activity.
- Refer to social services for placement of the infant after hospitalization, as well as follow-up of the mother or other caretaker.

Nursing Considerations
Assessment
- Suspect maternal substance abuse with:
  — A history of no prenatal care.
  — Unusual behaviors during labor and delivery.
  — Abruptio placentae (may occur after cocaine use).
- Use scoring sheets to follow the number, frequency, and severity of behaviors indicating neonatal abstinence syndrome.

Feeding
- Determine the infant's ability to coordinate sucking and swallowing.
- Prevent distractions by feeding in a quiet area of the nursery.
- Swaddle during feedings to prevent excessive activity.
- Gavage-feed infants with excessive agitation, poor suck and swallow, or rapid respirations.
- Give chin and cheek support to help the infant suck more efficiently.
- Position the infant on the right side with the head of the bed elevated 30 to 45 degrees after feedings.

Rest
- Assess effect of agitation and irritability on rest and sleep patterns.
- Prevent overstimulation by reducing noise, bright lights, and excessive handling. Organize care to prevent disturbances.

- Swaddle the infant in a flexed position to prevent startling and agitation. Use slow, smooth movements during care.
- Provide nonnutritive suckling to help quiet the infant.

   Bonding. The mother may be required to enter a drug rehabilitation program before she can obtain custody of the infant. She will probably obtain custody eventually if she desires, and attachment should be facilitated. Until that time the infant may be placed with alternative caregivers.

- Assess the frequency of maternal visits and evidence of bonding behavior.
- Help the mother feel welcome when she visits. Avoid being judgmental of the mother's past behavior.
- Help the mother participate actively in infant care during her visits.
- Assess the mother's infant care skills and teach where needed.
- Teach the parents about the infant's characteristics.
- Model parenting skills and methods of interacting with the infant.
- Provide positive feedback.
- Teach the parent or caregiver the techniques needed for care of drug-exposed infants.
    — Swaddling the infant in a flexed position to prevent excessive tremors
    — Signs of overstimulation and how to treat
    — Usual methods of interaction by drug-exposed infants (avoiding eye contact, able to tolerate only brief periods of interaction)
    — Teach measures to prevent frantic crying such as gentle handling, soft voices, swaddling with hands brought to midline, pacifier use, avoiding simultaneous visual and auditory stimuli, and rocking with the infant upright.
- Refer to programs for parenting drug-exposed infants.
- Acknowledge feelings of frustration and rejection that caregivers often feel when they are unable to console or feed the infant without difficulty.

NEURAL TUBE DEFECTS

Neural tube defects result from a failure of the vertebral arch to close.

Etiology and Predisposing Factors

- Genetic predisposition
- Associated with folic acid deficiency in the mother near the time of conception

Clinical Signs

- Spina bifida occulta: A dimple on the back where the vertebral arch did not close; often has a tuft of hair over it; usually no other abnormalities. The opening may be palpated.
- Meningocele: Protrusion of meninges and spinal fluid through the spina bifida, covered by skin or thin membrane; no paralysis because the spinal cord is not involved.
- Myelomeningocele: Protrusion of meninges, spinal cord, nerve roots, and spinal fluid covered with membrane through the spina bifida. The degree of paralysis depends on the location of the defect. The infant may also have hydrocephalus before or after surgery.

Therapeutic Management

- Folic acid before conception and during pregnancy
- Surgery for meningocele and myelomeningocele
- Shunt to divert cerebrospinal fluid if hydrocephalus develops
- Antibiotics
- Long-term follow-up with physical therapy
- Fetal surgery may be performed

Nursing Considerations

- Assessments
  — Position and covering of the defect at birth
  — Movement below the level of the defect
  — Relaxation of the anal sphincter or dribbling of stool and urine

- — Integrity of the sac
- — Signs of infection
- — Signs of increasing intracranial pressure. See Hydrocephalus, p. 255.
- Place the infant's torso in a sterile plastic bag or cover the defect with a sterile saline dressing and plastic to prevent drying.
- Handle the infant carefully to prevent trauma to the sac.
- Position on the side or prone.
- Keep the site free of contamination with urine or feces.

OMPHALOCELE AND GASTROSCHISIS
Omphalocele and gastroschisis are abdominal wall defects resulting in protrusion of abdominal contents outside the abdominal cavity.

Etiology and Predisposing Factors. Weakness of the abdominal wall. In omphalocele, the intestines protrude into the base of the umbilical cord. In gastroschisis, there is a defect in the lateral abdominal wall that does not involve the cord. Other anomalies may be present in omphalocele.

Clinical Signs
- Omphalocele: Enlarged cord with intestines visible through it
- Gastroschisis: Intestines outside the abdominal wall without a sac or other covering

Therapeutic Management
- Diagnosis may be made by elevated alpha-fetoprotein and prenatal ultrasound
- Intubation at delivery
- Gastric suction
- Surgery as soon as possible
- A Silastic silo (pouch) may be used to replace the intestines gradually over days

- Parenteral nutrition
- Antibiotics

Nursing Considerations
- Cover the intestines with sterile saline dressings and plastic or place the infant's torso in a sterile plastic bag to prevent drying.
- Prevent infection and trauma.
- Explain to parents.
- Provide postsurgical care.

PERIVENTRICULAR-INTRAVENTRICULAR HEMORRHAGE (PIVH)
Periventricular-intraventricular hemorrhage is bleeding around and into the ventricles of the brain. Severity of effects depends on the degree of hemorrhage.

Etiology and Predisposing Factors
- Rupture of blood vessels in the germinal matrix around the ventricles
- Gestation less than 32 weeks
- Weight less than 1500 g (3 lb, 7 oz)
- Hypoxic injury to the vessels
- Increased blood pressure
- Increased or fluctuating cerebral blood flow

Clinical Signs. Signs vary according to the severity of the hemorrhage.

- Lethargy
- Poor muscle tone
- Deterioration of respiratory status (cyanosis, apnea)
- Decreased hematocrit level
- Decreased reflexes
- Full or bulging fontanel
- Seizures

Therapeutic Management
- Early and repeated ultrasonography to diagnose and determine progression in infants younger than 32 weeks

- Maintenance of respiratory function
- Treatment of complications such as hydrocephalus
- Lumbar taps or a ventriculoperitoneal shunt to drain fluid

Nursing Considerations
- Measure the head circumference daily.
- Assess for changes in neurologic status, which may be subtle.
- Avoid increases in blood pressure from excessive handling or environmental stresses
- Parental teaching for long term follow-up

PERSISTENT FETAL CIRCULATION
See Persistent Pulmonary Hypertension of the Newborn, following.

PERSISTENT PULMONARY HYPERTENSION OF THE NEWBORN (PPHN)
In *persistent pulmonary hypertension of the newborn* (also called *persistent fetal circulation*) the vascular resistance of the lungs remains high after birth. There is vasoconstriction of the pulmonary artery and the ductus arteriosus remains dilated. A right-to-left shunt of blood through the foramen ovale and patent ductus arteriosus occurs.

Etiology and Predisposing Factors
- Hypoxia, asphyxia
- Abnormal lung development
- Maternal use of nonsteroidal antiinflammatory agents or aspirin
- Acidosis
- Meconium aspiration
- Sepsis
- Respiratory distress syndrome
- Polycythemia
- Diaphragmatic hernia
- Unknown causes

Clinical Signs
- Signs develop within 12 hours after birth
- Tachypnea, respiratory distress, and progressive cyanosis
- Decreased oxygen saturation and Pao_2
- Acidosis
- Hypoxia that increases with handling and stimuli

Therapeutic Management. Management involves treating the underlying cause of poor oxygenation.

- Sedation
- High-frequency ventilation or surfactant therapy
- Inhaled nitric oxide
- ECMO therapy

Nursing Considerations. Nursing care is similar to that for other severe respiratory disease.

PHENYLKETONURIA

Phenylketonuria (PKU) is a genetic disorder that causes damage to the central nervous system from toxic levels of phenylalanine in the blood. Early identification can prevent mental retardation.

Etiology and Predisposing Factors
- Deficiency of the liver enzyme phenylalanine hydroxylase, which converts phenylalanine to tyrosine
- Autosomal recessive disorder

Clinical Signs. Signs begin at 3 months if infants do not receive treatment.

- Feeding difficulty
- Vomiting
- Hypertonia
- Irritability
- Eczema
- Musty odor to the urine

- Mental retardation
- Hypopigmentation of the hair, skin, and irises

Therapeutic Management
- Screening of all infants shortly after birth
- Low phenylalanine diet for life

Nursing Considerations
- Ensure that all newborns are screened at the appropriate time.
- Teach parents the importance of screening and care of infants with the condition.

POLYCYTHEMIA
In polycythemia, the hemoglobin is greater than 22 g/dL and the hematocrit is higher than 65% due to an excessive number of erythrocytes. This may cause organ damage from decreased blood flow, pulmonary hypertension, renal vein thrombosis, necrotizing enterocolitis, congestive heart failure, and hyperbilirubinemia.

Etiology and Predisposing Factors
- Conditions in which the fetus produces more erythrocytes than normal due to poor oxygenation
- Intrauterine growth restriction
- Postterm infant
- Large or small infant for gestational age
- Delayed clamping of the umbilical cord
- Transfusion from one twin to another
- Maternal diabetes, preeclampsia, or smoking

Clinical Signs. Signs vary depending on the areas affected by the viscous blood flow.

- Ruddy skin tone
- Respiratory distress
- Hypoglycemia, hypocalcemia
- Lethargy

- Poor feeding
- Tremors

Therapeutic Management
- Monitoring of bilirubin levels
- Partial exchange transfusion to decrease RBCs

Nursing Considerations
- Check hematocrit in infants with ruddy color.
- Adequate hydration to prevent sluggish blood flow and ischemia to vital organs
- Observe for jaundice or other complications.

POSTMATURITY SYNDROME
Postterm infants are born after the 42nd week of gestation. Some postterm infants have postmaturity syndrome because of decreased placental functioning causing hypoxia and malnourishment.

Etiology and Predisposing Factors
- Unknown

Clinical Signs
- During pregnancy and birth
  - Diminished fetal growth
  - Oligohydramnios
  - Meconium passage
- After birth
  - Alert, wide-eyed, worried look
  - Thin, loose skin with little subcutaneous fat
  - Little or no lanugo or vernix caseosa
  - Wrinkled, cracked, peeling skin
  - Thin umbilical cord
  - Polycythemia

Therapeutic Management. Treatment varies according to the problems presented (asphyxia, meconium aspiration). Tests of fetal well-being are performed before labor.

Nursing Considerations
- Check blood glucose soon after birth. Repeat at 1 hour of age and as indicated.
- Feed early and frequently.
- Assess temperature regulation ability and adapt nursing care as needed.
- Observe for other complications.

PRETERM INFANTS

Preterm infants (also called *premature infants*) are born before the beginning of the 38th week of gestation. They may have complications such as respiratory distress syndrome, bronchopulmonary dysplasia, periventricular-intraventricular hemorrhage, retinopathy of prematurity, and necrotizing enterocolitis, which are discussed separately. Care is focused on the following discussed problem areas.

Predisposing/Etiologic Factors. See Preterm Labor, p. 192.

Characteristics. Characteristics depend on gestational age but may include:

- Frail, weak appearance with poor muscle tone.
- Limp, extended extremities.
- Large head in comparison to the body.
- Thin skin with visible blood vessels.
- Abundant vernix caseosa and lanugo.
- Immature genitalia.

Respiratory Problems. The lungs are underdeveloped. Surfactant production may be inadequate and may lead to respiratory distress syndrome.

Clinical Signs
- Tachypnea
- Nasal flaring
- Grunting
- Periodic breathing and apneic spells

- Asymmetry or decreased chest expansion
- Intercostal or xiphoid retractions

Therapeutic Management. Respiratory assistance needed may vary from oxygen in a hood to mechanical ventilation.

Nursing Considerations
- Assess the respiratory status. Use the Silverman-Andersen Index to evaluate the degree of respiratory distress.
- Monitor the infant's blood oxygen levels and adjust oxygen as needed for activity.
- Place the infant in a side-lying or prone position to facilitate oxygenation. Use the supine position when the infant can tolerate it.
- Increase oxygen before and after suctioning and suction gently to avoid trauma.
- Maintain adequate hydration to keep secretions thin.

Thermoregulatory Problems
Clinical Signs
- Axillary temperature less than 36.3° C (97.3° F) or greater than 36.9° C (98.4° F)
- Abdominal skin temperature less than 36° C (96.8° F) or greater than 36.5° C (97.7° F)
- Poor feeding or intolerance to feedings
- Lethargy
- Irritability
- Decreased muscle tone
- Cool skin temperature
- Mottled skin
- Signs of hypoglycemia
- Signs of respiratory difficulty
- Poor weight gain

Therapeutic Management
- Maintain a neutral thermal environment using radiant warmers, incubators, or open cribs as appropriate.
- Place a transparent plastic blanket over the infant to allow heat from the radiant warmer to reach the infant, decrease

insensible water loss, and maintain visibility of the infant's body parts.

- Consider weaning to an open crib when infants reach about 1500 g (3 lb, 7 oz), gain weight consistently for 5 days, and are tolerating feedings.

Nursing Considerations

- Ensure that all heating devices are properly set to prevent over- or underheating.
- Use an open radiant warmer for procedures.
- Warm oxygen before administering.
- Keep portholes and doors of incubators closed as much as possible to prevent heat loss.
- Use heated blankets and a head covering when removing infants from heat sources.
- Consider infection in infants whose temperature remains unstable.
- Be alert for overheating from warming device controls set too high.
- When infants are ready to be weaned to an open crib:
  — Decrease the incubator temperature gradually each day. Raise the temperature if the infant's temperature falls below normal.
  — When ready to transfer to an open crib, double-wrap the infant with warm blankets and assess the temperature frequently.
  — Watch for hypoglycemia or respiratory distress if the temperature falls.

Fluid and Electrolyte Balance Problems. Infants younger than 35 weeks of gestation have immature kidneys and are prone to fluid and electrolyte balance problems. Radiant warmers and phototherapy cause increased fluid losses through the infant's thin skin.

Clinical Signs

- Dehydration
  — Urine output <2 mL/kg/hr
  — Urine specific gravity >1.010

- — Weight loss greater than expected
- — Dry skin and mucous membranes
- — Sunken anterior fontanel
- — Poor tissue turgor
- — Blood: Elevated sodium, protein, and hematocrit levels
- — Hypotension
- Overhydration
  - — Urine output >5 mL/kg/hr
  - — Urine specific gravity <1.002
  - — Edema
  - — Weight gain greater than expected
  - — Bulging fontanels
  - — Blood: Decreased sodium, protein, and hematocrit levels
  - — Moist breath sounds
  - — Difficulty breathing
- Electrolyte imbalances: Signs vary according to specific electrolytes involved.

Therapeutic Management
- Fluid and electrolytes are carefully calculated and prescribed according to gestational age.
- Average fluid need is 80 to 120 mL/kg/day on the first day, 90 to 140 mL/kg/day on the second and third days, and 100 to 175 mL/kg/day by the end of the first week depending on gestational age and weight.

Nursing Considerations
- Measure and record all intake and output: parenteral, feeding tube, oral fluids; output from urine, drainage tubes, and blood specimens taken for laboratory tests.
- Weigh diapers to measure urine output (1 g equals 1 mL of urine). Normal urinary output is 2 to 5 mL/kg/hr.
- Check specific gravity as indicated. Normal range is 1.002 to 1.010.
- Assess weight daily.
- Use infusion control devices to help prevent fluid volume overload.

- Assess IV sites at least every hour for infiltration, infection signs, or position changes.
- Dilute intravenous medications with as little fluid as is consistent with safe administration of the drug.
- Observe for signs of dehydration, overhydration, or specific electrolyte imbalances.

Problems with the Skin. The skin is fragile, permeable, and easily damaged.

Clinical Signs. Any redness, rash, or break in the skin

Therapeutic Management. Treat as necessary.

Nursing Considerations
- Assess the skin frequently for changes.
- Restrict use of adhesives to prevent damage to the skin. Use nontraumatizing tape and adhesives that are easy to remove.
- Avoid the use of chemicals that may be absorbed or damage the skin.
- Bathe infants only as necessary. Consider immersion in water for stable infants.
- Use skin emollients to decrease transepidermal water loss.
- Position infants and equipment to avoid undue pressure on the skin.

Problems with Infection. Many preterm infants have one or more episodes of sepsis during their hospital stay because of their lack of passive immunity from the mother, immature immune response, and exposure to hospital organisms.

Clinical Signs. See Sepsis Neonatorum, Clinical Signs, p. 298.

Therapeutic Management. See Sepsis Neonatorum, p. 292.

Nursing Considerations

- Have parents and staff scrub their hands and arms before handling infants. Teach family members to avoid exposing infants to contagious diseases.
- Assess for signs of infection to treat early.
- Assess response to treatment.

Problems with Pain. Infants in the NICU setting undergo many painful procedures that cause physiologic and behavioral changes.

Clinical Signs

- High-pitched, intense, harsh cry
- Whimpering, moaning
- "Cry face": eyes squeezed shut, mouth open
- Grimacing
- Furrowing or bulging of the brow
- Tense, rigid muscles or flaccid muscle tone
- Rigidity or flailing of extremities
- Color changes: red, dusky, pale
- Heart rate or respiratory changes
- Increased BP
- Decreased oxygen saturation
- Sleep-wake pattern changes

Therapeutic Management. Medication should be provided for the infant during painful procedures and for long-term pain. Dosage should be changed according to the infant's response.

Nursing Considerations

- Prepare infants for potentially painful procedures.
  - Minimize handling before and after procedures to provide rest.
  - Wake infants slowly and gently.
  - Give ordered pain medications before procedures.
  - Use containment—swaddling, positioning devices, or the nurse's hands—to keep the extremities in a

flexed position with the hands near the mouth for sucking.
* Use an assessment tool to measure the infant's pain during procedures and at other times.
* Use comfort measures during and after procedures
  — Nonnutritive sucking
  — Sucrose, when appropriate
  — Soft talking
  — Holding, rocking
  — Ordered pain medication as needed

Environmentally Caused Stress.   Noise, lights, and handling cause stress, increase energy expenditure, and increase complications in preterm infants. Efforts to avoid overstimulation and to provide developmentally appropriate care are essential.

Clinical Signs
* Oxygenation changes
  — Increase or decrease in pulse and respiratory rate
  — Cyanosis, pallor, or mottling
  — Flaring nares
  — Decreased oxygen saturation levels
* Behavior changes
  — Stiff, extended arms and legs
  — Fisting of the hands or splaying of the fingers
  — Alert, worried expression
  — Turning away from eye contact (gaze aversion)
  — Hiccuping
  — Regurgitation
  — Fatigue
  — Coughing
  — Yawning

Nursing Considerations.   The nurse must provide developmentally supportive nursing care.

* Assess the level of environmental stimuli and the infant's response.

- Schedule activities when the infant is awake, when possible.
- Group activities to allow rest between, but watch for signs of stress.
- Avoid routine care that is not essential, such as frequent vital signs or bathing.
- Coordinate activities of different health care workers to prevent overstimulation.
- Keep environmental noise as low as possible.
  — Avoid talking near the incubator.
  — Use incubator covers to reduce noise inside.
  — Set alarm volumes on low; respond quickly when they sound.
  — Open and close doors on incubators and cupboards gently.
  — Do not place objects on top of the incubator.
- Decrease light stimulation to help develop sleep cycles.
  — Position incubators away from bright lights.
  — Place infants so they are not facing lights.
  — Drape a blanket or incubator cover over one end to decrease light.
  — Use a dimmer switch to vary the intensity of lights.
- Schedule "quiet periods" of undisturbed rest when lights and noise in the unit are kept to a minimum.
- Schedule daytime, evening, and night naps.
- Avoid musculoskeletal problems and promote rest by keeping infants in flexed positions using positioning devices.
- Use a side-lying or prone position with flexion and the hands near midline.

Problems with Nutrition. Preterm infants need 105 to 130 kcal/kg/day depending on their gestational age, activity, and illnesses. Their small stomach capacity limits the volume that they can tolerate at each feeding.

Clinical Signs
- Absent or uncoordinated suck, swallow, and gag reflexes
- Low blood glucose levels

- Lack of expected growth
- Excessive gastric residuals

Therapeutic Management
- Administer intravenous or gavage feedings until the infant is ready for oral feedings.
- Calories, amino acids, fatty acids, vitamins, and minerals are calculated according to the infant's gestational age, weight, and tolerance to feedings.
- When the infant is ready for oral feeding special formulas or fortified breast milk are needed to meet the preterm infant's special requirements.

Nursing Considerations
- Administer intravenous and gavage feedings as ordered. See Procedure: Gavage Feeding Administration, p. 430.
- Use nonnutritive sucking during feedings.
- Note signs that the infant is not yet ready for nipple feedings.
  — Respiratory rate >60 breaths/min
  — No rooting, sucking, or gag reflex
  — Excessive gastric residuals
- Note signs of readiness for nipple feedings, especially when infants reach 32 to 34 weeks corrected gestational age.
  — Rooting
  — Sucking on gavage tube, finger, or pacifier
  — Able to tolerate holding
  — Respiratory rate <60 breaths/min
  — Presence of gag reflex
- Assist interested mothers with breastfeeding.
  — Explain the benefits of breastfeeding: helps increase feeding tolerance, reduces infection, enhances neurologic development, helps prevent necrotizing enterocolitis, oxygenation is better.
  — Teach the use of a breast pump and milk storage.
  — Provide privacy as the mother breastfeeds the infant.
  — Demonstrate kangaroo care for very small infants.
  — Demonstrate breastfeeding techniques for small infants.

- Provide a period of rest before and after feedings.
- Use a pacifier just before feedings.
- Begin oral feedings with just a few milliliters once a day and advance slowly. Complete feedings with gavage.
- Position the infant at a 45- to 60-degree angle with the head and neck in a neutral position.
- Place a finger on each cheek and one under the jaw at the base of the tongue to provide support during feeding, if necessary.
- Feed slowly with frequent stops to burp and rest.
- Experiment with different types of nipples to find one that works best.
- Teach mothers signs of fatigue during breast- or bottle feeding.
- Finish feedings by gavage if the infant becomes too fatigued.
- Position on the right side or prone with a 30-degree head elevation after feedings.
- Note and report adverse responses to nipple feedings.
  - Tachycardia or bradycardia
  - Increased respiratory rate
  - Cyanosis, apnea
  - Markedly decreased oxygen saturation level
  - Coughing or gagging
  - Falling asleep early in the feeding
  - Feeding time beyond 20 to 30 minutes
- Observe for signs of intestinal complications.
  - Measure abdominal girth with tape at the level of the umbilicus to check for abdominal distention.
  - Test stools for reducing substance and occult blood.

Parenting. The extended hospitalization of the preterm infant results in separation from parents and may interfere with parenting.

   Clinical Signs. Parental behaviors that may indicate delayed bonding include:

- Using negative terms to describe the infant.
- Discussing the infant in impersonal or technical terms.

- Failing to give the infant a name or to use the name.
- Visiting or calling infrequently or not at all.
- Decreasing the number and length of visits.
- Showing interest in other infants equal to that in their own infant.
- Refusing offers to hold and learn to care for the infant.
- Showing a decrease in or lack of eye contact
- Spending less time talking to or smiling at the infant.

Nursing Considerations
- Allow the parents to see and touch the infant immediately after delivery if possible.
- Allow the father/support person to be present for initial care of the infant, if possible.
- Explain all nursing care, its purpose, and the expected response.
- Use therapeutic communication techniques to support parents.
- Prepare parents for what they will see in the NICU before the first visit (equipment, sounds, how the infant will look).
- Show parents how to touch the infant appropriately to promote development of attachment.
- Offer realistic reassurance about the infant's condition.
- Begin kangaroo care as soon as possible. Place the infant, wearing only a diaper and hat, under the mother's clothes between her breasts. Encourage fathers to participate in kangaroo care, too.
- Explain the infant's socialization abilities based on the gestational age.
- Teach parents signs of overstimulation and signs the infant is ready for more interaction.
- Involve the parents in care as soon as possible.
- Allow parents to participate in decisions about the infant.
- Refer to parent groups for contact with other parents of preterm infants.
- Assess for gradual increase in comfort and participation in care of the infant.

- Help parents prepare for discharge.
  — Give them a copy of the critical pathway, if used.
  — Teach medication administration, special procedures, and other care the infant will need after discharge.
  — Observe the parents perform care until they feel comfortable and are safe.
  — Discuss adaptations necessary in the home for care of the infant.
  — Arrange for home nursing services.

RESPIRATORY DISTRESS SYNDROME (RDS)
Respiratory distress syndrome is most often seen in preterm infants. Immature lungs and lack of adequate surfactant production cause atelectasis and severe respiratory difficulty.

Etiology and Predisposing Factors
- Insufficient surfactant production in the lungs
- Birth asphyxia
- Cesarean birth
- Maternal diabetes

Clinical Signs. Signs begin within hours of birth, peak at 2 to 3 days, and then begin to improve.

- Tachypnea, tachycardia
- Nasal flaring
- Retractions
- Cyanosis
- Grunting on expiration
- Rales, decreased breath sounds
- Acidosis
- Chest radiograph: "ground glass" appearance of the lungs with areas of atelectasis

Therapeutic Management
- Surfactant replacement therapy at birth or when signs occur. Repeat doses if necessary.

- Mechanical ventilation
- Correction of acidosis
- Intravenous feedings
- Other treatment as appropriate

Nursing Considerations
- Observe for signs of developing respiratory distress syndrome at birth and during the early hours after the delivery.
- Observe for changes in the infant's condition and other complications.
- Other nursing care is supportive and depends on the infant's condition.

RETINOPATHY OF PREMATURITY

Retinopathy of prematurity (ROP), or *retrolental fibroplasia* (RLF), may result in visual impairment or blindness in preterm infants.

Etiology and Predisposing Factors
- Exact cause unknown
- Damage to retinal blood vessels and scarring
- Preterm birth, especially low birth weight
- Birth weight less than 1500 g (3 lb, 5 oz)
- Exposure to oxygen

Clinical Signs. Signs can be seen only on ophthalmic examination.

- Constriction of blood vessels of the eye
- Proliferation of new blood vessels in the retina and into the vitreous
- Hemorrhage and scarring
- Retinal detachment

Therapeutic Management
- Screening of LBW infants between 4 and 8 weeks after birth

- Laser surgery, cryotherapy, or reattachment of the retina, if necessary

Nursing Considerations
- Adjust oxygen to the smallest amounts possible to maintain the infant.
- Arrange for ophthalmic examinations.
- Explain the condition and the need for eye exams to parents.

SEPSIS NEONATORUM

Sepsis neonatorum is a systemic infection with bacteria in the bloodstream. Early-onset sepsis usually begins in the first 24 hours after birth and has a more rapid progression than late-onset sepsis. It often causes pneumonia or meningitis. Late-onset sepsis generally develops after the first week of life and usually involves the central nervous system.

Etiology
- Group B streptococci (GBS) and *Escherichia coli* are the most common causes.
- *Staphylococcus epidermidis, Staphylococcus aureus, Haemophilus influenzae, and Listeria monocytogenes*
- Coagulase-negative staphylococci and *Candida albicans* are common causes of nosocomial infections of hospitalized low-birthweight (LBW) infants.
- Vertical infection
  — Transplacental
  — Transmitted from the mother during birth
  — Common vertical infections and their effects on the neonate are listed in Table 3-3.
- Horizontal infection: Contact with infected people or objects

Predisposing Factors
- Prolonged rupture of membranes
- Prolonged labor
- Chorioamnionitis
- Preterm birth

Text continued on p. 298.

Table 3-3	Common Vertical Infections in the Newborn	
Transmission	**Effect on Newborn**	**Nursing Considerations***
Viral Infections		
	Cytomegalovirus	
Transplacental, during birth, in breast milk.	Most infants asymptomatic at birth. LBW, IUGR, enlarged liver and spleen, jaundice, mental retardation, hearing loss, purpura, blindness, and seizures. May have no signs for months or years.	May shed virus in saliva and urine for months or years. No effective drug therapy.
	Hepatitis B	
Usually during birth through contact with maternal blood. Also transplacental and in breast milk.	Asymptomatic at birth. LBW, prematurity. Most become chronic carriers. Risk of later liver cancer.	Wash well to remove all blood before skin is punctured for any reason. After cleaning, administer hepatitis B immune globulin and hepatitis B vaccine to prevent infection.

*Standard precautions for infection control apply to all patients and are not listed above.

Continued

Table 3-3	Common Vertical Infections in the Newborn—cont'd	
Transmission	Effect on Newborn	Nursing Considerations
Viral Infections—cont'd		
	Herpes	
Usually during birth through infected vagina or ascending infection after rupture of membranes. Transplacental rarely. Transmission highest with primary infection.	Clusters of vesicles, temperature instability, lethargy; poor suck, seizures, encephalitis, jaundice, purpura. Death or severe neurologic impairment is high with disseminated infection.	Contact precautions. Obtain lesion specimens for culture. High mortality and morbidity rate if untreated. Antiviral drug therapy improves outcome.
	Human Immunodeficiency Virus and Acquired Immunodeficiency Syndrome	
Transplacental, during birth from infected blood and secretions, or from breast milk. Transmission rate is greatly decreased if mother takes antiretroviral drugs during pregnancy and birth.	Asymptomatic at birth, signs usually apparent at 4 to 12 months. Enlarged liver and spleen, lymphadenopathy, failure to thrive, pneumonia, persistent *Candida* and bacterial infections.	Diagnosis may be delayed because of maternal antibodies. Some early tests available. Wash early and before skin is punctured to remove blood. Treat with antiretroviral drugs and prophylaxis against other infections. Advise against breastfeeding.

Rubella

Transplacental.	Asymptomatic or IUGR, cataracts, cardiac defects, mental retardation. Damage greatest if infected in first trimester.	Contact precautions. Infant may shed virus for months after birth. Diagnosed by presence of antibody. No treatment.

Varicella Zoster Virus (Chickenpox)

Transplacental.	Congenital varicella syndrome (skin scarring, IUGR, limb hypoplasia, CNS involvement), rash, eye damage, death. Damage greatest before the 20th week of gestation.	Immune globulin for pregnant woman exposed in pregnancy or for infants of mothers infected just before or after delivery. Airborne isolation precautions for infants with lesions.

Other Infections

Group B Streptococcal Infection

During birth or ascending after rupture of membranes.	Sudden onset of respiratory distress in infant usually well at birth, pneumonia, shock, meningitis. May have early or late onset.	Early identification essential to prevent death. Treatment of infected mothers during labor has decreased neonatal infection. IV antibiotics given to infected infants.

Continued

CNS, Central nervous system; *IUGR*, intrauterine growth restriction; *IV*, intravenous.

Table 3-3	Common Vertical Infections in the Newborn*—cont'd	
Transmission	**Effect on Newborn**	**Nursing Considerations**
	Gonorrhea	
Usually during birth.	Conjunctivitis (ophthalmia neonatorum), with red, edematous lids and purulent eye drainage. May result in blindness if untreated.	All infants receive prophylactic treatment. Erythromycin eye ointment is most common. Infected infants are treated with antibiotics.
	Chlamydial Infection	
During birth.	Conjunctivitis, pneumonia, otitis media.	Erythromycin or tetracycline eye ointment for prevention of conjunctivitis. Infection treated with erythromycin.
	Candidiasis	
During birth.	White patches in mouth (thrush) that bleed if removed. Rash on perineum. May be systemic.	Administer antifungal drops or cream and teach parents how to administer them. Assess mother for vaginal or breast infection. IV antibiotics for systemic infection.

Toxoplasmosis

Transplacental.	Asymptomatic, or LBW, thrombocytopenia, enlarged liver and spleen, jaundice, anemia, seizures, microcephaly, hydrocephalus, chorioretinitis. Signs may not develop for years.	Consider in infants with IUGR. Confirmed by serum tests. Treatment: spiramycin during pregnancy, pyrimethamine, sulfadiazine, folinic acid, and steroids.

Syphilis

Transplacental.	Asymptomatic or enlarged liver and spleen, jaundice, lymphadenopathy, anemia, rhinitis, pink or copper-colored peeling rash, pneumonitis, osteochondritis, CNS involvement.	Diagnosed by blood and cerebrospinal fluid testing. Administer penicillin as ordered.

CNS, Central nervous system; *IUGR,* intrauterine growth restriction; *LBW,* low birth weight.

Text continued from p. 292.

Clinical Signs. Signs tend to be subtle and may indicate other conditions.

- General signs
  — Temperature instability (low or fever)
  — The nurse's feeling that the infant is not doing well
  — Rash
- Respiratory signs
  — Tachypnea
  — Respiratory distress—nasal flaring, retractions, grunting
  — Apnea
- Cardiovascular signs
  — Color changes—cyanosis, pallor, mottling
  — Tachycardia
  — Hypotension
  — Decreased peripheral perfusion
- Gastrointestinal signs
  — Decreased oral intake
  — Vomiting
  — Excessive gastric residuals
  — Diarrhea
  — Abdominal distention
  — Hypoglycemia or hyperglycemia
- Neurologic signs
  — Decreased or increased muscle tone
  — Lethargy
  — Jitteriness
  — Irritability
  — Bulging fontanel
- Signs that may indicate advanced infection
  — Jaundice
  — Evidence of hemorrhage (petechiae, purpura, pulmonary bleeding)
  — Anemia
  — Enlarged liver and spleen
  — Respiratory failure

— Shock
— Seizures

Therapeutic Management
- Cultures of the blood, urine, skin lesions, cerebrospinal fluid
- Blood analysis: decreased neutrophils, increased bands (immature neutrophils), and decreased platelets. Elevated IgM levels in cord blood or shortly after birth indicates in utero infection.
- C-reactive protein
- Chest radiograph
- Intravenous antibiotics, usually for 10 to 14 or more days
- Other supportive care as needed

Nursing Considerations
- Identify infants at risk.
- Emphasize handwashing to prevent infections.
- Prevent spread of infection to other infants by scrupulous use of medical asepsis.
- Ensure that medications are administered on time.
- Plan with the laboratory for analysis of antibiotic peak and trough levels.
- Maintain fluid balance and hourly urine output
- Monitor vital signs
- Observe for complications such as shock, hypoglycemia, hyperglycemia, electrolyte imbalances, and problems in temperature regulation.
- Gavage feed if necessary.
- Support parents, who may be shocked at the sudden illness of their infant.

SMALL-FOR-GESTATIONAL-AGE (SGA) INFANTS
Small-for-gestational-age infants are below the 10th percentile in size because of intrauterine growth restriction (IUGR). Infants may be preterm, full-term, or postterm.

Etiology and Predisposing Factors
- Congenital malformations
- Chromosomal anomalies

- Fetal infections
- Poor placental function
- Maternal preeclampsia, severe diabetes
- Maternal substance abuse

Clinical Signs

- Symmetric growth restriction: Entire body is proportionately small.
- Asymmetric growth restriction
  - Normal size head that appears large
  - Normal length
  - Abdominal circumference decreased
  - Weight below that expected for gestational age
  - Long, thin appearance
  - Loose skin with longitudinal thigh creases
  - Sparse hair
  - Thin cord
  - Dry skin

Therapeutic Management

- Prevention by good prenatal care
- Treatment as problems occur
- Treat complications such as asphyxia, meconium aspiration, hypoglycemia, polycythemia

Nursing Considerations

- Assess for hypoglycemia.
- Feed frequently to provide extra calories.
- Assess temperature regulation.
- Assess for complications.
- Other care depends on complications.

SPINA BIFIDA OCCULTA

See Neural Tube Defects, p. 272.

TRACHEOESOPHAGEAL FISTULA (TEF)

See Esophageal Atresia and Tracheoesophageal Fistula, p. 254.

TRANSIENT TACHYPNEA OF THE NEWBORN (TTN)

Transient tachypnea of the newborn, also called *retained lung fluid* and *respiratory distress syndrome, type II,* is a condition of rapid respirations with decreased lung compliance and air trapping in full or preterm infants. The condition usually resolves in 1 to 5 days.

Etiology
- Exact cause unknown
- May be due to a delay in absorption of fetal lung fluid
- May be mild immaturity of surfactant production

Predisposing Factors
- Cesarean birth without labor
- Asphyxia
- Precipitous or breach delivery
- Macrosomia
- Maternal analgesia
- Bleeding
- Diabetes

Clinical Signs
- Respirations as high as 120/min
- Grunting
- Retractions
- Nasal flaring
- Mild cyanosis
- Chest radiograph: Hyperinflation and presence of fluid along bronchovascular spaces, in the fissures between the lobes, and in the pleural space

Therapeutic Management
- Treatment is supportive.
- Administer sufficient oxygen to prevent cyanosis.
- Feed intravenously or by gavage, while the respiratory rate is high to prevent aspiration and conserve energy.

- Observation for RDS and sepsis because the signs are similar.
- Administer ordered antibiotics until sepsis is ruled out.

Nursing Considerations
- Identify signs and report to the provider
- Carry out treatment as ordered

COMMON NURSING DIAGNOSES FOR NEWBORN COMPLICATIONS

- Activity Intolerance related to weakness, fatigue, and possible overstimulation
- Disturbed Sleep Pattern related to agitation from own activity and irritability
- Impaired Parenting related to lack of understanding of the infant's characteristics and how to relate to the infant
- Ineffective Infant Feeding Pattern related to muscle weakness and fatigue during feedings
- Risk for Disorganized Infant Behavior related to stress from an overstimulating environment
- Risk for Imbalanced Fluid Volume related to inadequate oral intake to meet needs of increased insensible water loss and frequent loose stools
- Risk for Imbalanced Nutrition: Less Than Body Requirements related to uncoordinated suck and swallow and fatigue during feedings
- Risk for Impaired Parent-Infant Attachment related to separation of parents from infant and lack of understanding about the infant's condition and characteristics

Section 4

Postpartum

POSTPARTUM ADAPTATIONS
REPRODUCTIVE SYSTEM

Uterus. Involution begins when muscle fibers contract around maternal blood vessels at the site left denuded by placental separation.

- The fundus is palpable in the midline of the abdomen and at about the level of the umbilicus shortly after childbirth.
- The uterus becomes smaller, and the fundus descends about 1 cm (one fingerbreadth) a day.
- The uterus is in the pelvic cavity and no longer palpable above the symphysis pubis by approximately 10 days after birth (Figure 4-1).

Afterpains
- Multiparas have more severe afterpains because of intermittent contraction of uterine muscles that have been stretched repeatedly.
- Afterpains may also be strong during breastfeeding when oxytocin, which causes the milk-ejection reflex, brings about strong contraction of uterine muscles.

Lochia. Lochia decreases in amount and changes color over time.

- Lochia rubra is dark red and lasts 3 days.
- Lochia serosa, a serosanguineous discharge that is pink or brown, lasts from about days 4 to 10.
- Lochia alba, the final discharge, is white, cream, or light yellow and generally lasts until the third week after childbirth. It may persist until 6 weeks for some women.

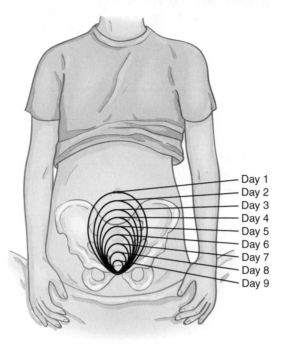

Figure 4-1 Involution of the uterus. Height of the uterine fundus decreases by approximately 1 cm per day.

- The odor of lochia is "musty," "earthy," or "fleshy." A foul odor suggests infection.
- Bright red lochia in the presence of a firm fundus suggests a laceration.
- The amount of lochia may be described as:
  — Scant: Less than a 2.5-cm (1-inch) stain on the peripad
  — Light: 2.5- to 10-cm (1- to 4-inch) stain
  — Moderate: 10- to 15-cm (4- to 6-inch) stain
  — Heavy: Saturated peripad in 1 hour
  — Excessive: Saturated peripad in 15 minutes

Perineum. Some edema and bruising of the perineum can be expected following childbirth. An episiotomy may be performed to provide additional room at the introitus.

Lacerations may also occur and require suturing. Lacerations and episiotomies are classified according to the amount of tissue involved.

- *First degree* involves superficial vaginal mucosa or perineal skin.
- *Second degree* involves deeper tissue and may include perineal muscles.
- *Third degree* extends into the rectal sphincter.
- *Fourth degree* extends through the sphincter and into the rectal mucosa.

CARDIOVASCULAR SYSTEM
Blood Volume. On the average, up to 500 mL of blood is lost during vaginal births and up to 1000 mL in cesarean births. The woman can tolerate this loss without ill effects because:

- Increases in vascular volume occur during pregnancy.
- Blood from the uteroplacental unit returns to central circulation when the placenta is expelled.

Blood Values
- The increase in clotting factors puts the new mother at risk for thrombus formation.
- White blood cell count increases to as high as 30,000/mm^3 with an average increase to 14,000 to 16,000/mm^3. Neutrophils, which rise in response to inflammation, pain, and stress, account for most of the increase. Leukocyte count returns to normal values by 4 to 7 days after birth.
- Hemoglobin and hematocrit are difficult to interpret because of remobilization and excretion of excess body fluid.

VITAL SIGNS
Blood Pressure. Blood pressure should remain near prepregnancy levels. It should be measured with the

mother in the same position and using the same arm each time.

- Orthostatic hypotension occurs due to a rapid reduction in intra-abdominal pressure after childbirth that results in dilation of visceral blood vessels.
- Engorgement of abdominal blood vessels causes a blood pressure fall of 15 to 20 mm Hg when the woman moves from a recumbent to an upright position.
- The woman may feel dizzy or lightheaded on standing, and may faint
- Hypotension may also indicate excessive blood loss.

Pulse and Respirations
- Pulse and respirations should remain within normal limits.
- Bradycardia may occur as a result of increased vascular volume from an increase in cardiac return and a consequent rise in stroke volume.
- Tachycardia may be the first indication of hypovolemia. It may also indicate excitement, pain, fatigue, infection, dehydration, or anemia.

Temperature
- Temperature of up to 38° C (100.4° F) is common the first 24 hours following childbirth and may be caused by dehydration or the normal stress response.
- Infection should be suspected if the elevation persists for longer than 24 hours or if it exceeds 38° C.

BREASTS
Following childbirth, levels of estrogen and progesterone decline. This decrease allows prolactin, which stimulates milk production, to rise. Although colostrum is present from the second trimester of pregnancy, milk is generally not produced until 2 to 3 days following childbirth. A second hormone, oxytocin, stimulates the milk-ejection (let-down) reflex.

CHANGES IN ELIMINATION
Bladder and Kidneys
- Decreased sensitivity to fluid pressure in the bladder due to loss of muscle tone, plus trauma to the urethra, bladder, and urinary meatus that often occurs during childbirth, interfere with emptying the bladder.
- The bladder fills quickly because of diuresis.
- The woman may be completely unaware of a distended bladder.
- A distended bladder lifts and displaces the uterus and is one of the major causes of excessive bleeding.
- Signs of a distended bladder
  — Fundus is located above baseline level (i.e., when the bladder is empty)
  — Fundus displaced from midline
  — Excessive lochia
  — Bladder discomfort
  — Bulge of bladder above symphysis pubis
  — Frequent voidings of less than 150 mL of urine (indicating urinary retention with overflow)
- Acetone in the urine in the early postpartum period suggests dehydration that may occur during labor.
- Mild proteinuria is usually the result of catabolic processes of involution.

Bowel. Constipation and painful defecation may occur in the postpartal period because:

- Bowel tone remains sluggish for several days as a result of progesterone.
- Food and fluid intake are restricted during labor.
- Pain from perineal trauma, episiotomies, and hemorrhoids interferes with effective bowel elimination.

MUSCLES, JOINTS, SKIN, AND HAIR
- Exertion in labor may result in muscle fatigue and aches, particularly of the shoulders, neck, and arms.

- Relaxin levels gradually subside and ligaments and cartilage of the pelvis return to their prepregnancy position, causing temporary hip or joint pain.
- Skin changes, such as the "mask of pregnancy," spider nevi, and palmar erythema, disappear when the hormones of pregnancy decline following childbirth.
- Striae gravidarum (stretch marks) fade to silvery lines but do not disappear altogether.
- Increased hair loss which peaks at 3 to 4 months after birth occurs because less hair was lost during pregnancy. Regrowth generally occurs by 9 months after childbirth.

PSYCHOSOCIAL ADAPTATIONS
BONDING AND ATTACHMENT

- Bonding is the initial attraction felt by the parents and the development of an emotional tie to the infant.
- Attachment is a process that forms an enduring bond between a parent and a child over time. It is facilitated by:
  — Positive feedback, such as mutual gazing of parents and infant, the ability to console the infant, and the infant's response to parental touch and voice.
  — Close and prolonged contact between parents and infant.

RECIPROCAL ATTACHMENT BEHAVIORS

Infants actively participate in communication through signals or cues called reciprocal attachment behaviors. Infant cues can be verbal or nonverbal. Verbal cues include crying and cooing. Nonverbal cues include:

- Making eye contact and engaging in prolonged mutual gazing.
- Moving the eyes and attempting to "track" the parent's face.
- Grasping and holding the parent's fingers.
- Moving in rhythm to the parent's pattern of speech (entrainment).

- Rooting, latching on to the nipple, and suckling.
- Being comforted by the parent's voice or touch.

MATERNAL TOUCH AND VERBAL INTERACTION

Maternal touch progresses from "fingertipping" as the mother becomes acquainted with her child to enfolding as she becomes more comfortable with the infant. Verbal behaviors also indicate maternal attachment. Most mothers:

- Speak to the infant in a high-pitched voice.
- Progress from calling the baby "it" to "he" or "she" and then to using the given name. This may occur before birth if the mother has seen her infant on an ultrasound.
- Paternal behaviors parallel those of the mother during the initial contact with the infant.

PUERPERAL PHASES

Following childbirth, the mother passes through three phases as she replenishes her energy and gains confidence in her role as mother.

- *Taking-in* occurs during the first hours after childbirth and is characterized by passive, dependent behavior. The mother is often focused on her own care rather than the infant. She "takes in" attention and physical care. Her primary needs are for fluid, food, and sleep. She integrates the childbirth experience into reality by talking about it to others.
- *Taking-hold* occurs as the mother becomes more independent and assumes care of herself. She gradually shifts her attention from her needs to those of the infant. She is concerned about her mothering skills and is interested in teaching about care of herself and the infant.
- *Letting-go* is a time of relinquishment as the mother gives up idealized expectations of the birth experience and the infant of her fantasies. She is then able to accept this infant, who may be very different from the infant she dreamed of during pregnancy. She must also give up her lifestyle as a childless woman if this is the first baby.

ROLE ATTAINMENT

Role attainment is the process by which the mother becomes comfortable with the mother role. There are four stages.

- Anticipatory Stage: Begins during pregnancy as the woman prepares for birth by choosing a health care provider and seeks out role models to help her learn the role of parent.
- Formal Stage: Begins after birth and lasts 4 to 6 weeks. Becomes acquainted with the infant but relies on others for guidance.
- Informal Stage: Has learned the infant's cues and responds to meet them, developing the maternal role to fit herself.
- Personal Stage: Occurs when the parental role is internalized and the mother feels comfortable in the role.

FACTORS THAT AFFECT ADAPTATION

Factors that can interfere with family adaptation to the birth of an infant include:

- Lingering fatigue or discomfort (perineal, incisional, etc.).
- Lack of knowledge of infant needs.
- Previous experience with infants.
- Expectations of the newborn.
- Maternal age (adolescents usually require more assistance).
- Maternal temperament (calm, secure mother has an easier time).
- Temperament of the infant (easily consoled, enjoys cuddling versus irritable, difficult to console).
- Availability of strong support system.
- Other events (cesarean birth, preterm or ill infant, birth of multiple infants)

NURSING ASSESSMENTS

Because of the risk of postpartal hemorrhage, frequent and thorough physical assessments are a priority during the first hours following childbirth. When physical safety of the mother is ensured, psychosocial assessments become equally important. See Table 4-1, Postpartum Nursing Assessment.

Text continued on p. 317

Postpartum Nursing Assessment	

Table 4-1

Assessment	Expected Findings	Nursing Actions
	Physiologic Adaptation	
	Uterus	
Assess the uterine fundus. See Procedure: Uterine Fundus Assessment, p. 443.	The fundus should be firm, midline, and located midway between the symphysis pubis and the umbilicus immediately after the placenta is expelled. It then rises to the level of the umbilicus. It should remain firm and begin to decrease in size by the second postpartal day.	Help the woman empty her bladder so the uterus can contract firmly. Begin at the umbilicus and palpate gently until the fundus is located. If the fundus is boggy, massage until firm and express clots. Reassess to be sure the uterus remains contracted when massage is stopped.
	Lochia	
Evaluate lochia for amount, character, and odor. Note how often pads are saturated and observe the perineum for a constant trickle or dribble that indicates excessive flow.	The amount should be moderate. Women who had cesarean births will have less lochia. A few small clots are normal during the first day or two. Odor should not be foul.	If excessive flow is suspected, weigh all pads and bedliners to accurately estimate blood loss (1 g = 1 mL).

Continued

Table 4-1	Postpartum Nursing Assessment—cont'd	
Assessment	**Expected Findings**	**Nursing Actions**
Note: Blood can pool under the woman's hips. Ask her to turn so linen and bedliners can be seen. Excessive flow in the presence of a contracted fundus suggests a laceration of the cervix or vagina.		
	Perineum	
Observe the perineum and episiotomy; see Procedure: Perineal Assessment, p. 439.	Slight edema or bruising is normal. There should be no redness or drainage. Edges of the episiotomy should be approximated.	Notify the primary caregiver if there are signs of infection, excessive pain, or bulging of tissue that indicates formation of a hematoma.
	Vital Signs	
	Blood Pressure (BP)	
Measure the BP in the same arm with the mother in the	BP should remain near the prepregnancy level. Elevation	Review the chart to determine prepregnancy BP. Help the mother

same position each time to avoid inaccurate data. Be consistent in use of Korotkoff's 4th or 5th sound to determine diastolic pressure.	suggests preeclampsia. Decline may indicate excessive bleeding.	ambulate for the first few times to prevent injury from orthostatic hypotension.

Pulse

Count the radial or apical pulse with the mother at rest.	A pulse rate of 50-90 is normal. Bradycardia is not unusual.	Tachycardia, which may result from hypovolemia, excitement, pain, fatigue, infection, anemia, or dehydration, requires additional assessments.

Respirations

Count with the mother at rest.	Normally 12-20 per minute.	If decreased, assess for effects of medication; if increased, check for other signs of respiratory difficulty or for source of anxiety.

Temperature

	Up to 38° C (100.4° F) is considered normal for the first 24 hours if there are no other signs of infection.	Report a higher elevation or one that persists for longer than 24 hours.

Continued

Table 4-1	Postpartum Nursing Assessment—cont'd	
Assessment	**Expected Findings**	**Nursing Actions**
Pain		
Assess pain type, location, and severity along with vital signs.	Pain may occur from an episiotomy or lacerations, afterpains, or nipple tenderness.	Encourage the woman to take prescribed pain medications. Assess effectiveness of medications.
Breasts		
Palpate the breasts and inspect the skin and areolae. Observe the nipples for tenderness, redness, fissures, bruises, or blisters. Observe breastfeeding techniques.	The breasts should be soft (initially), somewhat firm (filling), or firm (full of milk). Protruding nipples facilitate breastfeeding.	Women with flat or inverted nipples or signs of nipple trauma need special assistance with breastfeeding. Fissures may allow microorganisms to enter and cause infection.
Elimination		
Bladder		
Observe and measure the first voidings. Palpate the fundus and note the amount of	The first voiding should be more than 150 mL. The fundus should be firm, near the level of the umbilicus, and	Review signs of a distended bladder (p. 307). Assist the mother to void; catheterize her if necessary.

lochia. Observe for a palpable bulge above the symphysis pubis.	midline. Lochia should be no more than moderate.	

Bowel

Ask about the usual pattern of bowel elimination and determine when she had the last bowel movement. Observe the number and size of hemorrhoids.	The first stool should occur by 2 to 3 days postpartum.	Infrequent, hard stools or painful defecation may require administration of stool softeners. Teach measures to reduce the pain of hemorrhoids and to prevent constipation.

Lower Extremities

Inspect the legs for areas of redness, heat, or tenderness. Palpate pedal pulses.	The legs should be free of reddened areas, heat, or tenderness. Pedal pulses should be equal bilaterally.	Help the mother ambulate as soon as possible. Apply antiembolism stockings as indicated. Report any abnormal signs.

Laboratory Values

Check hemoglobin, hematocrit, RBC, WBC, blood type, Rh factor, rubella titer, hepatitis B status, syphilis screen, and group B streptococcus status.	A hematocrit decrease of 10% or more is considered hemorrhage. WBC may be elevated.	Administer RhoGAM to unsensitized Rh-negative mother with Rh-positive infant. Administer rubella vaccine to mother who is not immune (titer <1:8).

Continued

Table 4-1	Postpartum Nursing Assessment—cont'd	
Assessment	**Expected Findings**	**Nursing Actions**
	Psychologic Adaptation	
	Puerperal Phases	
Taking-in	Passive, depends on nurses for assistance; recounts birth experience over and over; does not initiate care of the infant.	This is a time to "mother the mother." Provide nourishment and time for rest.
Taking-hold	More autonomous, assumes self-care; seeks information about infant care.	Foster independence; promote attachment by involving mother in infant care.
Letting-go	Relinquishes the role of childless person; gives up the "fantasy baby" of pregnancy and accepts her own infant.	Provide anticipatory guidance for this phase, which may occur after discharge from birth facility.
	Interaction with Infant	
Maternal touch	Fingertipping, palming, enfolding, consoling behaviors, holding in "en face" position.	Provide ample opportunity for contact with the infant.
Verbal interaction	Speaks in high voice; uses given name; coos to attract and hold attention of the infant.	Model how to make eye contact and interact with the infant.
Response to infant cues	Prompt, gentle, consistent response.	Point out infant signals and model appropriate responses.

Text continued from p. 310.

RISK ASSESSMENT

Two of the most common complications of the puerperium are hemorrhage and infection. Nurses must be aware of factors that increase the risk of these complications so they can expand their vigilance to protect the mother.

Risk Factors for Hemorrhage

- Grand multiparity (5 or more)
- Overdistention of the uterus
- Precipitous labor (<3 hours)
- Prolonged labor
- Retained placenta
- Placenta previa or abruptio placentae
- Induction or augmentation of labor
- Administration of tocolytics to stop uterine contractions
- Operative procedures (vacuum extraction, forceps, cesarean birth)

Risk Factors for Infection

- Operative procedures
- Multiple cervical examinations
- Prolonged labor (>24 hours)
- Prolonged rupture of membranes
- Manual extraction of the placenta
- Diabetes
- Catheterization
- Anemia

COMMON NURSING DIAGNOSES

- Acute Pain related to uterine contractions (afterpains), perineal trauma, breast engorgement, or hemorrhoids
- Impaired Skin Integrity (nipple) related to incorrect positioning during breastfeeding
- Impaired Urinary Elimination related to temporary loss of sensation and decreased muscle tone of the bladder
- Constipation related to knowledge deficit of measures to promote bowel elimination

- Risk for Ineffective Health Maintenance related to knowledge deficit of self-care or signs of complication
- Risk for Infection related to impaired tissue integrity and tissue trauma from childbirth
- Health-Seeking Behaviors regarding self-care, newborn care, health maintenance, prevention of complications
- Risk for Impaired Parenting related to fatigue, discomfort, lack of knowledge of infant care
- Risk for Interrupted Family Processes related to lack of knowledge of infant needs and behaviors
- Sleep Deprivation related to anxiety, postpartum discomfort, and infant needs
- Risk for Injury related to vertigo secondary to orthostatic hypotension
- Imbalanced Nutrition: More (or Less) Than Body Requirements related to lack of understanding of nutritional needs of the postpartum period

NURSING INTERVENTIONS
Nursing interventions focus on preventing hemorrhage or injury, promoting comfort, and providing health education.

PREVENTING HEMORRHAGE
Initial Assessments
- Every 15 minutes for the first hour following childbirth:
  — Palpate the fundus for uterine tone and position.
  — Assess the amount and color of lochia.
  — Determine vital signs.
- Repeat assessments every 30 minutes for the next hour (more frequently if condition warrants).
- Continue assessments every 4 hours for 24 hours (or according to facility protocol).
- Assess every 8 hours after 24 hours

Massaging the Uterus. If the uterus is soft or boggy, massage the uterus to stimulate uterine contraction and restore firm tone.

- Place the nondominant hand above the symphysis pubis to anchor and support the lower segment of the uterus.

- Compress and massage the fundus with the dominant hand.
- Attempt to express clots only when the uterus is firm (pushing against a boggy uterus could cause uterine inversion).
- Stop massage when the uterus becomes firm.
- Reevaluate the fundus frequently to be sure it remains firm.

Administering Oxytocin. If massage fails to restore uterine tone, expect to administer intravenous (IV) oxytocin preparation, methylergonovine maleate, or prostaglandin to control bleeding. See p. 331 for further information about management of postpartum hemorrhage.

Ensuring Bladder Elimination. Several measures help the perineal muscles relax and stimulate the sensation of needing to void.

- Assist the woman to the bathroom as soon as she can ambulate. Allow plenty of time and provide privacy.
- Medicate the woman to promote relaxation.
- Run water in the sink or shower.
- Place the mother's hands in water.
- Pour warm water over the mother's vulva.
- Encourage urination in the shower or sitz bath.
- Provide hot tea or fluids of choice.
- Ask the mother to blow bubbles through a straw.
- Catheterize if there are signs of bladder distention and she is unable to void.

PREVENTING INJURY
Women may be dizzy or lightheaded because of medication, blood loss, fatigue, or orthostatic hypotension. To prevent falls that can result in injury, nurses should:

- Advise the mother to call for assistance before getting out of bed for the first time.
- Keep the bed in a locked position with the side rails up until she is fully recovered from anesthesia or analgesia.

- Elevate the head of the bed for a few minutes before the mother attempts to stand.
- Help her sit on the side of the bed, and then to stand slowly to allow blood pressure to stabilize before she is fully upright.
- Instruct her to move her feet constantly when she first stands to increase venous return from the lower extremities.
- Remain accessible and provide emergency signals during showers or sitz baths, when heat may add to the problem.
- Lower her to a sitting or lying position if she becomes lightheaded. This increases blood flow to the brain and prevents fainting. Call for added help.

PROMOTING COMFORT
Perineal Trauma and Hemorrhoids
- Use a plastic bag or glove filled with ice or a chemical cold pack for the first 12 hours following childbirth.
  - Wrap ice pack in paper before applying to the perineum.
  - Leave in place until the ice melts; then remove it for 10 minutes before applying another pack.
- Teach the mother to use topical medications to decrease perineal discomfort. Instruct her to hold the nozzle of anesthetic spray 6 to 12 inches from her body and direct it toward the perineum.
- Advise the mother to squeeze her buttocks together before sitting and to lower her weight slowly to lessen pain in the perineal area.
- Apply soothing witch-hazel compresses or an anesthetic cream to hemorrhoids or insert antihemorrhoidal suppositories for relief of discomfort.
- Begin sitz baths according to facility protocol. Cool water reduces pain caused by edema; warm water increases circulation and promotes healing.
- Encourage the woman to take prescribed analgesics as needed.

Afterpains
- Suggest that the woman lie in a prone position with a small pillow under the abdomen. This constant pressure

causes the uterus to remain contracted and relieves pain of intermittent contractions.
- Instruct her that analgesics take one-half hour or more to reach the milk so medicating just before breastfeeding is helpful. Reassure the woman that the medication will not harm the infant.

PROVIDING HEALTH EDUCATION
Process of Involution
- Teach the mother how to locate and palpate the fundus and how to estimate the amount of lochia.
- Demonstrate the expected rate of uterine descent.
- Instruct in expected color, quantity, and duration of lochia.

Handwashing. Emphasize the importance of thorough handwashing before touching the breasts, after diaper changes, after bladder or bowel elimination, and always before handling the infant.

Breast Care. This discussion is for nonlactating mothers. See pp. 247-249 for breast care for lactating mothers.

- Explain that the woman must avoid breast stimulation to suppress lactation. For instance, when showering, she should protect her breasts from the cascade of warm water and should not pump or massage the breasts.
- Remind her to wear a snug support bra or breast binder to reduce circulation and filling of the breasts.
- Recommend that she apply ice to reduce discomfort if her breasts become engorged.

Perineal Care. Teach a method for perineal cleansing as soon as possible.

- Fill a squeeze bottle with warm water and spray over the perineum from front to back.
- Avoid separating the labia so water does not enter the vagina.

- Pat dry with toilet paper or a moist antiseptic towelette.
- Dry from front to back to prevent contamination from the anal area toward the vaginal introitus.
- Cleanse the perineum after each voiding or defecation, and change the perineal pads at the same time.
- Wash the hands thoroughly before and after elimination and changing peripads.

Kegel Exercise
- Teach the mother to contract muscles around the vagina (as though stopping the flow of urine) for 10 seconds, then relax the muscles for 10 seconds.
- Encourage the mother to work up to 30 contraction-relaxation cycles each day.

Bowel Elimination
- Emphasize the importance of adequate fluid, dietary fiber, and progressive exercise.
- Encourage the mother to establish a regular pattern of bowel elimination.
- Teach measures to reduce perineal or hemorrhoidal pain (sitz baths, witch-hazel compresses, or appropriate ointments).
- Advise her to act on any urge to defecate and to take adequate time.
- Reassure her that she will not damage the repaired episiotomy wound by bearing down gently.
- The physician may order a stool softener to make elimination easier.

Body Mechanics
- Encourage the mother and father to find a location for infant care that does not require bending.
- Suggest mild exercises, such as abdominal breathing, head lifts, and knee rolls to improve muscle tone. She may begin these exercises within a few days of childbirth.
- Advise her to reduce or stop exercising if lochial flow increases or if she becomes uncomfortable or fatigued.

Sexual Activity

- Suggest that she avoid sexual intercourse until the perineum is healed, usually about 3 weeks, or consult her health care provider.
- Advise her that intercourse should be gentle because the vaginal and perineal areas may remain tender.
- Recommend that she use a lubricant if vaginal dryness is a problem.
- Caution her that she can become pregnant during the puerperium, whether or not she is breastfeeding.
- Identify the need for family planning (see p. 346).

Return of Menstruation

- Nonlactating women resume menses within 7 to 9 weeks after giving birth, on average.
- Lactating women resume menses as early as 12 weeks or as late as 18 months postpartum.
- The first cycles for lactating and nonlactating women are often anovulatory, but ovulation may occur before the first menses.
- Ovulation and menses become more likely by 6 months in breastfeeding women, and contraception should be used by that time.

Nutrition

- Recommend the breastfeeding woman consume:
  - 330 calories per day above her normal needs during the first 6 months of lactation.
  - 400 calories per day above her normal needs during the second 6 months of lactation.
  - The same amount of protein as required for pregnancy.
- Explain that breastfeeding mothers can eat any food unless they are allergic to it. A food eaten in the previous 8 to 12 hours may cause fussiness in some infants. The mother can eliminate the food for a few days and then try it again to determine if it was the cause.
- The nonlactating woman should resume her prepregnancy diet if it met her Recommended Dietary Allowances.

It should contain enough protein and vitamin C to promote healing.

- All postpartum women should have a diet high in fresh fruits and vegetables to meet their needs for vitamins and minerals.
- The woman can continue her vitamin-mineral supplement from pregnancy until the supply is finished.

Weight Loss
- The woman will lose approximately 4.5 to 5.5 kg (10-12 lb) during childbirth.
- She will lose another 2.3 to 3.6 kg (5-8 lb) during the early postpartum period.
- If pregnancy weight gain was not excessive, most women are near their pre-pregnancy weight by 6 to 12 months after childbirth.

Signs and Symptoms That Should Be Reported. New mothers and at least one member of the family should know the signs and symptoms that should be reported to the health care provider as soon as possible.

- Fever
- Localized area of redness, swelling, or pain in either breast that is not relieved by support or analgesics
- Persistent abdominal tenderness
- Feelings of pelvic fullness or pelvic pressure
- Persistent perineal pain
- Frequency, urgency, or burning on urination
- Abnormal changes in character of lochia (increased amount, resumption of bright red color, passage of clots, foul odor)
- Localized tenderness, redness, or warmth of the legs
- Swelling, redness, drainage from, or separation of an incision

Promoting Bonding and Attachment
- Provide early, unlimited contact between the parents and newborn.

- Position the infant so that eye contact with the parent is possible.
- Point out reciprocal attachment behaviors of the infant.
- Help breastfeeding mothers put the infant to breast.
- Model appropriate behaviors (holding close, using high-pitched, soothing tones).
- Point out infant characteristics in a positive way.
- Provide comfort and ample time for rest so the mother can replenish her energy and be free of discomfort as she assumes care of the newborn.

NURSING CARE FOLLOWING CESAREAN BIRTH
NURSING ASSESSMENT
Assessments must be modified and expanded when the mother has a cesarean birth. See Table 4-2, Nursing Assessments Following Cesarean Birth, on p. 326.

MOST COMMON NURSING DIAGNOSES
- Acute Pain related to surgical incision or abdominal distention
- Activity Intolerance related to incisional pain, effects of anesthesia
- Ineffective Airway Clearance related to immobility and depressed respirations
- Risk for Impaired Parenting related to discomfort, difficulty in moving or positioning infant

NURSING INTERVENTIONS
Providing Comfort. PCA and epidural analgesia are two methods used for pain relief. Respiratory depression may occur if opioids are used for analgesia. Some women experience nausea or itching, which may be relieved by antiemetics or antihistamines.

Overcoming Effects of Immobility
- Splint the abdomen with a small pillow to reduce discomfort.

Text continued on p. 328

Table 4-2	Nursing Assessments Following Cesarean Birth	
Physiologic Changes: Expected Findings	**How to Assess Expected Findings**	**Abnormal Findings: Nursing Actions**
	Respiratory Effort	
Epidural narcotics, which can cause respiratory depression, may be used for pain relief. Immobility and decreased respirations may result in pooling of bronchial secretions.	If a pulse oximeter or apnea monitor is not used, evaluate respiratory rate and depth every 30 minutes for 3-6 hours and every 30-60 minutes until 24 hours postoperatively. Auscultate breath sounds.	Respiratory rate <12 per minute. Diminished depth or adventitious breath sounds. Notify anesthesiologist; elevate head of bed, administer oxygen and follow protocol regarding administration of a narcotic antagonist.
	Pain Relief	
Pain relief should be sufficient to allow comfort and prevent immobility.	Determine pain level frequently. If patient-controlled analgesia (PCA) is used, assess frequency of use and effectiveness. Observe side effects of all analgesia.	Offer pain relief as needed. Report adverse effects. Give oxygen and prescribed narcotic antagonists if necessary.

Surgical Incision

A transverse incision in the lower uterine segment is most common.

Use the acronym REEDA (redness, ecchymosis, edema, drainage, approximation) to assess the surgical wound.

Report any signs of infection.

Abdomen

Decreased peristalsis occurs as a result of operative procedures.

Auscultate for bowel sounds. Palpate the fundus gently to decrease discomfort. The abdomen should be soft, bowel sounds present, flatus passed with in 1-2 days.

Abdominal distention, no bowel sounds (listen in all four quadrants), unable to pass flatus. Increase ambulation, report.

Intake and Output

IV fluids are usually given, and an indwelling urinary catheter is left in place for the first 24 hours.

Monitor the rate of IV flow and condition of the IV site. Evaluate the amount, color, and clarity of urine.

Adjust IV rate as directed. Restarting the IV may be necessary if edema, redness, or pain at the IV site occurs.

Text continued from p. 325.

- Help the mother turn, cough, and breathe deeply every 2 hours to prevent pooling of bronchial secretions.
- Explain use of an incentive spirometer, if prescribed.
- Apply antiembolism stockings or sequential compression devices, if prescribed to improve peripheral circulation.
- Help her sit and dangle the legs after about 8 hours and walk as soon as possible to prevent thromboembolic complications and to prevent abdominal distention.

Resuming Normal Activities. After 24 hours, several normal functions usually return, and mothers are able to participate more actively in their own care.

- Discontinue the IV infusion.
- Provide fluids and food according to agency protocol.
- Remove the indwelling urinary catheter and monitor first voidings to be sure the bladder is empty.
- Remove the dressing and staples, if present, according to facility protocol.
- Encourage ambulation and as much self-care as is comfortable for the mother.
- Provide ample opportunity for parent-infant contact.

Relieving Abdominal Distention
- Encourage early, frequent ambulation.
- Advise mother to avoid carbonated beverages, use of straws, and gas-forming foods.
- Teach pelvic lifts (a flat, supine position with knees bent, lifting the pelvis from the bed) to reduce distention.
- Teach tightening and relaxing the abdominal muscles.
- Insert suppositories, as prescribed, to help expel flatus from the distal colon.
- Obtain an order for simethicone to help disperse flatulence.

Assisting with Infant Feeding
- Find a comfortable position for holding the infant.
  — Suggest a football hold or side-lying position for breastfeeding.

— Place a pillow on the mother's lap to protect the incisional area from the weight of the infant.
— Help the mother change position to breastfeed on both sides.

POSTPARTUM COMPLICATIONS
POSTPARTUM HEMORRHAGE

Postpartum hemorrhage is loss of more than 500 mL of blood following vaginal childbirth or loss of more than 1000 mL following cesarean birth. Because estimating blood loss is difficult, the definition of hemorrhage as a decrease in hematocrit of 10% or more since admission or a need for a blood transfusion is often used. Early hemorrhage occurs in the first 24 hours after childbirth. Late postpartum hemorrhage occurs after the first 24 hours.

Etiology
• Early postpartum hemorrhage (most common type)
— Uterine atony
— Trauma to the birth canal
• Late postpartum hemorrhage
— Retained placental fragments
— Subinvolution or infection

Predisposing Factors
• Overdistention of the uterus (multiple gestation, large infant, hydramnios)
• Multiparity (5 or more)
• Precipitate labor or delivery
• Prolonged labor
• Use of assistive devices (forceps, vacuum extractor)
• Cesarean birth
• Manual removal of the placenta
• Previous postpartum hemorrhage
• Placenta previa or accreta
• Drugs: oxytocin, prostaglandins, tocolytics or magnesium sulfate
• General anesthesia

- Chorioamnionitis
- Clotting disorders
- Previous postpartum hemorrhage or uterine surgery
- Disseminated intravascular coagulation

Clinical Signs
- A fundus that is soft, "boggy," or difficult to locate
- A uterus that does not remain firm when massage is stopped
- A fundus that is located above the expected level or displaced from the midline
- Excessive lochia (especially if it is bright red)
- Excessive clots
- Tachycardia, tachypnea
- Falling blood pressure
- Skin cool and pale

Priority Nursing Assessments
- Review chart for history of predisposing factors.
- Evaluate firmness and location of fundus. Excessive bleeding when the fundus is firm suggests cervical or vaginal laceration.
- Assess blood loss; weigh pads, bedliners, and linen (1 g = 1 mL).
- Examine the perineum for bluish discoloration, bulging, or tender areas that might indicate a hematoma. Deep, unrelieved pelvic pain implies vaginal or retroperitoneal hematoma that cannot be seen.
- Measure vital signs every 15 minutes or more often if necessary. Tachycardia and falling pulse pressure are early signs of hypovolemia. Blood pressure may remain normal as hypovolemia develops because vasoconstriction shunts blood to the vital organs during the initial phase of hypovolemic shock.
- Evaluate the bladder (a distended bladder hinders effective uterine contraction) and urinary output (less than 30 mL per hour suggests inadequate vascular volume).
- Analyze laboratory reports (decreasing hematocrit and hemoglobin indicate blood loss).

Therapeutic Management

- Massage the uterus while supporting the lower uterine segment. Express clots. See Figure 4-2.
- Insert an indwelling catheter to empty the bladder and allow accurate measurement of output.
- Place the woman in supine position. Avoid Trendelenburg position, which may interfere with respiratory and cardiac function.
- Maintain IV access and start a second IV with a large-bore catheter capable of carrying whole blood.
- Administer IV fluids, volume expanders, and blood as directed.
- Draw blood (per protocol or orders) for hemoglobin and hematocrit, type and crossmatch, platelets, prothrombin time, activated partial thromboplastin time (aPTT), fibrinogen, fibrin degradation products, and fibrin split products.
- Administer prescribed drugs, such as oxytocin, prostaglandins, or methylergonovine maleate.
- Apply a pulse oximeter to determine the oxygen saturation; administer oxygen by snug face mask at 8 to 10 L/min or as directed by the physician or facility protocol.
- Anticipate further medical interventions (uterine packing, ligation or embolization of uterine, ovarian, or hypogastric

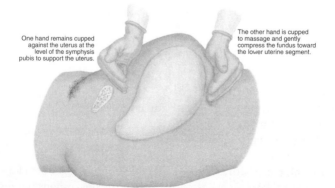

One hand remains cupped against the uterus at the level of the symphysis pubis to support the uterus.

The other hand is cupped to massage and gently compress the fundus toward the lower uterine segment.

Figure 4-2 Technique for fundal massage.

arteries, or hysterectomy if other measures fail to control bleeding.

Nursing Considerations. In addition to the above, the nurse will:

- Monitor the condition of the woman, and communicate with the health care provider.
- Provide explanations and emotional support for the woman and her family.
- Obtain signed consents for specific surgical procedures or blood transfusions.

SUBINVOLUTION

Subinvolution refers to a slower than expected return of the uterus to its prepregnancy size after childbirth.

Etiology. The most common causes of subinvolution are:

- Retained placental fragments.
- Pelvic infection.

Clinical Signs and Symptoms
- Prolonged lochial discharge.
- Irregular or excessive uterine bleeding.
- Pelvic pain or feelings of pelvic heaviness.
- Backache, fatigue, persistent malaise.
- A uterus that feels larger and softer than expected for a particular time.

Therapeutic Management
- Methylergonovine maleate for 24 to 48 hours to provide sustained contraction of the uterus.
- Antimicrobial therapy for infection.

Nursing Considerations. Because subinvolution develops well after the mother has gone home, nursing responsibilities focus on providing education.

- Teach the mother (and a significant other) how to palpate the fundus and where it should be located in relation to the umbilicus.
- Remind the mother that the uterus should get smaller and should descend by about one fingerbreadth every day.
- Explain normal duration and changes in lochia (from rubra to serosa to alba).
- Instruct woman to report if the uterus does not become smaller, if there is a deviation from expected pattern or duration of lochia, or if a foul odor (suggesting infection) is noted.

THROMBOEMBOLIC DISORDERS

The three most common thromboembolic disorders are (1) superficial venous thrombosis, (2) deep vein thrombosis, and (3) pulmonary embolism. A *thrombus* is a collection of blood factors, primarily platelets and fibrin, on a vessel wall. Once started, the thrombus can enlarge, with successive layering of platelets, fibrin, and blood cells as blood flows past the clot. When an inflammatory process also occurs in the vessel wall, it is termed *thrombophlebitis*.

Etiology.   Three major causes of thrombosis

- Venous stasis
- Hypercoagulable blood
- Injury to the endothelial surface of the blood vessel.

Predisposing Factors for Thrombosis
- Inactivity
- Obesity
- Cesarean birth
- Smoking
- History of previous thrombosis
- Varicose veins
- Diabetes mellitus
- Prolonged bed rest
- Prolonged time in stirrups in second stage of labor
- Age >35 years

- Parity greater than 3
- Dehydration

Superficial Venous Thrombosis

Clinical Signs and Symptoms. Signs and symptoms include swelling, tenderness, redness, warmth, pain on walking, or no signs at all. It may be possible to palpate the enlarged, hardened vein.

Therapeutic Management. Treatment includes analgesics, rest, and elastic support hose. Elevate the lower extremity to improve venous return, and apply warm packs to promote healing. After symptoms disappear, allow the woman to ambulate gradually. Recommend that she avoid standing for long periods and continue to wear support hose to prevent venous stasis. Anticoagulant therapy is usually not required and there is little chance of pulmonary embolism if the thrombosis remains in the superficial veins of the lower leg.

Deep Vein Thrombosis (DVT)

Clinical Signs and Symptoms
- Leg swelling (more than 2 cm larger than the other leg)
- Erythema and heat or pallor and coolness of the affected leg
- Tenderness, stiffness, pain on ambulation
- Pedal edema
- Chills, tachycardia
- Positive Homans' sign may or may not be present
- Signs may be absent or diffuse.

Diagnosis is usually based on ultrasonography with vein compression and Doppler flow studies, magnetic resonance imaging (MRI) for pelvic veins, or impedance plethysmography (used less often).

Therapeutic Management. In addition to treatment for superficial thrombophlebitis, anticoagulant therapy is needed for DVT.

- Administer either standard unfractionated heparin (UH) or low-molecular-weight heparin (LMWH) as directed.
- Monitor aPTT so that the heparin dose can be adjusted to maintain a therapeutic level of 1.5 to 2.5 times control. Antifactor Xa may also be monitored if LMWH is used.
- Have protamine sulfate on hand for heparin overdose.

After several days, anticoagulation therapy for the postpartum woman may be changed to warfarin (Coumadin). Prothrombin time and international normalized ratio (INR) are used to monitor coagulation time when warfarin is used. An appropriate INR for DVT is 2 or 3. Vitamin K is the antidote for warfarin overdose.

Nursing Considerations
- Help prevent thrombus formation.
  - Prevent prolonged time in stirrups and pad stirrups during childbirth to prevent excess pressure against the popliteal space during the second stage of labor.
  - Help the mother ambulate frequently and as early as possible.
  - Perform range of motion and assist with passive exercises if the mother is unable to ambulate.
  - Instruct the mother to avoid using pillows or the knee gatch to prevent pressure on the popliteal space and consequent pooling of blood in the lower legs.
  - Obtain an order for antiembolism stockings or sequential compression devices for women with varicose veins, a history of thrombophlebitis, or cesarean birth.
- Provide information to prevent hemorrhage when anticoagulant therapy is used for a prolonged time.
  - Instruct the mother to report bleeding, including bruises, petechiae, epistaxis, blood in the urine or stools, bleeding gums, or increased vaginal bleeding.

— Teach measures to prevent excessive anticoagulation, such as the appropriate schedule of medication, side effects, the importance of taking medication as directed and not to "double up" on medications if a dose has been missed.

— Caution that over-the-counter medications, such as aspirin and nonsteroidal antiinflammatory drugs, increase the risk of hemorrhage.

— Recommend that she take only medications prescribed by a physician who is aware that she is taking anticoagulants.

— Suggest that she use a soft toothbrush, floss her teeth gently, and postpone dental appointments until therapy is completed.

— Recommend a depilatory, which is safer than a razor, to remove unwanted hair while she is on anticoagulant therapy.

— Instruct the woman to report bleeding, unexplained fever, unusual fatigue, or sore throat to the health care provider.

— Advise women taking warfarin to use effective contraception to prevent fetal defects.

— Instruct the woman to avoid excessive intake of vitamin K foods (broccoli, cabbage, lettuce, spinach, lentils) when taking warfarin.

Pulmonary Embolism. Pulmonary embolism is a rare but potentially life-threatening complication of DVT. It occurs when fragments of a blood clot or amniotic fluid and its debris are carried to the pulmonary artery or one of its branches. This occludes the vessel and obstructs the flow of blood into the lungs.

Clinical Signs and Symptoms. Signs and symptoms depend on how much blood flow is obstructed. The most common signs and symptoms are dyspnea; sudden, sharp chest pain; tachycardia; tachypnea; syncope, pulmonary rales; cough; and hemoptysis.

Therapeutic Management. Treatment is aimed at dissolving the clot and maintaining pulmonary circulation.

- Give oxygen (8-10 L/min) to decrease hypoxia.
- Administer analgesics to relieve pain.
- Elevate the head of the bed slightly to reduce dyspnea.
- Initiate pulse oximetry to evaluate oxygen saturation.
- Administer intravenous heparin or thrombolytic drugs, such as streptokinase or urokinase. Embolectomy may be performed.
- Obtain critical care nursing for support of ventilation and cardiovascular status.

Nursing Considerations
- Be aware of the signs and symptoms of pulmonary embolism and be vigilant in assessments of women with thrombosis.
- Report any sign of embolism to the health care provider.
- When signs of embolism are present, obtain assistance, position the woman to reduce dyspnea, and begin oxygen administration.
- The nurse should remain with the woman and provide information and support to a family that usually becomes increasingly fearful.

PUERPERAL INFECTIONS
The definition of puerperal infection is a fever of 38° C (100.4° F) or higher after the first 24 hours and occurring on at least 2 days during the first 10 days after childbirth. The most common puerperal infections are metritis, wound infections, urinary tract infections, mastitis, and septic pelvic thrombophlebitis.

Predisposing Factors. Factors that increase the risk of puerperal infection are:

- History of previous infections
- Colonization of lower genital tract by pathogenic organisms

- Cesarean birth
- Trauma
- Prolonged rupture of membranes
- Prolonged labor
- Catheterization
- Excessive number of vaginal examinations
- Retained placental fragments
- Hemorrhage
- Poor general health (anemia, excessive fatigue, frequent illnesses)
- Poor nutrition (inadequate intake of protein, vitamin C)
- Poor hygiene
- Other medical conditions such as diabetes mellitus
- Low socioeconomic status

Endometritis

Etiology. Endometritis is infection of the endometrium or inner lining of the uterus. If the surrounding tissues are involved, the infection may be called metritis. Organisms involved ascend to the uterus from the lower genital tract. Common organisms include Group B streptococci, enterococci, *Escherichia coli*, *Klebsiella pneumoniae*, *Proteus*, *Bacteroides*, *Prevotella*, and *Chlamydia trachomatis*.

Clinical Signs and Symptoms
- Fever
- Chills
- Malaise, lethargy, anorexia
- Abdominal pain, cramping, and uterine tenderness
- Purulent, foul-smelling lochia (depending on the responsible organism)
- Tachycardia
- Subinvolution

Therapeutic Management. Initial medical management includes intravenous administration of broad-spectrum antibiotics. Specimens from the blood, endocervix, and uterine cavity are cultured to determine specific second-line antibiotic therapy. Oral antibiotics may be used to complete the course of treatment. Antipyretics are often administered for fever, and oxytocics are administered to promote involution.

Nursing Considerations

- Place the mother in Fowler's position to promote drainage of lochia.
- Give medications as directed, and observe for signs of improvement or the development of new symptoms, such as nausea and vomiting, abdominal distention, absent bowel sounds, or severe abdominal pain, that indicate the development of complications.
- Provide comfort measures such as pain medication, warm blankets, cool compresses, sponge baths, cold or warm drinks.
- Help the mother pump her breasts to maintain her milk supply if she is unable to breastfeed.
- Instruct the mother (and family) in measures to prevent the spread of infection.

Wound Infections. Any break in the skin or mucous membranes provides a portal of entry for bacteria. The most common sites for wound infections include:

- Cesarean incisions
- Episiotomies
- Perineal lacerations

Clinical Signs and Symptoms. Signs of infection include localized areas of edema, warmth, redness, tenderness, and pain. In addition, the edges of the wound may pull apart, and there may be seropurulent drainage from the wound. If untreated, systemic signs such as fever and malaise may develop.

Therapeutic Management. Initial medical management includes administration of broad-spectrum antibiotics until a report of the antibiotic-sensitive organism is determined. An incision and drainage may be necessary.

Nursing Considerations. Wound infections may require readmittance to the hospital or home health care visits. Mothers require reassurance, supportive care, and comfort measures.

- Administer analgesics as necessary.
- Provide warm compresses, frequent perineal care, and sitz baths for comfort.
- Teach importance of wiping front to back and good hand-washing.
- Instruct in intake of adequate fluid and good diet.

Urinary Tract Infections
Etiology
- Trauma to the bladder and urethra
- Catheterization
- Urinary stasis, retention, reflux
- Asymptomatic bacteriuria during pregnancy

Clinical Signs and Symptoms
- Dysuria
- Urgency, frequency of urination
- Suprapubic pain
- Low-grade fever
- Signs of pyelonephritis
  — Chills
  — Spiking fever
  — Costovertebral angle tenderness
  — Flank pain
  — Nausea and vomiting

Therapeutic Management. Medical management involves oral or intravenous antibiotics. Generally treated on an out-patient basis.

Nursing Considerations
- Instruct the mother to take all medication.
- Explain the need for 2500 to 3000 mL fluid daily.

- Suggest she drink apricot, plum, prune, or cranberry juices to acidify the urine, and avoid carbonated drinks. Instruct her to take adequate fluid and food necessary for healing.
- Explain perineal care and the need to urinate frequently.

Mastitis. *Mastitis,* an infection of the lactating breast, usually affects only one breast. It occurs most often in the second and third weeks following birth. If untreated, it may lead to a breast abscess.

Etiology
- *Staphylococcus aureus* entering an injured area of the nipple from the infant's mouth or carried on the hands of the mother or the medical or nursing staff.
- Engorgement and stasis of milk frequently precede mastitis.

Clinical Signs and Symptoms
- Localized area of pain, redness, inflammation
- Fatigue, malaise, aching muscles
- Fever, chills
- Headache

Therapeutic Management
- Antibiotics
- Analgesics
- Moist heat or ice packs, breast support
- Emptying the breast by breastfeeding or breast pump
- Bed rest
- Surgical drainage for breast abscess

Nursing Considerations. A major responsibility for nurses is to teach measures that prevent mastitis.

- Demonstrate how to position the infant correctly for breastfeeding.
- Encourage breastfeeding at least every 2 to 3 hours.
- Recommend that the woman avoid formula supplements, which may make the infant less interested in breastfeeding.

- Suggest that she change nursing pads as soon as they are wet.
- Instruct her to avoid continuous pressure on the breasts from tight bras or infant carriers.

Once mastitis occurs, nursing measures are aimed at increasing comfort and helping the mother maintain lactation.

- Recommend that the woman apply moist heat to increase comfort and circulation.
- Suggest cold packs between feedings to reduce edema.
- Emphasize that breasts should be emptied completely at each feeding to prevent stasis of milk.
- Teach her how to express milk or to use a breast pump if breastfeeding must be temporarily curtailed on the affected side.
- Recommend that she drink 2500 to 3000 mL of fluid each day.
- Discourage weaning, which may cause engorgement and lead to a breast abscess

Septic Pelvic Thrombophlebitis. *Septic pelvic thrombophlebitis* occurs when infection spreads along the venous system and thrombophlebitis develops. It occurs more often in women with wound infections, and it usually involves the ovarian, uterine, or hypogastric veins.

Clinical Signs and Symptoms
- Pain in the groin, abdomen, or flank
- Fever, tachycardia
- Gastrointestinal distress, decreased bowel sounds

Diagnostic testing includes CBC with differential, blood chemistries, coagulation studies, blood cultures, computed tomography or magnetic resonance imaging.

Therapeutic Management. Readmittance to the hospital is usually necessary. Treatment includes IV antibiotics and anticoagulation therapy with IV heparin. Other care is similar to that for DVT and includes monitoring for safe levels of anti-coagulation therapy and for signs of pulmonary embolism.

AFFECTIVE DISORDERS

Postpartum Blues. Postpartum blues, the so-called baby blues, is a common transient, self-limited, mild depression that usually begins in the first week following childbirth and usually lasts no longer than 2 weeks. It does not seriously affect the woman's ability to care for her infant.

Etiology

The cause is unknown; however, emotional letdown, discomfort, fatigue, anxiety, and feelings of unattractiveness may contribute. Hormonal fluctuations have not been proven to be a cause.

Clinical Signs and Symptoms
- Insomnia
- Irritability
- Fatigue
- Tearfulness
- Mood instability
- Anxiety

Nursing Considerations
- Acknowledge feelings and offer support.
- Explain that what the woman is experiencing is normal.
- Reassure her that the feeling will abate in less than 2 weeks.
- Encourage rest and time for herself.
- Distinguish between blues and postpartum depression or psychosis.

Postpartum Depression (PPD)

Etiology and Predisposing Factors.
The cause is unknown but predisposing factors are believed to be:

- Previous PPD or depression during pregnancy
- Hormonal fluctuations

- Medical problems, such as preeclampsia, preexisting diabetes mellitus, anemia, or thyroid dysfunction, during or after pregnancy
- A history of depression, mental illness, or alcoholism either in the woman or in her family
- Immaturity or low self-esteem
- Marital dysfunction or difficult relationship with significant other
- Anger or ambivalence about the pregnancy
- Feelings of isolation, lack of social support
- Fatigue, sleep deprivation, financial worries
- Birth of an infant with illness or anomalies
- Multifetal pregnancy

Clinical Signs and Symptoms. Postpartum depression is distinguished from the normal labile emotions of pregnancy and the puerperium by the number, intensity, and persistence of the symptoms. A majority of the symptoms mentioned are intensely and consistently experienced for at least 2 weeks. Common signs and symptoms include:

- Loss of interest in surroundings
- Loss of usual emotional response toward her family
- Intense feelings of unworthiness, guilt, and shame
- Generalized fatigue, irritability, difficulty concentrating
- Anorexia and sleep disturbances
- Tense, irritable appearance
- Panic attacks and obsessive thoughts
- Caring for the infant in a loving manner but without feeling pleasure or love

Therapeutic Management. Primary care is a combination of psychotherapy, social support, and medications such as antidepressants.

Nursing Considerations
- Assess all women for depression during pregnancy and after childbirth.

- Allow ample time to convey a caring attitude.
- Recommend that the woman acknowledge her feelings and insist that others acknowledge them also.
- Emphasize the need for continued communication with the partner.
- Encourage continued contact with other adults.
- Explain the importance of adequate rest and nutrition.
- Help the mother increase sensitivity to infant cues.
- Include family members in discussions.
- Help her identify and contact appropriate support groups.

Postpartum Psychosis. Postpartum psychosis is a rare condition occurring within 3 months of childbirth. A history of previous postpartum psychosis or bipolar disorder increases the risk.

Clinical Signs and Symptoms. Signs and symptoms include sleep disturbances, confusion, agitation, irritability, hallucinations, delusions, and the risk that the mother may kill herself or the infant. Other signs and symptoms include tearfulness, preoccupations of guilt, feelings of worthlessness, lack of appetite, and an inordinate concern with the baby's health. Delusions about the infant being dead or defective are common.

Therapeutic Management. The mother usually requires hospitalization, supportive psychotherapy, and antipsychotic or antidepressant drugs. The woman must be assessed for suicide potential.

Section 5

Reproductive Issues and Women's Health Care

FAMILY PLANNING

Nearly half of all pregnancies are unintended and of those, half are due to incorrect contraceptive use or contraceptive failure. Nurses have a major role in educating women about family planning.

CONSIDERATIONS WHEN TEACHING ABOUT CONTRACEPTION

- Offer teaching about contraception during any contact with women.
- Provide privacy for the discussion.
- Include the woman's partner, if she wishes.
- Assess the woman's knowledge, satisfaction, and concerns about her contraceptive method.
- Answer questions and correct misunderstandings.
- Help women/couples analyze various contraceptive methods if they wish (Table 5-1). Include:
  - Safety
  - Protection from sexually transmitted diseases
  - Effectiveness
  - Acceptability
  - Convenience
  - Education needed
  - Benefits
  - Side effects
  - Interference with spontaneity
  - Availability
  - Expense

Table 5-1	**Comparison of Pregnancy Rates among Common Contraceptive Methods**

Method	Pregnancy Rate: Actual or Typical Use (%)
Sterilization	
Vasectomy	0.15
Tubal ligation	0.5
Intrauterine devices	
Copper T 380A (Paragard)	0.8
LNG-IUS (Mirena)	0.1
Depo-Provera	3
Transdermal contraceptive patch	8
Vaginal contraceptive ring	8
Oral contraceptives	8
Condoms	
Male	15
Female	21
Diaphragm with spermicide	16
Sponge	
Nulliparous women	16
Parous women	32
Natural family planning (all types)	25
Coitus interruptus (withdrawal)	27
Spermicides, gel, foam, films, suppositories (used alone)	29
No contraceptive use	85

Data from Trussell, J. (2004). The essentials of contraception: Efficacy, safety, and personal considerations. In R.A. Hatcher, J. Trussell, F. Stewart, A.L. Nelson, W. Cates, F. Guest, & D. Kowal. (2004). *Contraceptive technology* (18th ed.). New York: Ardent Media.

- — Preference
- — Religious and personal beliefs
- — Culture
- Show examples of contraceptive devices, if possible.
- Provide demonstrations and ask for return demonstrations.
- Explain the need to use another contraceptive method immediately if the woman decides to change methods.

Table 5-2	Discontinuation of Various Types of Contraception

Method	Women Who Discontinue Use at 1 Year (%)
Intrauterine devices	
LNG-IUS (Mirena)	19
Copper T 380A (ParaGard)	22
Depo-Provera	44
Oral contraceptives	32
Contraceptive patch	32
Vaginal ring	32
Condoms	
Male	47
Female	51
Diaphragm	43
Spermicides, gel, foam, films, suppositories (used alone)	58
Natural family planning (all types)	49
Withdrawal	57

Data from Trussell, J. (2004). The essentials of contraception: Efficacy, safety, and personal considerations. In R.A. Hatcher, J. Trussell, F. Stewart, A.L. Nelson, W. Cates, F. Guest, & D. Kowal. (2004). *Contraceptive technology* (18th ed.). New York: Ardent Media.

Women sometimes have an interval of using no contraception before beginning a new method (Table 5-2).

ABSTINENCE

Abstinence, the avoidance of sexual intercourse or any activity that would allow sperm to enter the vagina, is the only completely effective method of preventing pregnancy and sexually transmitted diseases (STDs).

Advantages

- Avoids drugs, hormones, and devices
- Inexpensive
- No side effects or complications

Disadvantages
- Requires perfect use to be effective
- Pregnancy rate with imperfect use as high as 85%
- Often difficult to achieve

Teaching
- May be practiced continuously or periodically
- Women should have information about contraception available if they decide to become sexually active at a later time

BREASTFEEDING

Breastfeeding inhibits ovulation but is a less reliable method of contraception because many things can alter hormone production. Another contraceptive method should be used by 6 months or before that time if the mother uses supplementary feedings or resumes her menses.

Advantages
- Avoids drugs, hormones, and devices.
- Inexpensive.
- No side effects or complications.

Disadvantages
- Infants must be totally breastfed with no supplements or solid foods.
- Breastfeeding must continue day and night.
- Ovulation could occur without the woman's knowledge.

Teaching
- Do not give solids or formula or skip feedings because ovulation may occur.
- Use another method of contraception by 6 months or before if menses occurs.

CERVICAL CAP

The cervical cap (FemCap) is a silicone cap that fits over the cervix to prevent sperm from entering. Spermicide is applied to both sides of the cap.

Advantages
- Avoids systemic hormones
- May fit women who are unable to use a diaphragm
- Has a loop to make insertion and removal easier
- No need for added spermicide for repeated intercourse
- No pressure against the bladder
- Less noticeable than a diaphragm
- Can remain in place for 48 hours

Disadvantages
- Women with cervical abnormalities may not be able to use it
- Must be fitted by a health care provider
- Possibility of toxic shock syndrome
- Initially expensive
- Must be comfortable touching the genitalia

Teaching
- May be inserted ahead of time to decrease interference with spontaneity.
- Do not remove for 6 hours after last intercourse.
- Add spermicide for repeated intercourse.
- Feel the cervix to check placement before and after intercourse.
- Do not use during menses or with a history of toxic shock syndrome.
- Replace after 2 years or after pregnancy.

COITUS INTERRUPTUS
Coitus interruptus, or withdrawal, is the removal of the penis from the vagina before ejaculation.

Advantages
- Avoids drugs, hormones, and devices
- Inexpensive

Disadvantages
- Pregnancy rate: 27%
- Requires great control by the man
- May be unsatisfying to both partners

Teaching
- Not a reliable method of contraception.

CONDOM, FEMALE
The female condom is a polyurethane sheath inserted into the vagina with a flexible ring at each end. One ring fits over the cervix like a diaphragm and the other ring extends outside the vagina to partially cover the perineum.

Advantages
- Gives a woman some protection from STDs without relying on the male condom
- Avoids systemic hormones
- Easy to obtain and carry
- Relatively inexpensive per use

Disadvantages
- Less effective than male condoms (pregnancy rate 21%)
- Many women object to it on esthetic grounds
- Single use only
- Must be comfortable touching the genitalia

Teaching
- Hold the outer ring in place during insertion and removal of the penis.
- Do not use with a male condom as they may adhere to each other.

CONDOM, MALE
The male condom covers the penis during intercourse, preventing sperm from entering the vagina. Latex condoms provide the best protection available (other than abstinence) from STDs. Natural membrane condoms are less effective against STDs. Polyurethane condoms can be used by people allergic to latex.

Advantages
- Readily available without a prescription
- Inexpensive per use

- Can be carried inconspicuously by the man or the woman.
- Help protect against STDs
- Avoid use of systemic hormones
- Pregnancy rate: 15%

Disadvantages
- Interfere with spontaneity
- May interfere with sensation
- Latex allergies may occur
- May be affected by vaginal medications
- May break or slip off during intercourse or withdrawal
- For single use only

Teaching
- Use during any possible exposure to an STD, even if another contraceptive technique is practiced or if the woman is pregnant.
- Use reservoir tips and water-based lubricants to help prevent breakage.
- Check expiration dates; may deteriorate after 5 years.
- Use lubrication to increase comfort for the woman.
- Use water-soluble lubricants or spermicides. Oil-based products (such as petroleum jelly or baby oil) cause deterioration of the latex.
- Apply the condom prior to any contact between the penis and the vagina.
- Squeeze the air out of the tip of the condom.
- Leave a half inch of space at the tip as the condom is rolled onto the erect penis.
- Withdraw the penis from the vagina before it becomes soft while holding the condom in place.
- Use a new condom each time intercourse is repeated.

DEPO-PROVERA
See Hormone Injections, p. 357.

DIAPHRAGM

The diaphragm is a latex dome surrounded by a spring or coil that is inserted over the cervix. It prevents passage of sperm while holding spermicide in place.

Advantages
- Avoids systemic hormones
- Failure rate 16%
- May be inserted ahead of time to decrease interference with spontaneity

Disadvantages
- Pressure on the urethra may cause urinary tract infections
- Noticeable or uncomfortable when in place for some women
- Allergies to latex or history of toxic shock syndrome preclude use
- Must be fitted by a health care provider
- Initially expensive
- Requires education on insertion and removal
- Correct size may not be available for all women
- Some women have difficulty with insertion or removal
- Must be comfortable touching the genitalia
- Possibility of toxic shock syndrome

Teaching
- Inspect the diaphragm for small holes by holding it up to a light.
- Use spermicidal cream or gel inside the dome and around the rim with each use.
- Empty the bladder before insertion to decrease irritation and pressure.
- Use a squatting position or place one foot on a chair to make insertion and removal easier.
- Be sure the front rim fits behind the pubic bone, and the cervix can be felt through the center of the diaphragm.

- If more than 6 hours elapse between insertion and intercourse or if intercourse is repeated, insert more spermicide into the vagina without removing the diaphragm.
- Leave in place at least 6 hours after last intercourse but no more than a total of 24 hours to reduce risk of infection.
- Do not douche, because it is unnecessary and reduces effectiveness.
- Wash with mild soap and dry well after each use.
- Some medications used for vaginal *Candida* infections may damage the diaphragm.
- Get checked for size changes yearly and after pregnancy or abortion or weight gain or loss of more than 10 pounds.
- Replace every 2 years.

EMERGENCY CONTRACEPTION

Emergency contraception (EC), also called the "morning after pill," is used to prevent pregnancy after unprotected intercourse. The woman takes two tablets containing a large dose of progestin (Plan B) or a larger-than-usual dose of combined oral contraceptives (OCs). Action is to prevent or delay ovulation, thicken cervical mucus, and alter sperm transport. It is ineffective if implantation has occurred and will not harm a developing fetus. A copper T 380A intrauterine device may also be used for emergency and continuing contraception.

Advantages
- May be used for contraceptive failure, rape, or incorrect or lack of contraceptive use
- Reduces the risk of pregnancy by 75% (combined OCs) to 89% (Plan B) to 99% (IUD)

Disadvantages. Side effects include nausea and vomiting, especially with combined OCs.

Teaching
- Take EC as soon as possible after unprotected intercourse. It works best if taken within 72 hours but it may be taken as long as 120 hours after intercourse.

- Take Plan B tablets together or 12 hours apart.
- Antiemetics may be given for nausea.
- Some providers give women prescriptions to have on hand in case of need.
- May be obtained from pharmacists in some areas.
- Further information is available at 1-888-NOT-2-LATE or www.not-2-late.com.

HORMONE IMPLANT

The hormone implant Norplant is no longer available in the United States. A new single rod progestin implant (Implanon) is expected to be approved shortly. The implant will provide contraception for 3 years.

INTRAUTERINE DEVICES

Intrauterine devices (IUDs) are inserted into the uterus to provide continuous pregnancy prevention. Two types are available in the United States.

- Copper T 380A (ParaGard)
  — Has a copper wire on the device
  — Effective for 10 years
  — Pregnancy rate: 0.8%
- Levonorgestrel intrauterine system (Mirena)
  — Releases progestin continuously
  — Effective for 5 years
  — Pregnancy rate: 0.1%

Advantages

- Safe for use during lactation
- Low long-term cost
- In place at all times to provide continuous contraception
- Unrelated to coitus
- Often inserted at 6-week postpartum visit

Disadvantages

- Expensive at the time of insertion
- Should be used only by women in mutually monogamous relationships and at low risk for STDs

- Complications
  — Infection may occur with insertion or during the first few weeks. Then the risk of infection is low in women with low risk for STDs
  — Expulsion
  — Perforation of uterus at the time of insertion
  — If pregnancy occurs, may have ectopic pregnancy, spontaneous abortion, or preterm delivery
- Contraindications
  — Nulliparous women
  — Recurrent pelvic infections
  — History of ectopic pregnancy
  — Bleeding disorders
  — Uterine abnormalities

Teaching
- Side effects.
  — Cramping and bleeding with insertion
  — Irregular periods and spotting followed by amenorrhea (Mirena)
  — Menorrhagia (increased bleeding during menstruation)
  — Dysmenorrhea (painful menstruation)
- Use ibuprofen for cramping.
- Check for the plastic strings weekly during the first 4 weeks, then monthly after menses, and if signs of expulsion (cramping or unexpected bleeding) occur.
- Use only if in a mutually monogamous relationship and with a low risk for STDs.
- See a health care provider if signs of infection occur.
  — Unusual vaginal pain, discharge, or itching
  — Low pelvic pain
  — Fever
- Report signs of pregnancy to rule out ectopic pregnancy and remove the IUD.
- Schedule a yearly Pap smear.
- Get checked for anemia if menses are heavy. May need to take iron.

HORMONE INJECTIONS

Depo-Provera (medroxyprogesterone acetate, or DMPA) is an injectable progestin that is given by deep intramuscular injection. The site should not be massaged after injection, as this accelerates absorption. The injection should be given within 5 days of the beginning of the menstrual period.

Advantages
- Prevents ovulation for 12 weeks
- Only four doses a year are needed
- Pregnancy rate: 3%
- Convenient
- No estrogen
- Unrelated to coitus
- May cause amenorrhea

Disadvantages
- Must be repeated on time to keep up effectiveness
- Should not be used by women with contraindications for other hormone contraceptives
- Delay in return of fertility may be 10 to 18 months after discontinuation
- No protection from STDs
- Menstrual irregularities may cause discontinuation
- Should not be used in adolescents; other women should not use for more than 2 years

Teaching
- Side effects
  - Menstrual irregularities: spotting, breakthrough bleeding
  - Amenorrhea in 30% to 50% of women at 1 year
  - Decrease in bone density
  - Weight gain: approximately 1.8 kg (4 lb/year) for some women
  - Headaches
  - Decreased libido
  - Nervousness

— Breast discomfort
— Depression
- If received after the first 5 days of the menstrual cycle, use another contraceptive for the first week.
- Usually not started until 6 weeks after delivery for breast-feeding women.
- Return for injections every 12 weeks.
- Take calcium and vitamin D and get adequate exercise to decrease bone density loss.

MEDROXYPROGESTERONE ACETATE
See Hormone Injections, p. 357.

LEA'S SHIELD
This silicone device fits over the cervix like a diaphragm or cap. It is used with spermicide.

Advantages
- Avoids systemic hormones
- A loop aids in removal

Disadvantages
- Requires a prescription
- Possibility of toxic shock syndrome
- Must be comfortable touching the genitalia

Teaching
- Insert ahead of time to decrease interference with spontaneity.
- Do not remove for 8 hours after last intercourse.
- Remove within 24 hours.
- Add spermicide for repeated intercourse.
- Feel around the cervix to check placement before intercourse.

NATURAL FAMILY PLANNING METHODS
Natural family planning methods are also called *fertility awareness* or *periodic abstinence* methods. They are based on

predicting ovulation by physiologic changes and avoiding coitus or using another contraceptive method when the woman is fertile. They also may be used to help women become pregnant.

Advantages
- Acceptable to most religions
- Help women learn about normal body changes
- Avoid the use of drugs, chemicals, and devices
- Pregnancy rate 2% to 5% if used perfectly

Disadvantages
- Couples must be highly motivated
- Couples must avoid intercourse for as much as half the menstrual cycle
- Extensive education required
- Typical use pregnancy rate: 25%
- Very unforgiving method; errors likely to result in pregnancy
- No protection against STDs

Teaching
- Teaching must be specific to the individual method.
- Method may be used to determine fertile period and another contraceptive method can be used at that time.
- See Table 5-3 for specific methods.

Table 5-3	**Natural Family Planning Methods**
Instructions	**Cautions**
Calendar Method	
Keep track of menstrual cycles for 6 months. Subtract 18 days from the shortest cycle and 11 days from the longest cycle. Avoid intercourse on those days.	Least reliable of all natural methods; many factors, such as stress or illness, may affect time of ovulation.

Continued

Table 5-3	**Natural Family Planning Methods—cont'd**

Instructions	Cautions

Standard Days Method

Instructions	Cautions
Use a color-coded string of beads. Intercourse allowed on days 1-7 and 20 to the end of the cycle.	Use a barrier method or abstain on days 8-19; ineffective for cycles less than 26 days or longer than 32 days.

Basal Body Temperature (BBT) Method

Instructions	Cautions
Chart the oral temperature each morning before getting up or increasing activity. Watch for a rise of approximately 0.2°-0.4° C (0.4°-0.8° F), indicating ovulation has occurred.	Unreliable because BBT can be affected by stress, illness, interrupted sleep, etc.; difficult to know when the temperature will rise; avoid intercourse until the third day after the temperature rise.

Cervical Mucus (Billings or Ovulation) Method

Instructions	Cautions
Assess the cervical mucus daily by wiping the vaginal orifice with tissue. Watch for clear, slippery, stretchy (spinnbarkeit) mucus (like egg white). Avoid intercourse during menses and from the time of thick, sticky mucus until 4 days after the last day of clear, stretchy mucus.	Intercourse allowed only every other day from menses until the fertile period because semen interferes with mucus assessment.

Symptothermal Method

Instructions	Cautions
Combines calendar, BBT, and cervical mucus methods. Notes symptoms of ovulation (weight gain, abdominal bloating, mittelschmerz, increased libido).	More effective than other methods used alone, if cautions for all methods are followed.

ORAL CONTRACEPTIVES

OCs contain estrogen and progestin or progestin alone. Combination contraceptives cause cervical mucus to become too thick for sperm to penetrate, inhibit ovulation, impair sperm capacitation, slow tubal motility, and make the endometrium less hospitable to implantation. Progestin-only oral contraceptives are useful for women who must avoid estrogen, but they are less effective at inhibiting ovulation.

Advantages
- Pregnancy rate: 8%
- Can be used by healthy women who do not smoke until menopause
- Unrelated to coitus
- Reduce ovarian and endometrial cancer
- Regulate menstrual cycles and reduce blood loss
- Decrease incidence of benign breast disease, ovarian cysts, pelvic inflammatory disease, ectopic pregnancy
- Improve acne, premenstrual symptoms, dysmenorrhea, and other conditions

Disadvantages
- No protection against STDs
- Must be taken daily near the same time of day
- Return of fertility may take 3 to 6 months after discontinuation
- Increases incidence of some conditions (see following)

Teaching
- Should not be used by women with a history of:
  — Thrombophlebitis or thromboembolic disorders
  — Cerebrovascular or cardiovascular diseases
  — Any estrogen-dependent cancer or breast cancer
  — Benign or malignant liver tumors
  — Hypertension
  — Migraines with focal aura
  — Diabetes with vascular involvement or of more than 10 years' duration

- Should not be used by women who currently have:
  - Any of the above conditions
  - Impaired liver function
  - Suspected or known pregnancy
  - Undiagnosed vaginal bleeding
  - Heavy cigarette smoking (more than 15/day in women older than 35; any smoking over age 40. Any use of cigarettes is discouraged and should be evaluated individually)
  - Major surgery requiring prolonged immobilization
- Side effects
  - Nausea
  - Headaches
  - Breast tenderness
  - Breakthrough bleeding
  - Weight gain or loss
  - Fluid retention
  - Amenorrhea
  - Mood swings
  - Melasma
- Maintain hormone levels by taking the pills at the same time each day
- Use another contraceptive method during the first week of the first cycle unless the pills are begun on the first day of menses
- Side effects often decrease after the first few months of use. Changing the dose of estrogen or progestin may help
- Follow specific instructions from the health care provider for what to do when OCs are missed
- Progestin-only contraceptives do not affect milk production and are more appropriate during lactation than combination OCs. They are often started at 6 weeks postpartum.
- Inform the health care provider of all medications being used. OC interaction with other drugs may decrease effectiveness of both (e.g., some anticonvulsant, anti-tuberculosis, and antifungal drugs, St. John's wort, some antiviral drugs). Antibiotics such as ampicillin or tetracycline do not affect effectiveness.

- Obtain a yearly breast examination and blood pressure measurement. Papanicolaou test recommendations are the same as for other women.
- Use the acronym ACHES to help remember signs that should be reported immediately.
  - A: Abdominal pain (severe)
  - C: Chest pain, dyspnea, hemoptysis
  - H: Headache (severe), weakness or numbness of extremities, hypertension
  - E: Eye problems: visual changes such as blurred or double vision or visual loss, speech disturbance
  - S: Severe leg pain or swelling (calf or thigh)

PATCH (TRANSDERMAL)
The transdermal contraceptive patch (Ortho Evra) is applied to the skin once weekly for 3 weeks and left off during the fourth week, during which menses occurs. The patch releases small amounts of estrogen and progestin.

Advantages
- Applied only once a week, so is easier to remember than pills
- Unrelated to coitus
- Regulates menstrual cycles
- Pregnancy rate: 8%
- Convenient

Disadvantages
- Requires a prescription
- Must be applied on the right day
- Less effective in women greater than 90 kg (198 lb)
- May cause skin irritation
- Side effects similar to oral contraceptives
- Visible on the skin
- Does not protect from STDs

Teaching
- Apply to clean dry skin on the abdomen, upper torso (except the breasts), buttock, or upper outer arm.

- Avoid oil or lotion in the area.
- Use a different site each week and apply on the same day of the week.
- Wear continuously for 7 days.
- Begin a new cycle after the seventh day of the patch-free week.

SPERMICIDES

Spermicides (chemicals that kill sperm) come in many forms. Creams and gels are used with mechanical barriers such as the diaphragm or cervical cap. Foams, foaming tablets, suppositories, and vaginal film may be used alone. They are inserted into the vagina just before sexual intercourse and are effective for about 1 hour. Vaginal films and suppositories must melt, which takes approximately 15 minutes, before they become effective.

Advantages
- Readily available without a prescription
- Inexpensive per use
- Easy to use
- Provide lubrication
- Avoid use of systemic hormones

Disadvantages
- Should be used with condoms
- Messy
- Some feel they interfere with sensation
- Pregnancy rate: 29% if used alone
- No protection against STDs
- May cause irritation
- Must be comfortable touching the genitalia

Teaching
- Sensitivity may cause genital irritation, which may increase risk of infection.
- Avoid douching for at least 6 hours after intercourse.
- Add more spermicide if coitus is repeated.

STERILIZATION

Male or female sterilization is permanent and effective. It should be used only by those who understand that reversal surgery is difficult, expensive, not always successful, and may not be covered by insurance. Both female and male sterilization end concern about pregnancy but do not offer protection against STDs.

Tubal Ligation. Tubal ligation involves cutting or mechanically occluding the fallopian tubes during a minilaparotomy, laparoscopy, or other abdominal surgery such as cesarean birth. May also be performed nonsurgically by insertion of a coil through the cervix and into the fallopian tubes (Essure).

Advantages
- Pregnancy rate 0.5%
- Can be performed with a cesarean birth
- Convenient if performed during the immediate postpartum period, when the fundus is near the umbilicus and the fallopian tubes are directly below the abdominal wall
- Can be performed at other times as outpatient surgery

Disadvantages
- Most methods require surgery. Coil method requires a hysterosalpingogram at 3 months to ensure the tubes are blocked.
- General anesthesia is most common for surgery, but regional or local anesthesia may be used.
- Initially expensive, but ends future contraception costs.

Teaching
- If tubal ligation is to be performed soon after childbirth, the consent forms must be signed well before labor.
- Rest for 24 hours after surgery and do not lift heavy objects for a week.
- Call the provider if there is fainting, severe pain, or incisional bleeding or discharge.

Vasectomy. Vasectomy involves cutting or cauterizing the vas deferens through a small incision in the scrotum so that semen no longer carries sperm.

Advantages
- Pregnancy rate: 0.15%
- Can be performed in a physician's office under local anesthesia
- Less expensive than tubal ligation

Disadvantages
- Requires surgery
- Expensive at the time of the surgery, but less expensive than tubal ligation and ends future contraception costs
- Requires another contraceptive method until the semen is free of sperm

Teaching
- Rest, apply ice to the area, and use a scrotal support for 2 days.
- Observe for excessive fever, severe pain, bleeding or discharge, a painful nodule, or swelling more than twice the normal size.
- Complete sterilization does not occur until no sperm are in the semen, which may be 3 months or more.
- Semen specimens should be analyzed until two specimens show no sperm present.

TUBAL LIGATION
See Sterilization, p. 365.

VASECTOMY
See Sterilization, above.

VAGINAL RING
The contraceptive ring (NuvaRing) is a soft flexible ring inserted into the vagina and left in place for 3 weeks. It is removed for 1 week during which menses occurs. The ring releases small amounts of estrogen and progestin.

Advantages
- Requires action only twice a month (insertion or removal)
- Unrelated to coitus
- Pregnancy rate: 8%
- Convenient
- No fitting required
- Not visible to others
- Less spotting than with other hormonal methods

Disadvantages
- Requires a prescription
- Must remember when to insert and remove
- Side effects: expulsion, vaginitis, vaginal discomfort and others similar to oral contraceptives
- Must be comfortable touching the genitalia
- Some women or their partners feel the ring but this is not usually a problem

Teaching
- Insert within the first 5 days of the menstrual cycle.
- Use a backup method the first cycle unless a hormonal method was used the previous month.
- May be removed up to 3 hours without loss of effectiveness. If longer, use a backup method for 7 days.

WITHDRAWAL
See Coitus Interruptus p. 350.

INFERTILITY
Infertility is the inability to conceive after 1 year of unprotected regular sexual intercourse. A more workable definition is the inability to conceive at the time desired.

MALE FACTORS
- Sperm abnormalities
  - Low numbers (fewer than 20 million per milliliter of semen)
  - Excessive numbers of abnormally formed sperm

- Abnormal sperm movement
- Inability to penetrate the ovum
- Abnormal erections
- Abnormal ejaculation
  - Retrograde
  - Semen deposited near vaginal outlet
  - Premature ejaculation
- Abnormal seminal fluid
  - Does not liquefy
  - Abnormal amount
  - Abnormal composition

FEMALE FACTORS
- Ovulation disorders
  - Dysfunctional hormonal stimulation of the ovary to mature and release an ovum
  - Failure of the ovaries to respond to hormonal stimulation
  - Abnormal ova
- Fallopian tube abnormalities
  - Tubal obstruction
  - Abnormal tubal motility to move the ovum to the uterus
- Cervical abnormalities
  - Failure to secrete thin, slippery mucus at ovulation
  - Scarring from infections or surgery

REPEATED PREGNANCY LOSS
- Abnormal fetal chromosomes
- Abnormal cervix or uterus
  - Malformations
  - Scarring
  - Myomas (benign tumors)
- Endocrine abnormalities
  - Luteal phase defect
  - Hypo- or hyperthyroidism
  - Poorly controlled diabetes

- Immunologic abnormalities
  — Woman's body does not tolerate the foreign tissue of the embryo
  — Autoimmune disease
- Environmental agents
  — Radiation therapy
  — Alcohol
  — Isotretinoin (Accutane)
- Infections

INFERTILITY EVALUATION
Evaluation of infertility generally proceeds from the simpler tests to the more complex ones. If the woman is nearing the end of her reproductive years, testing may be accelerated.

INFERTILITY THERAPY
- Medications
- Surgery
  — Correct male varicocele
  — Relief of obstructions or adhesions
- Therapeutic insemination with the partner's or donor semen
- Egg donation
- Surrogate parenting
- Advanced reproductive technology
  — In vitro fertilization (IVF): Inducing ovulation and retrieving ova; mixing ova with sperm; returning fertilized ova to the uterus 2 days later
  — Gamete intrafallopian transfer (GIFT): Retrieving ova, placing ova and sperm in fallopian tube, where fertilization occurs
  — Zygote intrafallopian transfer (ZIFT), also called tubal embryo transfer (TET): Retrieving ova and fertilizing outside the body; replacing in fallopian tubes to enter uterus naturally
- Intracycloplasmic sperm injection (ICSI) using microsurgical techniques to obtain sperm and inject the spermatozoon into an ovum for fertilization

Text continued on p. 374

Table 5-4	Selected Diagnostic Tests in Infertility

Test/Purpose	Nursing Implications
Male *Semen Analysis* Evaluates structure and function of sperm and composition of seminal fluid. Semen volume: 2-6 mL pH: 7.2-7.8 Sperm concentration: 20 million/mL or more Motility: 50% or more with normal forms Morphology: 60% or more with normal forms Viability: 50% or more live Liquefaction: within 30 minutes Leukocytes (white blood cells): fewer than 1 million/mL Fructose: 150-600 mg/dL	Explain purpose of semen analysis: three or more specimens are usually collected over several weeks' time for accurate analysis. Explain to the man that he should collect the specimen by masturbation after a 2- to 3-day abstinence; semen may be collected in a condom if masturbation is unacceptable. Teach the man to note the time the specimen was obtained so the laboratory can evaluate liquefaction of the semen. To maintain warmth, the specimen should be transported near the body and should arrive in the laboratory within 1 hour.
Endocrine Tests Evaluate function of hypothalamus, pituitary gland, and the response of the testicles. Assays are made to determine testosterone, estradiol, luteinizing	Teach the man about the relationship between hypothalamic and pituitary function and sperm formation; LH stimulates testosterone production by

hormone (LH), and follicle-stimulating hormone (FSH) levels.
Additional tests may be done based on history and physical findings.

Leydig cells of the testes, and FSH stimulates Sertoli cells of the testes to produce sperm.

Ultrasonography

Evaluates structure of prostate gland, seminal vesicles, and ejaculatory ducts by use of a transrectal probe.

Teach the man that ultrasonography uses sound waves to evaluate these structures; no radiation is involved.

Testicular Biopsy

An invasive test for obtaining a sample of testicular tissue; identifies pathology and obstructions.

Explain the purpose of the test; a local anesthetic is used, and there should be little discomfort.

Sperm Penetration Assay

Evaluates fertilizing ability of sperm; assesses ability of sperm to undergo changes that allow penetration of a hamster ovum from which the zona pellucida has been removed.

Explain the purpose of the test; abnormal penetration does not necessarily mean that the sperm cannot fertilize a human ovum.

Female
Ovulation Prediction

Identifies the surge of LH, which precedes ovulation by 24 to 36 hours; improves ability to time intercourse to coincide with ovulation, and identifies the absence of ovulation.

Explain the purpose of the assessments.
Teach the woman to follow the instructions on commercial ovulation predictor.

Continued

Table 5-4	Selected Diagnostic Tests in Infertility—cont'd
Test/Purpose	**Nursing Implications**
Common prediction methods include commercial ovulation predictor kits, basal body temperature, and cervical mucus assessment (see Fertility Awareness, p. 421).	Teach her how to do the basal body temperature and cervical mucus assessment if that is used.
Ultrasonography	
Evaluates structure of pelvic organs. Identifies ovarian follicles and release of ova at ovulation. Evaluates for presence of ectopic or multifetal pregnancy.	Teach the woman that ultrasonography uses sound waves to evaluate these structures; no radiation is involved. Explain preparations needed for specific evaluations.
Postcoital Test	
Evaluates characteristics of cervical mucus and sperm function within that mucus at time of ovulation. Ultrasonography ensures proper timing for test.	Explain that the test is performed 6 to 12 hours after intercourse; the woman may have to rearrange her personal or work commitments each time this test is done. Use is becoming less frequent but remains a valid diagnostic tool.

Table 5-5	**Medications Used for Infertility Therapy**
Drug	**Primary Use**
Bromocriptine (Parlodel)	Corrects excess prolactin secretion by anterior pituitary, improving gonadotropin-releasing hormone (GnRH) secretion, in turn normalizing follicle-stimulating hormone (FSH) and luteinizing hormone (LH) release. These drug actions increase ovulation and support early pregnancy by stimulating progesterone secretion by the corpus luteum.
Chorionic gonadotropin, human (hCG; Pregnyl); recombinant deoxyribonucleic acid (DNA) origin (r-hCG; Ovidrel)	Used in conjunction with gonadotropins to stimulate ovulation in the female or sperm formation in the male. Stimulates progesterone production by corpus luteum.
Clomiphene citrate (Clomid)	Induction of ovulation in women who have specific types of ovulatory dysfunction. The drug increases frequency of GnRH secretion from the hypothalamus, thus increasing FSH and LH release and maturing the ovarian follicle and release of the ovum.
FSH, recombinant DNA origin (follitropin [Gonal-F])	Stimulation of ovarian follicle growth; ovulation-induction gonadotropin.
GnRH antagonists (e.g., cetrorelix [Cetrotide], ganirelix [Antagon])	Reduces endometriosis; adjunct to drugs given to stimulate ovulation by suppressing LH and FSH, reducing ovarian hyperstimulation. Depending on drug, doses may be given intranasally, subcutaneously, or intramuscularly.

Data from Leibowitz, D. & Hoffman, J. (2000). Fertility drug therapies: Past, present, and future. *Journal of Obstetric, Gynecologic, and Neonatal Nursing, 29*(2), 201-210; Richard-Davis, G. (2002). Ovulation induction for in vitro fertilization: The role of gonadotropin-releasing hormone antagonists. *Infertility and Reproductive Medicine Clinics of North America, 13*(3), 437-444; Thornton, K. L. (2002). Recombinant gonadotropins and IVF. *Infertility and Reproductive Medicine Clinics of North America, 13*(3), 445-458.

Continued

Table 5-5	**Medications Used for Infertility Therapy—cont'd**
Drug	**Primary Use**
GnRH agonists (goserelin [Zoladex], leuprolide [Lupron], nafarelin [Synarel])	Stimulates release of FSH and LH from the pituitary gland in men and women who have deficient GnRH secretion by their hypothalamus. FSH and LH, in turn, stimulate ovulation in the female and stimulate testosterone production and spermatogenesis in the male.
Gonadotropins, human (Bravelle, Humegon, Pergonal, Repronex)	Induction of ovulation with human-derived FSH and LH; brands may differ in the proportions of FSH to LH; recombinant DNA preparations are becoming more common because of their greater purity
LH, recombinant DNA origin	Replacement of LH; promotes ability of mature ovarian follicle to rupture and luteinize when hCG is secreted; usefulness of drug requires more study.
Progesterone (intramuscular or vaginal preparations)	Luteal phase support; prepares uterine lining and promotes implantation of embryo.
Erectile agents (sildenafil [Viagra], vardenafil [Levitra], tadalafil [Cialis])	Increase blood flow to the penis, improving erectile function.

Text continued from p. 369.

NURSING CARE OF THE INFERTILE COUPLE

- Assisting communication
  - Encourage expression of their feelings.
  - Encourage partners to accept their own feelings, both positive and negative.
  - Discuss differences in the partners' communication styles.
  - Encourage partners to be open with each other.

- Increasing the couple's sense of control
  - Encourage them to identify how their previous ways to deal with stresses can help them in this situation.
  - Reinforce positive coping skills that reduce stress.
  - Teach relaxation techniques (visualization, moderate exercise).
  - Explain procedures and purposes in understandable language. Reinforce any medical explanations already given. Encourage questions.
  - Help them explore their options at each decision point.
- Reducing isolation
  - Refer the couple to support groups.
  - Encourage reestablishment of ties with relatives and friends if these have been disrupted.
- Promoting a positive self-image
  - Explore areas of competence other than conception.
  - Encourage them to maintain activities such as hobbies.
  - Explore whether their careers are a source of stress or an avenue for positive self-perception.

WOMEN'S HEALTH CARE
HEALTH MAINTENANCE

Health maintenance refers to measures that can be taken to prevent or detect disorders. The most useful measures are individual health history, family history, physical examination, screening procedures, and immunizations.

Personal Health History. The health history should focus on particular habits and lifestyle factors that promote or interfere with long-term health.

- Menstrual and obstetric histories
- Usual medications and their uses (includes prescription and over-the-counter drugs; illicit drugs)
- Use of complementary or alternative therapies
- Habits (smoking, use of alcohol)
- Current and past state of health

- Elimination patterns, including current or previous problems
- Diet, typical food intake
- Exercise (type, frequency, duration)
- Sleep and rest patterns
- Degree of stress in life and how managed
- Safety and injury precautions (use of seat belts, nonskid area rugs, sunscreen, etc.)
- Sexual practices (age of first sexual experience, family planning methods, monogamous relationship, multiple partners or partner with multiple contacts, knowledge of how to prevent sexually transmitted diseases)

Family History. A family history may reveal a risk profile for specific diseases.

- Cardiovascular disease (heart attack, stroke, hypertension, clotting disorders, anemia)
- Osteoporosis
- Cancer (breast, ovarian, bowel, lung)

Physical Assessment. Although a physical examination should include every body system, particular emphasis is placed on the following:

- Height, weight, vital signs; allergies
  — Weight (should be within 10% of ideal weight for height according to weight charts)
  — Body mass index (BMI) helps identify underweight, overweight, and obesity as well as normal weight for height
  — Height and loss of height (associated with osteoporosis)
- Auscultation of heart sounds for rate and rhythm, and to detect murmurs
- Auscultation of lungs for adventitious sounds such as rales or wheezes
- Inspection and palpation of the breasts for lumps, masses, dimpling, or nipple discharge

- Observation and palpation of extremities for edema, varicosities, equality of pedal pulses
- Palpation of abdomen for tenderness, masses, or distention
- Common client explanation and instruction for pelvic examination
  — Schedule a pelvic examination between menstrual periods.
  — Do not have sexual intercourse for 48 hours prior to the exam.
  — Do not douche or use vaginal medications, sprays, or deodorants that might interfere with interpretation of cytology specimens that are collected.
  — Urinate just prior to the examination.
  — A lithotomy position with the head slightly elevated is necessary. Some practitioners offer the woman a mirror so she can observe the examination.
- Examination of external genitalia
  — Observation of the vulva for character and distribution of hair and the degree of development or atrophy of the labia
  — Evaluation of cysts, tumors, or inflammation of Bartholin's gland
  — Inspection of urethra and Skene's glands for exudate
  — Collection of any exudate for laboratory analysis
- Speculum examination to inspect the vagina and cervix
  — Warming and lubricating the speculum with warm water only to avoid interfering with the examination of cervical cytology or other vaginal exudate
  — Evaluation of the size, shape, and color of the cervix
  — Collection of purulent cervical discharge for culture
  — Collection of material for cervical cytologic smear (Pap smear) should be taken before speculum is withdrawn
- Bimanual examination for information about the uterus, fallopian tubes, and ovaries
  — Inspection of the anus for hemorrhoids, inflammation, or lesions
- Digital examination of the rectum to determine sphincter tone and to prepare a slide for detection of occult blood

Screening Procedures

- Breast self-examination (BSE) is a supplement to screening by professional examination and mammography. BSE should be performed monthly about a week following the onset of menses, when hormonal influences on the breasts are at a low level. See Procedure: Breast Self-Examination, p. 415)

- Clinical breast examination is similar to BSE; however, professional examiners may detect questionable areas that the woman misses. While the woman is in an upright position, the health professional should:
  - Inspect the breasts for size, symmetry, and color, or skin changes.
  - Observe the nipples and areola for differences in size, color, unilateral retraction of a nipple, or asymmetrical nipple direction.
  - Ask the woman to raise her hands above her head to inspect the sides and underneath portions of the breasts for asymmetry or color difference.
  - Direct the woman to place her hands on her hips and press down; this action may reveal skin dimpling or masses.
  - Palpate each axilla for enlarged or tender lymph nodes.

- Help the woman into a supine position and place a small pillow or folded towel under the shoulder to stretch and flatten the breast tissue on that side.
  - Use the flat part of the first three fingers to palpate the breast, rotate the fingers against the chest wall; palpate the tissue that extends into the axilla; repeat on opposite side.

Clinical Tip

Normal breast tissue may feel firm, lumpy, nodular, or tender. A discrete mass that can be felt or measured (often likened to a raisin, watermelon seed, or grape) is abnormal and requires further evaluation.

— Compress the nipples and collect a sample of any discharge for culture and examination of cells.

- Mammography is currently recommended every 1 to 2 years for women ages 40 to 49 and annually for women after the age of 50 (ACOG, 2003). American Cancer Society recommends a screening mammogram yearly beginning at age 40 (ACS, 2004). It is the only screening procedure that can detect breast lumps long before they are palpable.

- Vulvar self-examination (VSE) should be performed monthly by all women older than the age of 18 and by those younger than 18 years who are sexually active.
  — Instruct the woman to sit in a well-lighted area and use a handheld mirror to see the external genitalia.
  — Suggest that she inspect and palpate the area systematically, starting at the mons pubis and progressing to the labia, clitoris, and perineum. She should inspect the anus.
  — Emphasize that new moles, warts, or growths of any kind, as well as ulcers, sores, changes in skin color or itching should be reported to the health care provider as soon as possible.

- Papanicolaou (Pap) test is a reliable screening test for cervical cancer. Cytology findings are reported by the Bethesda system, which addresses three elements.
  — Specimen adequacy
  — General categorization (normal or abnormal)
  — Descriptive diagnosis of abnormal epithelial cell cytology that uses the following terminology: (a) atypical squamous cells of undetermined significance (ASCUS); (b) squamous intraepithelial lesion (SIL), which is subdivided into low-grade SIL and high-grade SIL (previously categorized as carcinoma in situ); and (c) squamous cell cancer
  — Glandular cell cytology may identify the following abnormalities using the Bethesda system: (a) atypical glandular cells of uncertain significance (AGCUS); (b) adenocarcinoma

- Fecal occult blood testing (FOBT) is a useful screening measure for colorectal cancer. To prevent false FOBT results, the woman should be advised to:
  - Maintain food restrictions as directed before and during the stool collection period.
  - Collect a specimen from three consecutive stools.
  - Return slides as directed.
- Laboratory screening tests depend on the history and risk assessment of the woman, but might include the following.
  - Testing for STDs is recommended for those with (a) a history of multiple sexual partners; (b) a sexual partner with multiple contacts; (c) sexual contact with people with culture-proven STD; (d) a history of repeated episodes of STDs.
  - HIV testing should be offered to those (a) seeking treatment for STDs; (b) who use IV drugs; (c) who have a bisexual partner or a partner who is HIV-positive; (d) who have been exposed to blood or other body fluids in their line of work.
  - Testing for rubella immunity if not known.
  - Tuberculosis screening
  - Cholesterol and lipid profile is appropriate for women with a family history or other risk factors for coronary artery disease, particularly after menopause.
  - Fasting glucose test should be performed every 3 years after age 45 or earlier if the woman has risk factors such as (a) obesity, (b) history of gestational diabetes, or (c) family history of diabetes mellitus.
  - Urinalysis is routinely performed to detect infection of urinary tract.
  - Thyroid function test is recommended if there are signs of thyroid dysfunction, such as heart palpitations or heat intolerance, or a family history of thyroid dysfunction.
  - Genetic testing for specific cancers such as the BRCA1, BRCA2, p53, CHEK-2 genes or other genes associated with breast or other cancers of concern
  - Serum CA 125 testing for the woman with a family history of ovarian cancer.

— Transvaginal ultrasound may be used to diagnose disorders of the ovaries or fallopian tubes.
— Colonoscopy or sigmoidoscopy every 5 to 10 years for women age 50 or older. More frequent evaluations may be recommended based on family and personal history.

Immunizations. Recommended immunizations are based on risk factors but may include:

• Tetanus-diphtheria booster every 10 years.
• Measles mumps rubella (MMR) for women of childbearing age with no evidence of immunity.
• Hepatitis B vaccine for high-risk groups (certain health care workers, IV drug use, current recipients of blood products, health-related job with exposure to blood products, household or sexual contact with hepatitis B carrier, sexual activity with multiple partners)
• Pneumococcal vaccine should be offered to those who have chronic disorders, are immunosuppressed or who have sickle cell disease, Hodgkin's disease, alcoholism, cirrhosis, or multiple myeloma
• Influenza vaccine is recommended annually for most ages

Updated immunization recommendations for adults and children may be found at www.cdc.gov.

BREAST DISORDERS
Diagnosis. Methods used to determine if a lesion or lump in the breast is benign or malignant include:

• Ultrasound examination to distinguish fluid-filled cysts from solid tissue that is potentially malignant.
• Fine-needle aspiration or core biopsy to remove fluid or tissue fragments for analysis of cells.
• Surgical biopsy is performed if:
— Suspicious mass persists through a menstrual cycle.
— Bloody fluid is removed from cyst.
— Cyst fails to disappear completely after aspiration.

— Cyst reoccurs after aspiration.
— Solid dominant mass is not diagnosed.
— Nipple discharge is bloody.
— Nipple is persistently ulcerated or crusted.
— Skin is swollen and red (suggests inflammatory breast cancer).
— Mammography, sonography, or other imaging findings are suspicious.

Risk Factors for Breast Cancer
- Female
- Age older than 50 years
- Early menarche (before age 10)
- Late menopause (after age 50)
- Previous history of breast cancer
- Nulliparity or delayed childbearing (after 30 years)
- Family history of breast cancer or other cancers such as colon or ovarian cancer
- Genetic factors (BRCA1 and BRCA2, p53, or other mutations)
- Previous irradiation of the chest area as a child or young woman to treat other cancers such as Hodgkin's disease or non-Hodgkin's lymphoma
- Some abnormal breast biopsy results other than malignant ones
- Long term hormone replacement therapy with estrogen and progesterone
- Physical inactivity

Psychosocial Implications of Breast Cancer. Common psychosocial concerns of women who have breast cancer and their families are:

- Fear of death
- Anxiety about treatment and quality of life
- Changes in body image
- The effect on sexuality
- Side effects of therapy
- The effect on family relationships and work responsibilities

Staging of Breast Cancer. Although confirmation of malignancy is the first step in evaluating a woman with cancer, staging is necessary to understand the extent of the cancer. Staging is based on a TNM (tumor, node, metastasis) system. Stages progress from stage 1, indicating a small tumor without lymphatic involvement or metastases, to stage 4, which indicates spread to lymph nodes and metastasis to distant organs.

Management. Treatment depends on many factors, including the location and size of the tumor, extension into surrounding tissue, and involvement of the lymphatic system. Body organs such as the bones, brain, and liver are scanned prior to treatment to detect metastasis. A combination of surgical excision and adjuvant therapy is often recommended. Sentinel lymph node (SLN) biopsy helps identify the degree of extension into lymph nodes.

Surgical Treatment
- Breast conservation treatment involves wide local excision (sometimes called lumpectomy) of the tumor to microscopically clean margins.
- Simple mastectomy is removal of the breast.
- Modified radical mastectomy is removal of breast tissue, axillary nodes, and some chest muscles; however, the pectoralis major is preserved.

Adjuvant Therapy. Adjuvant therapy is supportive therapy that includes radiation, chemotherapy, estrogen blocking therapy, and aromatase inhibitors. Immunotherapy is being studied as a means of blocking cancer cell growth.

Breast Reconstruction. Breast reconstruction may be immediate or delayed. The most common methods are listed if the woman chooses reconstruction.

- Tissue expansion is a method in which a prosthesis is filled with saline in small increments to slowly expand the tissue. An implant is inserted when the desired size is reached.

- Autogenous grafts, which carry their own blood supply, are recommended when radiation leaves the wound unsuitable for implants. They may be suited to the woman with large breasts or the woman who objects to implants. Thin women may not have sufficient tissue for transplant to the breast. Women who smoke or those who have a disorder such as diabetes that may cause poor circulation and healing of the transplanted tissue are not usually suitable.
- Nipple-areola reconstruction may use skin from the opposite nipple, skin that covers the prosthesis mound, or skin from other body tissue. Tattoo to color the areola and nipple reconstruction is often done.

Nursing Considerations. A woman who is diagnosed with breast cancer should be able to depend on nurses for accurate information and emotional support. Nurses must allow time for the woman to express her feelings and worries. Many women and their families experience a great deal of confusion and frustration as they try to coordinate appointments and information from a variety of specialists, such as surgeons, radiologists, and oncologists. Nurses must convey a sense of empathic understanding as they help the woman, and her family if she desires, participate in decisions about her care. Moreover, nurses are often responsible for providing information about the preoperative and postoperative periods.

- Usual time in the hospital or surgical facility (1-2 days; however, some surgical procedures including mastectomies, are performed in outpatient surgery centers)
- Function of pressure dressing and drainage tubes (to prevent further bleeding and edema)
- A description of the wound (may be red and raised for first few weeks); and when any sutures or staples should be removed if used

- How to minimize the risk of infection (keep wound dry and clean); signs of wound infection to report at once (purulent drainage, heat, tenderness)
- How the wound heals (redness and edema gradually subside, fluid from drainage tube lessens, wound gradually becomes a thin scar)
- Side effects of adjuvant therapy (nausea, fatigue, hair loss)
- Explanation of arm exercises that may be recommended to prevent lymphedema and to maintain mobility of the arm
- Information about groups that provide support (Reach to Recovery and Encore)

CARDIOVASCULAR DISEASE
RECOGNIZING CORONARY ARTERY DISEASE IN WOMEN

Risk Factors. Risk factors for coronary artery disease in women include:

- Cigarette smoking.
- Hypertension (including isolated systolic hypertension).
- Serum lipids (dyslipidemia):
  - Elevated total cholesterol (normal: ≤199 mg/dL; borderline: 200-239 mg/dL; elevated: ≥240 mg/dL)
  - Low levels of high-density lipoprotein (HDL) cholesterol: <35 mg/dL
  - Cholesterol ratio: The ratio of cholesterol to HDL cholesterol is often used instead of total blood cholesterol. The goal is to keep the ratio lower than 5 (total cholesterol): 1 (HDL cholesterol), with an optimum ratio of 3.5 to 1.
  - Triglyceride levels: >150 mg/dL
- Diabetes mellitus.
- Overweight and obesity.
- Sedentary lifestyle.
- Poor nutrition, especially a diet high in saturated fat and cholesterol but low in fiber and fruit.
- Age older than 60.

- Postmenopause status.
- Family history of coronary artery disease.

Prevention. Reducing a woman's risk for cardiovascular diseases and some cancers includes:

- Controlling hypertension with weight reduction, better nutrition, stress management, and antihypertensive medications.
- Smoking cessation, which also reduces the risk for lung cancer and other respiratory diseases.
- Cholesterol and glucose control.
- Aerobic exercise.
- Low-dose (81 mg) aspirin each day.

DYSFUNCTIONAL UTERINE BLEEDING

Normal menstruation occurs every 20 to 35 days and lasts 2 to 7 days. Abnormal bleeding occurs more frequently, lasts longer, or is excessive in amount.

Etiology. The most common causes of abnormal bleeding are:

- Pregnancy complications, such as spontaneous abortion.
- Anatomic lesions, such as cervical polyps or uterine myomas.
- "Break-through" bleeding that may occur when oral contraceptives are used.
- Systemic disorders, such as diabetes mellitus, fibroids, or hypothyroidism.
- Failure to ovulate.

Management. Management depends on the cause, but may include:

- Use of progestin-estrogen combination oral contraceptives that suppress ovulation and allow a more stable endometrial lining to form.

- Surgical therapy, such as dilation and curettage, to remove polyps or to diagnose endometrial hyperplasia.
- Myomectomy for uterine fibroids.
- Hysterectomy if fibroids are large, bleeding persists, and the woman no longer desires to become pregnant.
- Laser ablation to remove endometrial lining.
- Iron supplementation to treat iron deficiency anemia.

Nursing Considerations. Nurses are often responsible for encouraging women to seek medical attention promptly when abnormal bleeding occurs. Nurses may help the woman keep a record of bleeding episodes and the amount of blood lost. Moreover, nurses can emphasize the importance of adequate nutrition and provide information about diagnostic procedures that may be necessary, such as ultrasound examination and endometrial biopsy.

PAIN ASSOCIATED WITH MENSTRUAL CYCLE
Primary Dysmenorrhea. Primary dysmenorrhea ("cramps") refers to menstrual pain without identified pathology. It occurs during ovulatory cycles and most often affects young, nulliparous women.

Etiology
- Excessive production of prostaglandin during luteal phase of menstrual cycle
- Diffusion of prostaglandin into endometrial tissue, causing uterine ischemia, hypoxia, and muscle contraction

Signs and Symptoms
- Colicky, spasmodic pain of the lower abdomen that occurs within hours of the onset of menses
- Sharp pain may radiate from the abdomen to the lower back or down the legs
- Nausea, vomiting, or diarrhea may accompany discomfort

Management

- Oral contraceptives that decrease amount of endometrial growth and thus reduce the production of endometrial prostaglandins
- Prostaglandin inhibitors such as ibuprofen (Motrin, Advil) or naproxen (Naprosyn, Anaprox)

Nursing Considerations

- Recommend nonpharmacologic measures such as frequent rest periods, application of heat to lower abdomen, moderate exercise, and well-balanced diet.
- Instruct that prostaglandin inhibitors are more effective if taken before onset of menses.
- Suggest that they be taken with meals to decrease gastric irritation.

Endometriosis

Etiology. The cause of endometriosis is unknown, although various theories have been advanced, including the following:

- Menstrual discharge contains viable endometrial cells that can attach to sites outside the uterus.
- Endometrial cells are disseminated primarily by retrograde menstruation or reflux of menstrual flow through the fallopian tubes.
- Tissue that is identical to that in the endometrium is present outside the uterus. The tissue proliferates during the follicular and luteal phases of the menstrual cycle and then sloughs during menstruation. Unlike menstruation, however, the bleeding occurs in a closed cavity, causing pressure and pain. Cyclic bleeding initiates chronic inflammatory changes throughout the pelvis and can cause infertility.

Signs and Symptoms

- Abdominal pain that is deep and constant, unlike the spasmodic pain of primary dysmenorrhea
- Dyspareunia (especially with deep penetration)

- Rectal pain
- Diarrhea, constipation, feelings of rectal pressure
- Infertility

Management. Treatment is aimed at interrupting the menstrual cycle so that bleeding is impeded. Therapeutic measures may include:

- Oral contraceptives to induce a pseudopregnancy and prolonged amenorrhea.
- Gonadotropin inhibitor such as danazol (Danocrine) that causes atrophy of endometrial tissue, anovulation, and amenorrhea.
- Drugs that interfere with the production of hormones needed for ovulation, such as leuprolide (Lupron) and nafarelin (Synarel) inducing a *pseudomenopause* while taken.
- Laparoscopy for lysis of adhesions and laser vaporization of lesions.
- Hysterectomy with bilateral salpingo-oophorectomy if the woman no longer wishes to conceive; hormone replacement therapy may be indicated after removal of endometriosis lesions.

Nursing Considerations. Nurses must provide information and support for the woman who often lives with a great deal of cyclic pain and uncertainty about future fertility. Common nursing responsibilities include:

- Validation that the woman is not pregnant; therapy should begin during menstrual cycle.
- Education about expected side effects of medication, such as hot flashes, weight gain, oily skin.
- Instruction to notify health care provider of unusual side effects, such as headache, dizziness, rapid weight gain (>5 lb per week), swelling of fingers or feet, jaundice, dark urine, or clay-colored stools.
- Recommendation not to delay pregnancy if the woman wishes to conceive.

PREMENSTRUAL SYNDROME (PMS)

Signs and Symptoms. Complaints of PMS can be divided into behavioral and physical symptoms. See Table 5-6, Symptoms of Premenstrual Syndrome (PMS).

Criteria for Diagnosis

- Signs and symptoms must be cyclic and recur in the luteal phase of the menstrual cycle.
- The woman should be symptom-free during the follicular phase of the cycle, and there must be at least 7 symptom-free days.
- Symptoms must be severe enough to have an impact on work, lifestyle, and relationships.
- Diagnosis must be based on charting of symptoms as they occur rather than recall of symptoms that occurred in the past; see Figure 5-1 for one type of calendar on which symptoms may be recorded.

Table 5-6	Symptoms of Premenstrual Syndrome (PMS)
Physical Symptoms	**Psychologic Symptoms**
Headaches, dizziness	Depressed mood
Abdominal bloating or swelling; edema of the extremities	Feelings of hopelessness Marked anxiety
Breast tenderness	Confusion, forgetfulness,
Hot flashes	poor concentration
Abdominal cramps	Accident proneness
Generalized muscle and joint pain	Irritability and anger Emotional lability, tearfulness,
Fatigue	ready to cry, lonely, mood
Appetite changes such as binge eating, cravings	instability Reduced interest in activities
Sleep changes such as insomnia or excessive sleep	of living Social avoidance
Reduced sexual interest	Lethargy or high energy

Calendar for PMS symptoms

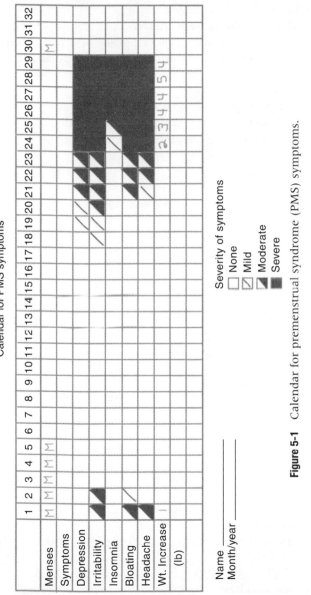

Figure 5-1 Calendar for premenstrual syndrome (PMS) symptoms.

Etiology

- Although the cause is unknown, there are several theories, such as biochemical responses of central hormones such as serotonin to normal hormone fluctuations that are part of the menstrual cycle.

Management. Treatment is based on the symptom profile of each individual woman, and there is little agreement on what is effective. Examples of therapy include:

- Relaxation therapy
- Exercise
- Reduction of salty foods, caffeine, chocolate, red meat, dairy products, and alcohol
- Small frequent meals
- Nutritional supplements such as calcium, magnesium, and vitamin E
- Evening primrose oil to reduce breast pain and tenderness
- Antianxiety drugs such as fluoxetine (Prozac), sertraline (Zoloft), or paroxetine (Paxil)

Nursing Considerations. Nurses can educate the family about lifestyle changes that may alleviate symptoms of PMS. The most common measures include the following:

- Decrease consumption of caffeine or other stimulants.
- Avoid simple sugars, which can cause rebound hypoglycemia.
- Restrict intake of salty foods, which increase fluid retention.
- Drink at least 2000 mL of water each day to maintain hydration.
- Eat six small meals per day to prevent episodes of hypoglycemia.
- Avoid alcohol, which can aggravate depression.
- Increase physical exercise for sense of well-being.

- Reduce stress by guided imagery, conscious relaxation techniques, warm baths, and massage.
- Adhere to a regular schedule for sleep and engage in relaxing activities before bedtime.
- Make concrete plans to obtain relief when she feels she is losing control or fears she may harm herself or a child.

MEDICAL TERMINATION OF PREGNANCY

Techniques used to terminate pregnancy depend on the length of gestation. Drugs may be used for medical abortion regimens during the first 7 weeks of pregnancy. Surgical techniques may be required for later pregnancy terminations.

- Drugs for medical abortion: mifepristone (RU486 or Mifeprex); misoprostol (Cytotec); methotrexate (Folex, Mexate)
- Surgical techniques to terminate pregnancy
  — Vacuum aspiration (to 13 weeks)
  — Dilation and evacuation (13-16 weeks)
  — Labor induction (after 16 weeks)

Nursing Considerations. Nurses must be knowledgeable about the current legal implications of medical termination of pregnancy in areas where they practice. For example, some states have laws that affect minors seeking an abortion. Other states have waiting periods and restrict abortion to specific periods of gestation. Moreover, nurses are often responsible for providing information about self-care measures following induced abortion. Major points of information include the following:

- Normal activities may be resumed, but strenuous work or exercise should be avoided for a few days.
- Bleeding or cramping may occur for a week or two; medical advice should be sought if either becomes severe.
- Sanitary pads, rather than tampons, should be used for the first week.

- Vaginal intercourse should be restricted for about a week or as ordered.
- Contraceptive measures when intercourse is resumed.
- Menstruation usually resumes in 4 to 6 weeks.
- Temperature should be taken twice a day; temperature above 37.8° C (100° F) should be reported to health care provider.
- $Rh_o(D)$ immune globulin (RhoGAM) as indicated.
- Follow-up appointment date and time.

MENOPAUSE

Menopause is the permanent cessation of menstruation after the loss of ovarian function. When the ovaries cease to function, the ovarian hormones, estrogen, and progesterone, fall. The average age of menopause in North America is 51½ years.

Signs and Symptoms of Menopause. Many of the signs and symptoms of menopause are due to a deficiency in estrogen.

- Amenorrhea
- Vasomotor instability (hot flashes, palpitations)
- Atrophic changes of the external genitalia, resulting in dyspareunia, atrophic vaginitis, or cystitis
- Adverse changes in serum lipids (increase in low-density lipoproteins, decrease in high-density lipoproteins) that increase the risk of coronary heart disease
- Decrease in bone density

Psychological responses to menopause vary widely, and a clear connection to estrogen deficiency has not been established.

- Depression
- Irritability
- Insomnia
- Fatigue
- Loss of libido

Hormone Replacement Therapy (HRT). Hormone replacement therapy may be recommended for women who have more severe physical and psychological problems during menopause. However, research results found in the Women's Health Initiative and other studies have demonstrated that some advantages thought to occur with HRT were not increased the risk for some disorders, primarily breast cancer and cardiovascular disease. A woman who may benefit from HRT to reduce menopausal symptoms must also consider risks associated with the specific therapy proposed.

If chosen, the type of hormone replacement depends on whether the woman has an intact uterus.

- Estrogen alone is prescribed for women who have had a hysterectomy and thus do not have the concern of endometrial hyperplasia.
- Estrogen and progesterone are prescribed for women who retain the uterus and are at risk for endometrial hyperplasia.

Contraindications and Cautions Related to Estrogen Replacement Therapy
- Previous breast cancer or other estrogen-dependent tumor
- Close family history of breast cancer
- Uterine cancer
- Unexplained abnormal vaginal bleeding
- Acute or chronic liver disease
- Gallbladder or pancreatic disease
- Recent vascular thrombosis or prior thromboembolic disorder when on estrogen
- Risk for cardiovascular disease
- Stroke
- Diabetes mellitus
- Conditions that may be worsened by fluid retention (migraine, epilepsy, cardiac, renal dysfunction, depression)

Nursing Considerations. Nurses are often the primary sources of information about measures to mitigate symptoms.

These measures are particularly helpful when the woman cannot or chooses not to take exogenous estrogen.

* Alternatives to estrogen such as botanical preparations should be discussed with the health care provider because they may interact with other drugs the woman takes. The website for more information on nonmedical therapies is the National Center for Complementary and Alternative Medicine of the National Institutes of Health (www. nccam.nih.gov)
* Water-soluble lubricants (Lubrin, Replens) for relief of vaginal dryness and dyspareunia
* Kegel exercises to increase tone in muscles around the vagina and urinary meatus that may atrophy without estrogen
* Drinking at least eight glasses of water a day to decrease urine concentration and reduce bacterial growth
* Wiping from front to back following urination or defecation to reduce transfer of bacteria from the anus to the urinary meatus
* Acknowledging symptoms, such as depression and irritability, that sometimes receive very little attention or sympathy

OSTEOPOROSIS

Osteoporosis is loss of bone density that leaves the bones porous, fragile, and susceptible to fractures. The vertebrae, wrists, and hips are the most common sites of fractures.

Risk Factors
* Slender, fair-skinned white and Asian women
* Family history of osteoporosis
* A sedentary lifestyle
* Early menopause (before 45 years)
* Alcoholism
* Smoking
* Anticonvulsants or corticosteroids
* Excessive amounts of caffeine
* Inadequate lifetime intake of calcium and vitamin D

Signs and Symptoms. Osteoporosis is sometimes called the "silent thief" because it takes place gradually without any signs or symptoms. The first noticeable signs are:

- Loss of height and back pain as vertebrae collapse.
- "Dowager's hump," which develops when vertebrae can no longer support the upper body. Disappearance of the waistline and protrusion of the abdomen as the ribs move toward the pelvis.
- Loss of bone mass demonstrated by dual energy x-ray absorptiometry (DEXA), ultrasound, or other methods of assessing bone density.

Prevention and Management
- Weight-bearing exercise (walking, aerobics)
- Adequate daily calcium intake by supplements (1200 mg/day for women older than 50, 1500 mg/day for women 65 years or older). Many young women need calcium supplements because of poor dietary calcium intake and other risk factors such as little exercise
- Vitamin D supplementation (400-800 mg/day for post-menopausal women or those with little exposure to direct sunlight)
- Decreasing risk factors (smoking, alcohol, caffeine)
- Estrogen replacement therapy (at least 0.625 mg/day)
- Calcitonin nasal spray (Calcimar, Miacalcin)
- Bisphosphonates (alendronate [Fosamax], risedronate [Actonel]) to inhibit bone resorption by osteoclasts
- Selective estrogen receptor modulator (raloxifene [Evista])

Nursing Considerations. In addition to providing information about diet, and exercise, and answering questions about medical regimen, nurses are also concerned about how to prevent falls. Teach the following important measures:

- Use ample lighting with easily available switches.
- Secure loose electrical cords.

- Area rugs should have nonskid backing.
- Install nonskid devices and grab bars by the bathtub.
- Install handrails by stairways.
- Keep loose items out of walking pathways.

PELVIC FLOOR DYSFUNCTION

When the muscles and ligaments of the pelvic floor become weakened, pelvic organs prolapse into the vagina. The most common problems are cystocele (the bladder protrudes downward into the vagina), rectocele (the rectum protrudes into the vagina), and uterine prolapse (the uterus sags backward and downward into the vagina). Enterocele (prolapse of the upper vaginal wall between the vagina and rectum) often accompanies uterine prolapse.

Etiology
- Genital atrophy that begins in the perimenopausal period
- Delayed result of traumatic childbirth
- Lifetime of lifting heavy objects
- Congenital defect of pelvic structures
- Coexistent medical disease (chronic respiratory disease, asthma) that may traumatize the pelvic supports

Signs and Symptoms
- Urinary incontinence
  - Stress incontinence (loss of urine with sudden increase in intraabdominal pressure, such as that generated by sneezing, coughing, lifting, or sudden jarring motions)
  - Urge incontinence (abrupt or strong desire to void)
  - Mixed incontinence (involuntary loss or "dribbling" of urine; associated with factors from both stress and urge incontinence patterns)
  - Overactive bladder (frequent sensations of urgency, nocturia)
- Constipation, flatulence, or difficulty defecating
- Feelings of pelvic fullness or pelvic pressure
- Low backache
- Fatigue

Management

- Surgical procedures such as anterior colporrhaphy (for cystocele), posterior colporrhaphy (for rectocele), and/or vaginal hysterectomy when other measures are unsuccessful
- Vaginal hysterectomy, often combined with anterior and posterior repair
- Rubber barrier insert for urethra for urinary incontinence
- Anticholinergic agents
- Bladder-neck support prosthesis to control stress incontinence
- Vaginal estrogen cream
- Vaginal pessary if surgery is not an option (pessary must be removed, cleaned, and replaced regularly)

Nursing Considerations

- Teach methods to strengthen pubococcygeal muscles (Kegel exercises, use of incrementally weighted vaginal cones).
- Initiate bladder retraining (gradually lengthen time between voiding) that enables women to accommodate greater volumes of urine.
- Suggest voiding according to a schedule that incorporates systematic delay of voiding by using distraction and relaxation techniques, self-monitoring, and positive reinforcement.
- Recommend drinking at least 2000 mL of fluid each day to prevent concentrated urine that can irritate the bladder.
- Advise to avoid or restrict alcohol and caffeine, which can aggravate bladder irritation.
- Provide information about practices to protect the skin and prevent odor (warm sitz baths, perineal care, thorough drying of genital area).
- Describe commercial products that trap urine and wick it away from the skin.
- Teach measures to prevent constipation.
  - Consume adequate dietary fiber and fluids.
  - Pay prompt attention to a feeling of rectal fullness.

— Use bulk producers, stool softeners, or stimulants as indicated or as recommended by health care provider.
— Exercise regularly.
- Instruct in measures to reduce discomfort, such as backache and pelvic pressure.
  — Lie down with legs elevated several times each day.
  — Assume knee-chest position for a few minutes as necessary.
  — Use biofeedback.
- Advise lifestyle changes (avoiding heavy lifting, weight reduction, cessation from smoking, and treatment of respiratory diseases).

BENIGN DISORDERS OF THE REPRODUCTIVE TRACT

Cervical Polyps. Polyps are small tumors, usually only a few millimeters in diameter, that are generally on a pedicle. They cause intermittent vaginal bleeding. They are surgically removed in an outpatient setting and sent for cytology examination to rule out the possibility of malignancy.

Uterine Leiomyomas (Fibroids). Fibroids develop from smooth muscle of the uterus. Growth is stimulated by estrogen and they may grow rapidly during the childbearing years. Fibroids may cause increased uterine size and excessive uterine bleeding. Treatment depends on size and may involve watchful waiting only. If abnormal bleeding is a problem, surgical intervention may be necessary and may include removal of the tumor (myomectomy), or removal of the uterus. Gonadotropin-releasing hormone agonists may reduce the size of the myoma and lessen the need for surgical removal.

Ovarian Cysts. Cysts are closed sacs filled with fluid or semifluids. They may be follicular (when the ovarian follicle fails to rupture during ovulation) or luteal (when the corpus luteum does not regress following ovulation). They are often asymptomatic, but may cause pain and some delay in the menstrual cycle. Treatment depends on differentiating a cyst from a solid tumor that may indicate cancer. Diagnosis may involve transvaginal ultrasound or laparoscopy.

If initial treatment involves watchful waiting, the woman should be instructed that

- Frequent pelvic examinations are necessary to monitor the size of the cyst.
- Oral contraceptives may be used for several months to suppress ovulation.
- Surgical removal may be necessary for large cysts or for cysts that do not shrink.
- Pain can usually be managed with analgesics and comfort measures such as application of heat to the abdomen.

MALIGNANT DISORDERS OF THE REPRODUCTIVE TRACT

The primary sites for cancer are the uterus, cervix, and ovaries.

Risk Factors. Risk factors vary according to the site of the cancer. See Table 5-7, Risk Factors for Cancer of the Reproductive Organs.

Signs and Symptoms. There are few signs and symptoms in the early stages of cancer of the female reproductive organs. Nurses must emphasize, however, that the following symptoms should *always* be reported:

- Irregular vaginal bleeding
- Unexplained postmenopausal bleeding
- Unusual vaginal discharge
- Dyspareunia
- Persistent vulvar or vaginal itching
- Elevated or discolored lesions on the vulva
- Persistent abdominal bloating or constipation
- Persistent anorexia or vomiting
- Blood in stools

Table 5-7	**Risk Factors for Cancer of the Reproductive Organs**

Uterus

African-Americans: higher risk for leiomyosarcoma
Obesity
Nulliparity
Middle-aged and elderly
Late menopause (>52 years)
Diabetes mellitus
Breast, colon, or ovarian cancer
Estrogen replacement therapy

Cervix

Human papillomavirus (HPV) infection
Sexual risks: young age at start of intercourse (<20 years), multiple sexual partners, uncircumcised male partners
Many pregnancies
Obesity
Diet low in fruits and vegetables
Smoking
Lower socioeconomic status (may be related to infrequent gynecologic examinations)
History of sexually transmitted diseases, such as chlamydia or human immunodeficiency virus (HIV) infection

Ovaries

Menses started at <12 years
No child or first child after 30 years
Late menopause (>55 years)
Infertility; infertility drugs
Family history of ovarian, breast, or colorectal cancer
Personal history of breast cancer

Diagnosis. Early diagnosis is strongly associated with long-term survival. In addition to screening procedures described earlier, a variety of diagnostic procedures are useful in early detection.

- Periodic pelvic examinations, Pap tests
- Testing for HPV that is linked to cervical cancer

- Serum tests, such as CA 125, for tumor markers. Genes linked to cancers of nonreproductive organs, such as BRCA1 or BRCA2, may lead to other diagnostic tests.
- Ultrasonography to distinguish fluid-filled cysts from solid tumors
- Endometrial biopsy to detect hyperplasia that may be associated with cancer
- Colposcopy that can identify patterns of abnormality near the cervical os where cancer often develops
- Conization (removal of a cone of tissue from the cervical canal) for diagnosis or for cure of preinvasive lesions of the cervix

Management. Treatment is based on the location and extent of the disease, as well as the age and desire of the woman to have children.

Cervical Cancer. Early treatment of cervical lesions may involve destruction of abnormal tissue.

- Cryosurgery to freeze abnormal cells, which then slough; normal tissue regenerates
- Laser surgery that allows for precise direction of a beam of light (heat) to remove diseased tissue
- Loop electrocautery excision procedure (LEEP), which often uses a wire-loop electrode that can excise tissue with minimal damage to surrounding tissue

Treatment of Invasive Cancer of the Cervix
- Hysterectomy
- Radiation therapy delivered by internal radium applications to the cervix or by external radiation therapy that includes lymphatics of the pelvis
- Chemotherapy

Endometrium. Treatment of uterine cancer depends on the extent of the cancer.

- Hysterectomy with bilateral salpingo-oophorectomy (BSO)

- Radical hysterectomy, BSO, and pelvic node dissection for more advanced disease
- Radiation therapy before or after surgery
- Chemotherapy for advanced or recurrent disease

Ovarian Cancer. Because the symptoms are vague and definitive screening tests do not exist, ovarian cancer is often diagnosed at an advanced stage. Palpation of an ovary in a postmenopausal woman or palpation of a pelvic mass is usually the first sign. Diagnostic and management procedures will vary according to the stage of cancer.

- Evaluation of bowel and urinary tract to detect invasion by ovarian cancer metastases
- Imaging and other diagnostic studies of the chest, liver, bone, and brain to detect metastasis to these organs
- Counseling regarding the possibility of temporary colostomy if tumor adheres to bowel
- Surgical removal of as much of the tumor as possible, plus excision of the uterus, fallopian tubes, and ovaries
- Chemotherapy plus counseling regarding the side effects and measures to control their adverse effects
- Posttherapy monitoring, which may include serial physical examinations, serum tumor marker determinations, and abdominal imaging
- Second-look surgery to determine the response of the disease to chemotherapy

Nursing Considerations. Most preoperative procedures are performed on an outpatient basis, and short hospital stays are common even for radical surgery. As a result, women need a great deal of information and support that nurses can provide and that often extends from diagnosis through home care. The extensiveness of surgery affects needed teaching. Nursing responsibilities may include providing information about the following:

- Preoperative procedures (ultrasonography, biopsies, etc.)

- Postoperative events and procedures (drainage tubes, suprapubic drains, intravenous fluids, nasogastric tube to prevent distention, and frequent evaluation of vital signs, wounds, urinary output, and bowel sounds)
- Postoperative care, such as pain management and measures to prevent hypostatic pneumonia (turning, coughing, breathing deeply)
- Discharge planning and teaching
  — Monitoring appetite and diet as well as bowel function and activity
  — Explaining that temporary vaginal discharge is expected even though uterus has been removed
  — Reminding her that she will no longer have menstrual periods
  — Encouraging questions about follow-up care such as chemotherapy or radiation
  — Facilitating a discussion about common fears that many women have such as fear of death or recurrence and concern about the effects on femininity or sexuality
  — Teaching measures to overcome anorexia, nausea, and diarrhea, which are common side effects of chemotherapy (frequent small meals, high-calorie snacks, protein shakes); to avoid rich fatty foods, alcohol, spicy foods, and carbonated drinks
  — Instructing about need and schedule for home follow-up appointments
  — Referring to appropriate support groups

SEXUALLY TRANSMITTED DISEASES (STDs)

Multiple diseases can be transmitted through sexual activity. For some diseases, such as syphilis, gonorrhea, or chlamydial infection, sexual activity is almost the only method of transmission. For other diseases, such as candidiasis or trichomoniasis, sexual activity may or may not be the mode of transmission. For information about signs and symptoms, diagnosis, and treatment, see Table 5-8. See pages 105-110 (Table 1-11) for impact of STDs on pregnancy and the fetus.

Text continued on p. 410

Table 5-8	Infections of the Reproductive Tract	

Some reproductive tract infections in this table are sexually transmitted, whereas others may or may not be transmitted sexually.

Signs and Symptoms	Diagnosis	Management
Syphilis (Spirochete *Treponema pallidum*)		
Primary stage: painless chancre of genitalia, lips, anus; Secondary stage: enlargement of spleen and liver, headache, generalized maculopapular rash; Tertiary stage: all body systems, including CNS, affected	Spirochete visible on dark-field examination. Positive serology (VDRL, RPR, or FTA-ABS) may not occur until after the primary stage.	Penicillin is the ideal antibiotic. A woman who is allergic to penicillin may be admitted to the hospital and desensitized prior to penicillin administration. Tetracycline is an alternative for those allergic to penicillin and not pregnant. Other effective antibiotics may include ceftriaxone or doxycycline.
Gonorrhea (*Neisseria gonorrhoeae*)		
May be asymptomatic in women; dysuria, purulent discharge, and dyspareunia are most common symptoms; pelvic pain indicates PID. Often coexists with chlamydial infection.	Identification of gonococci on culture of exudate from cervix, urethra, or other infected areas	Cefixime, ceftriaxone, ciprofloxacin. Many gonorrhea organisms have become resistant to penicillin and tetracycline. All sexual partners should be treated or the man should use a condom until a cure is confirmed.

Chlamydial Infection (*Chlamydia trachomatis*)

May be asymptomatic in women; dysuria, purulent discharge, abnormal vaginal bleeding, pelvic pain (PID). Often coexists with gonorrhea.	Tissue culture (most accurate but requires longer for results), antigen-antibody or ELISA tests	Azithromycin, doxycycline, clindamycin, ofloxacin, levofloxacin, or erythromycin should be used to treat all sexual partners.

Herpes Genitalis (Herpes simplex virus I or II [HSV])

Painful genital vesicles that ulcerate; fever, chills, muscle aches. More severe symptoms occur in a primary episode but all recurrences are as contagious as the primary episode.	Clinical signs and symptoms; culture of virus	No cure, but antiviral drugs include acyclovir, famciclovir, and valaciclovir. Sexual contact should be avoided while lesions are present and until a culture is negative. Prolonged viral shedding may occur, usually after the primary episode.

Condylomata Acuminata (Genital Warts) (Human papillomavirus [HPV])

Venereal or genital "warts" caused by HPV that may be small and discrete or may cluster and resemble a cauliflower. Sites include the vagina, labia, cervix, and perineal area.	Pap smear, colposcopy, or biopsy to identify abnormal tissue. Pap tests should be done more frequently because cervical cancer is more likely to occur when HPV infection has occurred.	Topical podophyllin, trichloroacetic acid (TCA) and bichloroacetic acid (BCA), or imiquimod cream. Cryotherapy, electrodessication, electrocautery, or laser therapy. The antineoplastic drug interferon may be used if there is no response to conventional therapy.

ELISA, Enzyme-linked immunosorbent assay; *FTA-ABS,* fluorescent treponemal antibody; absorption; *PID,* pelvic inflammatory disease; *RPR,* rapid plasma regain; *VDRL,* Venereal Disease Research Laboratory.

Continued

Table 5-8	Infections of the Reproductive Tract—cont'd	
Signs and Symptoms	Diagnosis	Management
Acquired Immunodeficiency Syndrome (AIDS) (Human Immunodeficiency Virus [HIV])		
Seroconversion usually within 6 months with flulike symptoms; asymptomatic period until there is destruction of cell-mediated immunity; opportunistic infections develop	Serology to detect antibodies (ELISA, IFA, Western blot)	Efavirenz, zidovudine, tenofovir, lamivudine, emtricitabine, didanosine, abacavir, stavudine, zalcitabine Protease inhibitors such as saquinavir, idinavir See http://aidsinfo.nih.gov/guidelines for updated information.
Hepatitis B (Hepatitis B Virus)		
Anorexia, nausea, vomiting, arthralgia, rash, jaundice, enlarged liver	HBsAg, HBeAg positive	Vaccine available
Candidiasis (*Candida albicans*)		
Vaginal and perineal itching and inflammation; thick white vaginal	Clinical signs and symptoms; visualization of organism	Nonprescription vaginal medications include butoconazole, miconazole,

discharge. Not considered a sexually transmitted infection but the male sexual partner may have inflammation and itching of the penis.		clotrimazole, terconazole, or nystatin. Fluconazole is a prescription medication that may be prescribed for a single oral dose.

Trichomoniasis (*Trichomonas vaginalis*)

Thin, malodorous, greenish yellow vaginal discharge; edema, itching, redness of the vulva	Identification of organism in a wet mount preparation	Metronidazole 2 g in a single oral dose or 500 mg twice daily for 7 days. Clotrimazole may be preferred if the woman is in early pregnancy.

Bacterial Vaginosis (*Gardnerella vaginalis*)

Grayish white vaginal discharge with "fishy" odor	Identification of clue cells in saline wet mount of the vaginal discharge	Metronidazole, clindamycin. Woman should refrain from sexual intercourse or the partner should use a condom until the infection is cured.

ELISA, Enzyme-linked immunosorbent assay; *HBsAg*, hepatitis B surface antigen to detect onset of infection; *HBeAg*, hepatitis Be antigen to detect degree of infectivity; *IFA*, immunofluorescence assay.

Text continued from p. 405.

PELVIC INFLAMMATORY DISEASE (PID)

Etiology. Bacteria invade the endocervical canal and cause cervicitis. The bacteria ascend to infect the endometrium, fallopian tubes, and pelvic cavity. The most common organisms are:

- *Neisseria gonorrhoeae.*
- Chlamydia trachomatis.

Signs and Symptoms. Some women are asymptomatic; however, the most common signs and symptoms are:

- Pelvic pain.
- Fever.
- Purulent vaginal discharge, irregular vaginal bleeding.
- Nausea, anorexia.
- Adnexal tenderness during bimanual examination.
- Leukocytosis, increased sedimentation rate.

Management
- Intravenous administration of cefoxitin or cefotetan, plus doxycycline or clindamycin plus gentamicin for women with serious infection that is manifested by fever, pain, and leukocytosis. After 48 hours of IV antibiotics, treatment may be changed to oral administration. Total duration of antibiotic treatment should be 14 days.
- Outpatient oral administration of antibiotics for women who are less ill and are able to comply with recommended regimen

Nursing Considerations. Nurses play an important role in teaching women how to protect themselves from STDs. Teaching should include measures to avoid exposure.

- Limit number of sexual partners.
- Avoid intercourse with those who have multiple partners or high-risk behaviors such as injectable drug use.

- Use barrier methods (latex condoms with spermicide containing nonoxynol 9, diaphragm with spermicide) to prevent STDs.
- Seek medical attention promptly after having unprotected sex with one who is suspected of having an STD or when vaginal discharge or genital lesions are apparent.
- Take medication as directed.
- Return for follow-up evaluation.

TOXIC SHOCK SYNDROME (TSS)

TSS is a rare but potentially fatal condition caused by toxin-producing *Staphylococcus aureus*.

Risk Factors
- Poor perineal hygiene
- Lack of handwashing before touching perineal area
- Menstruation
- Chronic vaginal infection
- Previous *S. aureus* wound infections
- Use of high-absorbency tampons
- Use of diaphragm or cervical cap, which may trap and hold bacteria if left in place for a prolonged period of time

Signs and Symptoms
- Sudden spiking fever
- Flulike symptoms (headache, sore throat, vomiting, diarrhea)
- Hypotension due to intravascular fluid leaking from blood vessels as a result of increased capillary permeability
- Generalized rash resembling sunburn
- Skin peeling from the palms of the hands and soles of the feet

Management
- Fluid replacement
- Administration of vasopressor drugs
- Antimicrobial therapy
- Corticosteroids to treat skin changes

Nursing Considerations. Nurses are often responsible for teaching measures to prevent TSS.

- Wash hands thoroughly before inserting tampons, diaphragm, or cervical cap.
- Change tampons at least every 1 to 4 hours.
- Avoid superabsorbent tampons.
- Use pads rather than tampons during hours of sleep, which usually range from 6 to 8 hours
- Do not use diaphragm during menstrual periods.
- Remove diaphragm within time recommended by health care provider.

Section 6

Procedures

CONTENTS

BLOOD GLUCOSE ASSESSMENT IN THE NEWBORN

1. Wash hands.
2. If the infant has not received a bath after birth, bathe the infant or wash the area to be used before puncturing the skin to avoid contamination of the puncture site with maternal blood on the infant's skin. This is especially important should the mother have a known or unknown infection such as hepatitis B or human immunodeficiency virus.
3. Gather supplies needed. Supplies may vary with different glucometers and for different types of tests.

Common supplies include gloves, alcohol wipe, 2 × 2–inch gauze, microlancet or commercial lancing device, adhesive bandage, cotton balls, pipettes, blood collecting devices (glucose screening reagent strips, blotting paper for phenylketonuria (PKU) tests, capillary tubes), cloth or commercial warming pack to warm heel.

4. Calibrate or program the glucometer and use quality control measures according to the manufacturer's guidelines.

5. Warm the infant's foot for a few minutes if it is cold or if blood is needed for several tests. Dampen a cloth with warm water and fasten it over the heel, or use a heel-warming pack according to directions. Use caution to prevent burning the infant's skin!

6. Provide comforting measures such as swaddling, providing a pacifier, allowing the mother to hold, or giving oral sucrose (according to hospital policy). Rate the infant's pain level before the procedure using an infant pain scale according to hospital policy.

7. Apply gloves.

8. Hold the heel in one hand. Palpate the bone of the heel and place the thumb or finger over the walking surface of the foot to avoid puncturing the calcaneus bone, which could result in osteomyelitis and to avoid damage to nerves and arteries. Choose a puncture site that has not been used before to decrease the chance of infection and scarring (Figure 6-1).

9. Clean the lateral heel with alcohol. Allow to dry or wipe dry with sterile gauze to prevent irritation to the tissues and diluting the specimen with alcohol.

10. Puncture the side of the heel with a lancet that punctures to a depth of less than 2 mm. Place lancet in a sharps container.

11. If automatic puncture device is used, place over appropriate site and activate according to manufacturer's directions.

12. Follow agency policy or manufacturer's direction for the type of test being performed about whether to wipe away the first drop of blood, how to collect the sample,

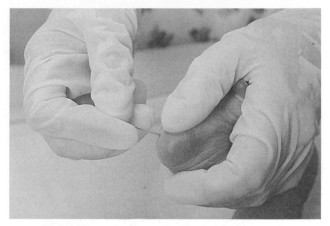

Figure 6-1 Correct site for heelstick in infants.

amount of blood to collect, proper handling, and reading of results.

13. Avoid excessive squeezing of the foot. Apply gentle pressure at a point higher than the puncture site if necessary. Obtain the blood sample.

14. Apply an adhesive bandage. Check the site frequently and remove the bandage when the bleeding stops.

15. Document the procedure and results. Send specimens to the laboratory as appropriate. Report abnormal readings and follow up according to agency policy.

BREAST SELF-EXAMINATION*

- Lie down. Flatten your right breast by placing a pillow under your right shoulder. If your breasts are large, use your right hand to hold your right breast while you do the examination with your left hand.

- Check the breast area from the collarbone at the top to the ribs on the bottom. Check your breast from the middle of your breast bone or sternum to an imaginary

*Modified from the American Cancer Society (ACS). (2003). *How to perform a breast self-exam.* Available at the ACS website: www.cancer.org.

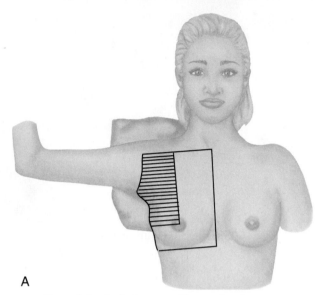

A

Figure 6-2 A-C, Breast self-examination.

line drawn straight down from the underarm. Check both breasts thoroughly in all directions until you feel ribs, the collarbone, and the breast bone.

- Use the sensitive pads of the middle three fingers on your left hand and a massaging motion to feel for lumps or changes in the breast tissue.
- Press firmly enough to distinguish different breast textures: light pressure to feel tissues near the skin, medium pressure to feel slightly deeper, and firm pressure to feel tissues near the chest and ribs.
- Completely palpate or feel all parts of the breast and chest area. Be sure to examine the breast tissue that extends toward the shoulder. The amount of time required to completely palpate all the breast tissue depends on the size of the breast. Women with small breasts need at least 2 minutes to examine each breast. Larger breasts take longer.

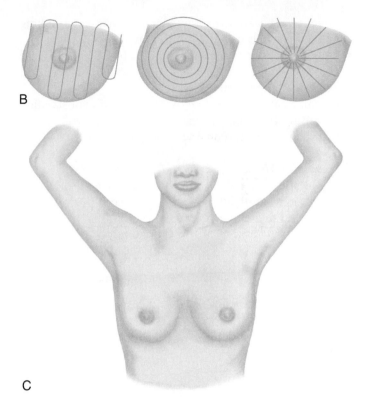

B

C

Figure 6-2   cont'd Breast self-examination.

- Use the same routine or pattern to feel every part of the breast tissue. Any of three patterns can help you make sure you have covered your entire breast: the vertical strip, the circular pattern, and the wedge. Choose the method you find easiest. Evidence suggests the up-and-down pattern is the most effective to avoid missing breast tissue.
- When you have completely examined your right breast, examine the left breast with your right hand using the same method. Compare what you feel in one breast with the other.

- You may also want to examine your breasts while bathing, when the skin is wet and lumps may be easily palpated.
- You can check your breasts in a mirror by raising your arms and looking for an unusual shape, dimpling of the skin, and any changes in the nipple.
- Examine each underarm, either when sitting or standing, by raising the arm. Raising your arm high will tighten tissues in the area, reducing what you can feel.

BULB SYRINGE USE

1. Position the infant's head to the side or hold the infant with the head slightly lower than the rest of the body.
2. Compress the bulb before inserting it into the mouth.
3. Gently insert the tip of the syringe into the side of the infant's mouth between the gum and the cheek. Do not insert it straight to the back of the throat because that could stimulate the gag reflex, causing regurgitation and could cause a vagal response resulting in bradycardia or apnea.
4. Release the bulb slowly to draw secretions into the mouth. Remove and empty it by compressing several times before using again.
5. Suction the nose, only if necessary, after the mouth is suctioned to prevent aspiration of secretions in the mouth if the infant gasps during nasal suction.
6. Suction the nose gently and avoid unnecessary suction because trauma could cause edema and obstruction of delicate nasal passages.

CONTRACTION PALPATION

Purpose: To determine whether a contraction pattern is typical of true labor. To identify abnormal contractions that may jeopardize the health of the mother or fetus.

1. Assess at least three contractions in a row at the time the fetal heart rate (FHR) is checked. Guidelines for minimal frequency of assessments are therefore:
   — Hourly during latent phase.
   — Every 30 minutes during active phase and transition.

    — Every 15 minutes during second stage.

Assess more frequently if abnormalities are identified.

2. Place fingertips of one hand on the uterine fundus, using light pressure. Keep fingertips relatively still rather than moving them over the uterus. The fingertips are more sensitive to the first tightening of the uterus. Contractions usually begin in the fundus, although the mother usually feels them in her lower abdomen and back. Constant moving of the hand over the uterus may stimulate contractions and give an inaccurate assessment of their true pattern.

3. Note the time when each contraction begins and ends.
   — Determine frequency by noting the average time that elapses from the beginning of one contraction to the beginning of the next one.
   — Determine duration by noting the average time in seconds from the beginning to the end of each contraction.
   — Determine interval by noting the average time between the end of one contraction and the beginning of the next one.

4. Estimate the average intensity of contractions by noting how easily the uterus can be indented during the peak of the contraction.
   — Mild contractions are easily indented with the fingertips. They feel similar to the tip of the nose.
   — Moderate contractions can be indented with more difficulty. They feel similar to the chin.
   — Firm contractions feel "woody" and cannot be readily indented. They feel similar to the forehead. Contractions during labor are expected to intensify progressively. If they do not the woman may not be in true labor or she may be experiencing dysfunctional labor.

5. Report hypertonic contractions.
   — Occurring less than 2 minutes apart, with a maximum number of no more than 5 contractions in 10 minutes

— Durations longer than 90 to 120 seconds
— Intervals shorter than 30 seconds
— Incomplete relaxation of the uterus between contractions

DEEP TENDON REFLEXES

Purpose: To determine if exaggerated reflexes (hyperreflexia) or diminished reflexes (hyporeflexia) exist

1. To assess the brachial reflex, support the woman's arm and instruct her to let it go totally limp while it is being held.
2. Place your thumb over the woman's tendon and strike the thumb with the small end of the reflex hammer. The normal response is slight flexion of the forearm.
3. The patellar reflex can be assessed in two positions, sitting or lying. When the woman is sitting, allow her lower legs to dangle freely to flex the knee and stretch the tendons. Strike the tendon with the reflex hammer just below the patella. The patellar reflex is less reliable in the woman who has had a recent epidural block and upper extremity reflexes should be assessed.
4. When the woman is in the supine position, the weight of her leg must be supported to flex the knee and stretch the tendons. Strike the partially stretched tendons just below the patella. Extension of the leg is the expected response.
5. Clonus should be tested, particularly when the reflexes are hyperactive. The woman's lower leg should be supported and the foot sharply dorsiflexed. Hold the stretch. With a normal response, no movement will be felt. When clonus is present, rapid rhythmic tapping motions of the foot are obvious.

DEEP TENDON REFLEX RATING SCALE

  0:   Reflex absent
+1:   Reflex present, hypoactive
+2:   Normal reflex

+3: Brisker than average reflex

+4: Hyperactive reflex; clonus may also be present

NOTE: The rating scales of some facilities omit the plus signs.

FERTILITY AWARENESS
Purposes:

- To identify whether ovulation occurs and the probable time of ovulation.
- To monitor therapeutic effects of drugs given to induce ovulation.

For additional information about fertility awareness, see the Planned Parenthood website (www.plannedparenthood.org).

BASAL BODY TEMPERATURE
The basal body temperature (BBT) is designed to detect the slight elevation in temperature that accompanies increased progesterone secretion in response to the luteinizing hormone (LH) surge and ovulation.

1. Teach the woman the relationship between her BBT and ovulation.
   — The BBT is the lowest, or resting, temperature of the body.
   — During the first half of a woman's menstrual cycle, her temperature is lower than during the second half of the cycle.
   — The basal temperature often drops slightly just before ovulation. Not all women experience this fall in basal temperature.
   — Progesterone is secreted during the second half of the cycle, rising just after ovulation. The BBT rises after the slight drop near ovulation and remains higher during the second half of the cycle.
   — The BBT remains higher if conception occurs and falls about 2 to 4 days before menstruation if conception does not occur.

2. Explain the occurrences that can interfere with the accuracy of her BBT. Examples include illness, restless or inadequate sleep (fewer than 6 hours), waking later than usual, traveling across time zones (jet lag), alcohol intake the evening before, sleeping under an electric blanket or on a heated waterbed, or performing any activity before taking the temperature.

3. Teach the woman how to take her basal temperature.
   — Show her an electronic thermometer that digitally displays tenths of a degree. Determine if she knows how to use it, and answer any questions.
   — Explain that she should place the thermometer under her tongue as soon as she awakens each morning and before any activity. It should remain in place until the electronic signal sounds because of the very slight rise in basal temperature at ovulation.

4. Show the woman the chart for recording her BBT and the symbols for marking relevant events, such as menstrual periods, intercourse, illness, or other occurrences that may alter her BBT. A string of colored beads may also be used, with different colors signifying whether the woman is having her menstrual flow (red), whether pregnancy is unlikely to occur (brown or tan), or if ovulation and fertility are likely (white).

5. Encourage the woman to demonstrate taking her temperature and recording the result. Ask her to list events other than ovulation that can alter the BBT.

6. As a method to avoid pregnancy: Explain that for the greatest effectiveness, a woman should avoid intercourse from the onset of the menstrual period through the second day of elevated temperature.

7. To enhance the chances of conception, this method has limited value because the rise in temperature indicates that ovulation has already occurred. It is helpful as a screening method to identify whether the woman is likely to be ovulating and if progesterone is secreted to prepare the endometrium for implantation.

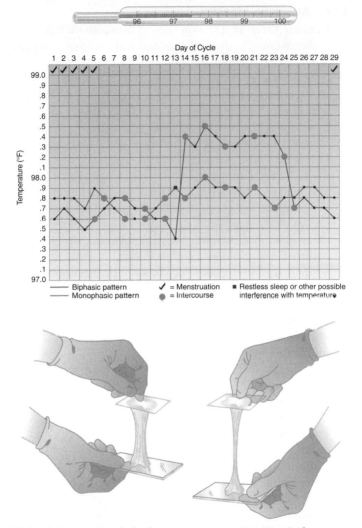

Figure 6-3   A, Basal body temperature. **B**, Cervical mucus assessment.

CERVICAL MUCUS ASSESSMENT

To facilitate survival of the sperm and promote their passage into the woman's uterus, the cervical mucus normally changes just before ovulation.

1. Teach the woman how her cervical mucus changes throughout the menstrual cycle. Spinnbarkeit describes how much the mucus can be stretched between her fingers or between a microscope slide and coverslip. Before and after ovulation, the cervical mucus is scant, thick, sticky, and opaque. It stretches less than 6 cm (2.3 inches). Just before and for 2 to 3 days after ovulation, the cervical mucus is thin, slippery, and clear and is similar to raw egg white. It stretches 6 cm or more. When this ovulatory mucus is present, the woman has probably ovulated and could become pregnant.

2. Explain common causes of changes in the mucus that are not related to fertility. It may be thicker if she takes antihistamines. Vaginal infections, contraceptive foams or jellies, sexual arousal, and semen can make the mucus thinner even if ovulation has not occurred. Tell her to record these factors.

3. Suggest that the woman simulate stretching mucus using raw egg white at home.

4. Teach the woman to wash her hands before and after assessing her mucus.

5. Teach the woman to use a tissue to obtain a small sample of mucus several times a day from just inside her vagina and to note the following:
   — The general sensation of wetness (around ovulation) or dryness (not near ovulation) on her labia
   — The appearance and consistency of the mucus: thick, sticky, and whitish; or thin, slippery, and clear or watery
   — The distance the mucus will stretch between her fingers, usually at least 6 cm (2.3 inches) at the time of ovulation.

6. Have the woman record the day's mucus characteristics (often combined with the BBT recording).

7. As a method of contraception, the woman should avoid intercourse from the time the thin, stretchy ovulatory mucus appears until 4 days after the end of the slippery mucus. *Avoiding intercourse reduces the chance that sperm are available for fertilization while the ovum is viable.*

8. To enhance chances of conception, the couple should have intercourse every 2 days during the period of ovulatory mucus (approximately days 12 to 16 if the woman has a 28-day cycle). Ovulation predictors available over-the-counter provide added predictive information that the woman trying to conceive may need.

FETAL HEART RATE AND CONTRACTION MONITORING, EXTERNAL
Purposes:

- To properly apply the external electronic fetal monitor.
- To perform a basic evaluation of the fetal heart rate (FHR) and uterine activity patterns.

1. Read instruction manual for equipment.

2. Perform a function test following manufacturer's instructions. Press TEST button and observe for result. Common correct test results are the following:
   - Fetal heart rate: The monitor prints a line at 120, 150, or 200 bpm, depending on the model.
   - Uterine activity: The monitor adds 50 to uterine activity display.

3. Explain the basic procedure of electronic fetal monitoring to the woman and her partner or family. Vary instructions according to equipment being used and hospital protocols. A sample is:
   - Using the electronic fetal monitor is the way we normally assess the baby's response to labor contractions.
   - Two belts go around your abdomen, one for the fetal heart rate sensor and one for contractions.
   - Feel free to move with the monitor on. If the tracing is poor, we can adjust the sensors.

4. Apply belts or stockinette if an adhesive ring is not used:
   — Slide both belts under the woman's back without the sensors attached. Be sure to keep the belts smooth under her back.
   — Cut a length of stockinette tubing about 15 to 18 inches long for the average-sized woman. Cut a longer length of wide stockinette for a heavier woman. Slide the stockinette up from her feet to her abdomen.
5. Use Leopold's maneuvers (see p. 435) to locate the fetal back as in Fetal Heart Rate Auscultation, p. 428.
6. Apply ultrasound gel to the Doppler ultrasound transducer and place it on the woman's abdomen at the approximate location of the fetus's back. Move the transducer until a clear signal is heard. Most bedside units have a green light or flashing heart shape to indicate a good signal.
7. Place the uterine activity sensor in the fundal area or the area where contractions feel the strongest when palpated. This is often near the umbilicus. When the woman has a contraction, observe the tracing for the bell shape. The line for uterine activity is jagged because it also senses the rise and fall of the abdomen with breathing. Fetal or maternal movement, coughing, or sneezing causes a spike in the line. Observe through several contractions.
8. Observe the strip for baseline FHR, presence of variability, periodic changes, and uterine activity (contraction duration, and frequency). Palpate contractions for intensity and relaxation between contractions. Notify the physician or nurse-midwife of nonreassuring patterns:
   — Contractions having a frequency greater than every 2 minutes or more than 5 contractions in a 10-minute time period
   — Contraction durations longer than 90 to 120 seconds
   — Resting intervals shorter than 30 seconds
   — Incomplete uterine relaxation between contractions

FETAL HEART RATE AND CONTRACTION MONITORING, INTERNAL

Purpose: To provide a record of the fetal heart rate and uterine contractions during labor that may be more accurate than external methods.

NOTE: Women often have a combination of external and internal electronic fetal monitoring, usually external contraction monitoring and internal fetal heart rate monitoring.

1. Perform steps 1 through 3 under the external monitoring procedure. Read also the directions for insertion on the packages of the intrauterine pressure catheter (IUPC) and the fetal scalp electrode.
2. The membranes must be ruptured to allow internal electronic monitoring. The cervix must be dilated enough to identify the fetal presenting part and to allow passage of the spiral electrode or IUPC.
3. Use sterile technique for insertion of internal monitor leads. Cleanse the woman's perineum according to the facility's protocol. Avoid iodine solutions if the woman is allergic to iodine, seafood, or x-ray contrast media.
4. Insert the IUPC, following specific directions on the package. Connect to the proper port on the fetal monitor. If a fluid-filled catheter is used, the transducer that joins it to the monitor should be at the height of the tip within the uterus. Both catheters must be "zeroed" to compensate for atmospheric pressure, and some solid catheters must be zeroed before insertion.
5. Apply the internal spiral electrode to the fetal presenting part. Avoid the face, fontanels, or genitalia. After locating the place for application (usually on the parietal bone), slide the electrode within its guide (outer) and drive (inner) tubes between the examining fingers to the presenting part. While maintaining pressure of the guide tube against the presenting part, turn the drive tube clockwise until the electrode wire catches in the skin. Release the electrode wires from the clamp on the outer

part of the tube and pull the drive tube, then the guide tube, out. Connect the wires to the leg plate on the woman's thigh and the leg plate to the monitor.
6. Documentation should be the same as for external monitoring.

FETAL HEART RATE AUSCULTATION*

Purpose: To evaluate the fetal condition and tolerance of labor.

1. Explain the procedure to give information to the woman and her partner. Wash your hands with warm water to reduce the transmission of microorganisms and to make your hands more comfortable when touching the woman's abdomen.
2. Use Leopold's maneuvers (p. 435) to identify the fetal back because it usually is closest to the surface of the maternal abdomen, where fetal heart sounds are clearest. Illustrations show approximate locations of the fetal heart rate in different presentations and positions.
3. Assess the fetal heart rate with a fetoscope or Doppler transducer. The external fetal monitor may be used but is more often used for intermittent electronic fetal monitoring (short periods of electronic monitoring interspersed with periods of no fetal surveillance, such as maternal ambulation).
4. Fetoscope: Place the bell of the fetoscope over the fetal back with the head plate pressed against your forehead to add bone conduction to the sound coming through the earpieces. Move the fetoscope until you locate where the sound is loudest. Use your forehead to maintain pressure during auscultation to enhance the faint fetal heart sounds.

*Modified from Feinstein, N.F., Torgersen, K.L., & Atterbury, J. (Eds.). (2003). *AWHONN's fetal heart monitoring: Principles and practices* (3rd ed.). Dubuque, IA: Kendall/Hunt.

LOA

ROA

LOP

ROP

LSA

RSA

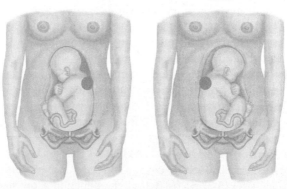

Figure 6-4 Auscultating the fetal heart rate.

5. Doppler transducer: Review the manufacturer's instructions for operating the Doppler device. Place water-soluble conducting gel over the transducer to make an interface for clear signal transmission, and turn it on. Place the transducer over the fetal back and move it until you hear clear sounds that represent the fetal heart motion.

6. With one hand, palpate the mother's radial pulse to verify that the fetal heart rate is what is actually heard. If her pulse is synchronized with the sounds from the fetoscope or Doppler transducer, try another location for the fetal heart. Other sounds that may be represented by the Doppler are the funic souffle (blood flowing through the umbilical cord) or uterine souffle (blood flowing through the uterine vessels). The funic souffle is synchronized with the fetal heart and is the same rate; the uterine souffle is synchronized with the mother's pulse.

7. Count the baseline fetal heart rate for 30 to 60 seconds between contractions. Assessment during a contraction may clarify findings, but auscultation is difficult during contractions. Note accelerations or slowing of the rate.

8. Note reassuring signs that suggest the fetus is tolerating labor well.
   — An average rate of 110 to 160 bpm
   — Regular rhythm
   — Accelerations from the baseline rate
   — No decrease in rate from the baseline rate

9. Note nonreassuring signs, and make more frequent assessments. Notify the physician or nurse-midwife for further evaluation.
   — Heart rate outside normal limits. Unexplained tachycardia or bradycardia for 10 minutes or longer
   — Irregular rhythm
   — Gradual or abrupt decrease in rate

GAVAGE FEEDING ADMINISTRATION

1. Wash hands. Gather equipment: gavage catheter of proper size (3.5, 5, or 8 French, depending on size of the infant), measured container, and 20-mL syringe.

Warm breast milk or formula to room or body temperature. Check the chart to determine how previous feedings were tolerated. Add fortifier to breast milk if necessary.

2. Don gloves. Position the infant on the right side or prone if the infant tends to regurgitate when moved after feedings. If parents are present, they may hold the infant in their arms once the catheter is inserted or hold the hands if the infant cannot be held.

3. Determine the length of catheter to insert. For orogastric insertion, measure from the mouth to the ear to the xiphoid process. For nasogastric feedings, measure from the infant's nose to the earlobe and to the end of the xiphoid process and add 1 cm or measure from the ear to the nose and then to the midpoint between the xiphoid process and the umbilicus. Mark the catheter at the proper point with a piece of tape or indelible ink. If the tube is to be indwelling, check every 4 to 8 hours to see that the mark or tape remains in the same place.

4. Give the infant a pacifier. Moisten the tip of the catheter. Hold the infant's head steady and gently insert the catheter through the mouth or nose to the point marked. Remove the catheter immediately if persistent coughing, choking, cyanosis, apnea, or bradycardia occurs.

5. Check for placement when the catheter is first placed, before beginning bolus feedings, and at least once a shift for continuous feedings.
   — Attach a syringe to the catheter and insert 1 to 2 mL of air through the tube while listening over the stomach with a stethoscope. Gently draw back on the plunger to withdraw the inserted air. Hearing air enter the stomach may show the catheter is in place, but is not as accurate as pH testing of gastric aspirate.
   — Gently aspirate stomach contents. Move or rotate the catheter slightly if the plunger does not withdraw easily. Check the pH of the aspirate to be sure it is gastric content.

6. Secure the catheter in place with an adhesive dressing.
7. Withdraw the stomach contents. Observe the amount, color, and consistency of the aspirate. During continuous feedings, check the gastric residual every 2 to 4 hours. Do not feed the infant if the aspirate is abnormal. Report abnormal appearance or amount of stomach contents. The residual should not be more than the hourly volume or 2 to 4 mL/kg.
8. Replace the aspirate before beginning the feeding or discard according to agency policy. If it is replaced, subtract the amount of gastric residual from the amount of milk to be given.
9. Remove the plunger and attach the syringe to the feeding tube. Pour the correct amount of solution into the syringe. Attach to a feeding pump that will regulate the amount of flow.
10. If using gravity flow, raise or lower the syringe to increase or decrease the rate of flow so that the feeding moves slowly into stomach over 15 to 30 minutes.
11. For continuous feedings, place no more than a 2- to 4-hour supply of milk into a feeding bag or syringe. Set the pump to deliver the correct rate of flow. Change the equipment every 4 hours or according to hospital policy.
12. Give the infant a pacifier during the feeding to help prepare for nippling and to provide comfort.
13. For intermittent feedings with a catheter that remains in place, clear the catheter with air or sterile water according to agency policy and close off the end when the feeding is completed.
14. When the catheter is to be withdrawn, pinch the catheter and remove it quickly to prevent drops of milk from entering the trachea as the catheter is removed.
15. Burp the infant, and position on the right side or prone, with the head of the bed elevated 35 to 45 degrees. If movement tends to cause regurgitation, omit burping. Allow the infant to remain on the right side or prone.

16. Record time, amount, and characteristics of gastric residual, type and amount of feeding given, and how the infant tolerated it.

INFANT IDENTIFICATION

1. Always identify infants and mothers (or support persons) with identification (ID) bands when reuniting them, even after a brief separation.
2. When taking infants into mothers' rooms, unwrap the blankets to expose the ID band on the infant's wrist or ankle. Do *not* rely on memory of the number.
3. Explain the ID procedure and its purpose to the mother. Show her the imprinted ID number on her band and the matching number on the infant's bands.
4. Look at the number on the infant's band and ask the mother to read off the ID number on her band. Do *not* reverse the process by reading the infant's number to the mother because the mother might indicate that the numbers are correct when they are not.
5. An alternative procedure is for the nurse to compare the mother's and the infant's bands visually if the mother does not speak English well or might have difficulty with the process.
6. If the infant is to be released to a support person who is wearing an identification band, follow the same identification procedure.

INTRAMUSCULAR INJECTION ADMINISTRATION TO NEWBORNS

1. Wash the infant's thigh if the bath has not yet been given to remove maternal blood that may be present on the infant's skin.
2. Prepare the medication for injection. Use a 1-mL syringe and a filter needle to draw up medications in glass ampules to prevent particles of glass from being drawn into the syringe. Remove the filter needle and place a 25-gauge ⅝" needle on the syringe to give the injection.
3. Put on gloves.

4. Locate the correct site (Figure 6-5). The best site for intramuscular injections is the infant's vastus lateralis muscle. Divide the area between the greater trochanter of the femur and the knee into thirds. Give the injection in the middle third of the muscle, lateral to the midline of the anterior thigh. (Note: The gluteal muscles are never used until a child has been walking for at least a year. These muscles are poorly developed and dangerously near the sciatic nerve.)
5. Cleanse the area with an alcohol wipe.
6. Stabilize the leg firmly while grasping the thigh between the thumb and fingers.
7. Insert the needle at a 90-degree angle.
8. Aspirate and inject the medication slowly if no blood returns. If blood returns, withdraw the needle. Discard the medication and syringe and prepare new medication.

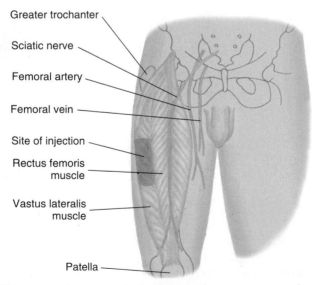

Greater trochanter

Sciatic nerve

Femoral artery

Femoral vein

Site of injection

Rectus femoris muscle

Vastus lateralis muscle

Patella

Figure 6-5   Correct site for intramuscular injection in infants.

9. Withdraw the needle and apply gentle pressure to the site with an alcohol wipe.

LEOPOLD'S MANEUVERS

Purpose: To determine presentation and position of the fetus and aid in location of fetal heart sounds.

1. Explain the procedure to the woman and the rationale for each step as it is performed. Tell her what is found at each step.
2. Ask the woman to empty her bladder if she has not done so recently. Have her lie on her back with her knees flexed slightly. Place a small pillow or folded towel under one hip.
3. Wash your hands with warm water. Wear gloves if contact with secretions is likely.
4. Stand beside the woman, facing her head, with your dominant hand nearest her.

First Maneuver
5. Palpate the uterine fundus. The breech (buttocks) is softer and more irregular in shape than the head. Moving the breech also moves the fetal trunk. The head is harder and has a round, uniform shape. The head can be moved without moving the entire fetal trunk.

Second Maneuver
6. Hold the left hand steady on one side of the uterus while palpating the opposite side of the uterus with the right hand. Then hold the right hand steady while palpating the opposite side of the uterus with the left hand. The fetal back is a smooth, convex surface. The fetal arms and legs feel nodular, and the fetus often moves them during palpation.

Third Maneuver
7. Palpate the suprapubic area. If a breech was palpated in the fundus, expect a hard, rounded head in this area.

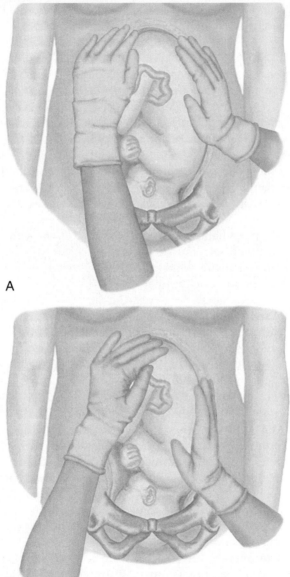

A

B

Figure 6-6 A, First maneuver. **B**, Second maneuver.

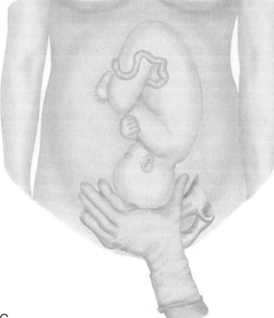

C

Figure 6-6 cont'd C, Third maneuver.

Continued

Attempt to grasp the presenting part gently between the thumb and fingers. If the presenting part is not engaged, the grasping movement of the fingers moves it upward in the uterus.

8. Omit the fourth maneuver if the fetus is in a breech presentation.

Fourth Maneuver
9. Turn so that you face the woman's feet.
10. Place your hands on each side of the uterus with fingers pointed toward the pelvic inlet. Slide hands downward on each side of the uterus. On one side, your fingers easily slide to the upper edge of the symphysis. On the other side, your fingers meet an obstruction, the cephalic

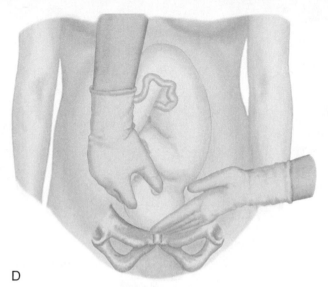

D

Figure 6-6 cont'd D, Fourth maneuver.

prominence. If the head is flexed, the cephalic prominence (the forehead in this case) is felt on the opposite side from the fetal back. If the head is extended, the cephalic prominence (the occiput in this case) is felt on the same side as the fetal back.

PEDIATRIC URINE COLLECTION BAG APPLICATION

1. Wash and dry the genitalia. Apply tincture of benzoin according to hospital policy. Allow to dry until tacky.
2. Remove the paper covering on the posterior adhesive tabs of the bag first. To apply to female infants, stretch the perineum (skin between the rectum and the vagina). Fold the bag in half and apply smoothly over the perineum, extending the tabs to the side. For male infants, place the penis and scrotum (if small) inside the bag and apply the posterior adhesive tabs to the perineum. If the scrotum will not fit in the bag easily, apply the tabs smoothly over the scrotum.

3. Remove the paper covering on the anterior adhesive tabs, and apply to cover the genitalia. Be sure that there are no wrinkles in the tabs.
4. Cut a slit in the diaper and gently pull the bag through the slit. Apply the diaper loosely.
5. Check the bag for urine frequently and remove it as soon as urine is present. Transfer the urine to a specimen cup by removing the tab over the hole in the bottom and pouring. The specimen also can be aspirated with a syringe after cleaning the puncture site with alcohol.
6. Clean the genitalia, and observe for irritation.
7. Label the specimen and transport to the lab or refrigerate if necessary. Record in the infant's chart.

PERINEAL ASSESSMENT
1. Provide privacy, and explain the purpose of the procedure.
2. Put on clean gloves.
3. Ask the mother to assume a Sims (side-lying) position and flex her upper leg; lower the perineal pads, and lift her superior buttock. Use a flashlight (if necessary) to inspect the perineal area.
4. Note the extent and location of edema or bruising.
5. Examine the episiotomy or laceration for redness, ecchymosis, edema, discharge, and approximation (REEDA).
6. Note the number and size of hemorrhoids.

RESUSCITATION IN NEWBORNS*
NOTE: Although this procedure is listed by steps, several steps may be performed at the same time. Because two people often are working together, more than one step can be performed at one time.

1. Place the infant under a preheated radiant warmer immediately.

---

*Data from Kattwinkel, J., American Academy of Pediatrics, & American Heart Association. (2000). *Textbook of neonatal resuscitation* (4th ed.). Elk Grove Village, IL: American Academy of Pediatrics and American Heart Association.

2. Position the infant with the neck in a neutral or slightly extended ("sniffing") position to open the airway. Avoid hyperextension or flexion of the neck. Place a small folded blanket under the shoulders.

3. Suction the mouth and then the nose. Endotracheal intubation may be necessary to clear the airway if meconium is present.

4. Dry and stimulate the infant if necessary. (Drying is often performed simultaneously with the previous steps.) Gently rub the infant's back or body, or flick or slap the soles of the feet.

5. If no response occurs after stimulating once or twice, stop and initiate immediate resuscitation. Do not delay resuscitation to continue stimulating or until the Apgar scores are given.

6. Remove wet linens and reposition the head as necessary.

7. Give 100% oxygen if the infant is breathing but cyanotic. Hold the oxygen mask or tubing close to the infant's nose (called "blow-by" oxygen).

8. Evaluate the respirations, heart rate, and color. Use a stethoscope or feel the pulsations at the base of the cord. Count for 6 seconds and multiply by 10 to obtain the heart rate per minute. Positioning, clearing the airway, drying, stimulating, and providing oxygen should take no more than 30 seconds.

9. Begin positive-pressure ventilation with an appropriately sized bag and mask if the infant fails to breathe spontaneously with initial stimulation, has gasping respirations, or the heart rate is 100 beats per minute or less when respirations have begun. The mask should fit well, covering the chin, mouth, and nose but not the eyes.

10. Attach the bag to an oxygen source with 100% oxygen. Place the mask snugly over the infant's nose and mouth. Squeeze the bag gently to force air into the infant's lungs. Use a bag with a manometer to show the amount of pressure being used and a flow-control valve that can

be adjusted to control the pressure delivered to the infant. Or use a bag with a pressure release valve that releases if the pressure is high enough to cause lung damage. The initial breaths require pressures of 30 to 40 cm H_2O to inflate the lungs. Less pressure is used for subsequent breaths but varies with the infant's condition.

11. If bag-and-mask ventilation is necessary for more than a few minutes a feeding tube is inserted through the mouth to the stomach and left open to the air.

12. Observe the rise and fall of the chest during ventilation. If the chest does not move, suction secretions and reposition the head and the mask. Ventilate the infant at a rate of 40 to 60 breaths per minute until the infant is breathing spontaneously and the heart rate is above 100 bpm.

13. If the heart rate is less than 60 bpm after 30 seconds of effective assisted ventilation, a second person should begin chest compressions while the first continues to ventilate the infant.

14. Compress the chest by placing the hands around the infant's chest with the fingers under the back to provide support and the thumbs over the lower third of the sternum (just below an imaginary line between the nipples and above the xiphoid process) (Figure 6-7). An alternate method is to use two fingers of one hand to compress the chest with the other hand under the back to provide support.

15. Compress the sternum to a depth of approximately one third of the anterior-posterior diameter of the chest and sufficient to cause a palpable pulse. Do not remove the fingers from the chest between compressions.

16. Use three compressions followed by one ventilation for a combined rate of compressions and ventilations of 120 each minute. This is 90 compressions and 30 ventilations each minute. Pause for $\frac{1}{2}$ second after every third compression for ventilation.

17. Check the heart rate after approximately 30 seconds. If it is 60 bpm or more, discontinue compressions but

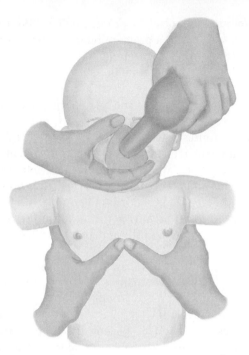

Figure 6-7 Performing resuscitation in newborns.

continue ventilation until the heart rate is greater than 100 bpm and spontaneous breathing begins. If the heart rate is less than 60 bpm after 30 seconds of effective assisted ventilation and compressions, epinephrine will be necessary. Endotracheal intubation may be performed at this point if not performed previously.

18. Prepare medications, if necessary. Epinephrine and naloxone may be given through an umbilical vein catheter or endotracheal tube. Intravenous volume expanders may include normal saline, Ringer's lactate, or type O-negative red blood cells. Sodium bicarbonate is given intravenously only after prolonged arrest and with effective ventilation.

RUPTURED MEMBRANES, TESTING FOR

Purpose: To help clarify if membranes are ruptured, or if the woman is having episodes of urinary incontinence.

1. Equipment
   — Disposable gloves (sterile if a vaginal exam will immediately follow)
   — Test to identify pH, such as nitrazine tape (about 5 cm [2 inches] long) or test swabs for this purpose
   — Slide and microscope if ferning will be tested.
2. Test for rupture of membranes *before* using lubricant for a vaginal examination.
3. Nitrazine tape: Touch the tape against wall of the vagina. Compare the color with the scale on the nitrazine tape or swab container. A color change to blue-green or dark blue (pH ≥6.5) suggests that the membranes are ruptured. A commercial swab test allows more accurate pH testing of a deeper pool of vaginal fluid.
4. Fern test: Spread a sample of vaginal secretions on a glass slide and allow it to dry. Examine the slide under a low-power microscope to identify the typical fern pattern of dry amniotic fluid.

UTERINE FUNDUS ASSESSMENT, POSTPARTUM

1. Explain the procedure and rationale for each step before beginning the procedure.
2. Ask the mother to empty her bladder if she has not voided recently.
3. Place the mother in a supine position with her knees slightly flexed to relax the abdominal muscles.
4. Put on clean gloves; lower the perineal pads to observe lochia as the fundus is palpated.
5. Place the nondominant hand above the woman's symphysis pubis.
6. Use the flat part of the fingers (not the fingertips) for palpation.

7. Begin palpation at the umbilicus and palpate gently until the fundus is located. Note firmness and location of the fundus. The fundus should be firm, in the midline, and approximately at the level of the umbilicus.

8. If the fundus is difficult to locate or is soft or "boggy," keep the nondominant hand above the symphysis pubis and massage the fundus with the dominant hand until the fundus is firm.

9. After the boggy fundus is massaged until it is firm, press down to expel clots. Keep one hand pressed firmly just above the symphysis to prevent uterine inversion while expelling clots. Never attempt to expel clots if the fundus is not firm.

10. If the fundus is above or below the umbilicus, use your fingers to determine the number of fingerbreadths or centimeters between the fundus and the umbilicus.

11. Document the consistency and location of the fundus. Consistency is recorded as "fundus firm," "firm with massage," or "boggy." Fundal height is recorded in fingerbreadths or centimeters above or below the umbilicus. Examples: "fundus firm, midline, ↓1" (1 fingerbreadth below the umbilicus); "fundus firm with light massage, U+2" (2 fingerbreadths above umbilicus), displaced to right.

VAGINAL EXAMINATION DURING LABOR
Purposes:

- To determine cervical effacement and dilation.
- To determine fetal presenting part, position, and station
- To determine status of amniotic membranes

NOTE: Vaginal examination should not be done if the woman is having active bleeding. Bloody show is not a contraindication.

1. Equipment:
   — Sterile gloves
   — Sterile water-soluble lubricant

— Nitrazine or other pH test if needed to check for ruptured membranes; slide to check for ferning under the microscope that indicates membrane rupture

2. Have the woman lie on her back with her head slightly elevated. Place a small pillow or wedge under one hip. Drape her to minimize exposure. Just before the examination, have her flex her thighs and abduct them, placing her heels together.

3. Open the gloves and lubricant. Place a small amount of lubricant on an unused part of the glove wrapper.

4. Obtaining fluid to detect membrane rupture or send for culture and sensitivity tests should be obtained without lubricant.

5. Separate the inner labia with the gloved nondominant hand to reveal the vaginal opening. Insert the lubricated and gloved index and middle fingers of the dominant hand into the vagina.

6. Gently move the fingers upward to locate the cervix. Have the woman take slow deep breaths if she tenses during the examination.

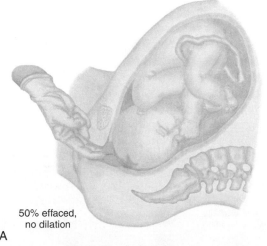

50% effaced,
no dilation

A

Figure 6-8   **A**, Hand position.

Continued

7. Determine if the amniotic sac is intact. It feels like a slippery membrane over the presenting part or a slick, fluid-filled balloon. The "balloon" has varying amounts of pressure behind it. If membranes have ruptured, manipulating the cervix often causes amniotic fluid to leak from the vagina. Note the color, odor, and amount of any fluid that leaks from the vagina during the exam.

8. Palpate the fetal presenting part to distinguish a vertex presentation from others. This is easier to do if the membranes are ruptured.

   — Vertex presentation: The nurse feels the hard, round surface of the fetal head. The triangular posterior fontanel is palpable if the head is well flexed. Caput (edema) may make it impossible to feel suture lines or fontanels.

   — Face presentation: The nurse feels an irregular surface and may elicit the fetal suck reflex as the finger is passed over the mouth.

   — Frank breech: The nurse feels a somewhat more irregular surface than the head, although the hip

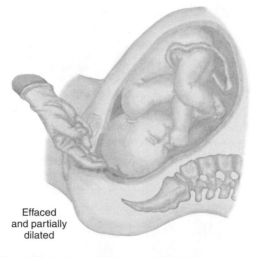

Effaced
and partially
dilated

B

Figure 6-8   cont'd B, Determining cervical effacement and dilation.

area may feel quite similar to the head. Fresh meconium stool (black and thick) is often passed during a frank breech labor.

— Footling breech: The nurse feels the small irregular surface of the fetal foot. Touching the foot often causes the fetus to curl it or draw it upward. The fetal hand will feel similar, but touching the hand may elicit the grasp reflex.

9. Palpate the cervix to identify:

— Dilation in centimeters. The dilation may range from closed to 10 cm (about 4 inches). A woman's index fingertip is about 1.5 cm.

— Effacement as a percentage of original length, or as actual length in centimeters. The noneffaced cervix is usually at least 2 cm long. When fully thinned (100%), it may feel like a delicate membrane that is almost indistinguishable from the fetal presenting part or amniotic sac when palpated.

— Fetal station in relation to the ischial spines. The ischial spines are prominences located on each side

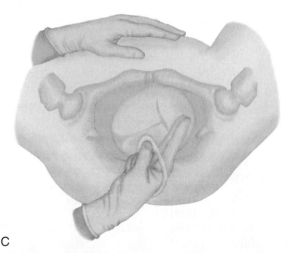

C

Figure 6-8   cont'd C, Determining the fetal position.

Continued

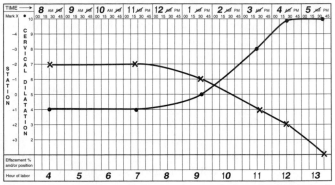

Findings of the vaginal examination may be recorded on a labor flow sheet, narrative, or a graph. The graph may be termed a *Friedman curve*, a *partogram*, or a *labor curve*.

D

Figure 6-8 cont'd D, Determining the station.

of the midpelvis. Station is recorded in minus numbers to signify centimeters above the ischial spines, a zero to signify that the widest part of the presenting part is at the level of the spines, and plus numbers to signify centimeters below the ischial spines.

10. Palpate the fetal head to identify fontanels and suture lines so that position (LOA, ROP, etc.) can be determined.
11. Remove the fingers, wipe excess lubricants or secretions from the woman's genitalia, and share the results of the examination with her.
12. Record the examination on the fetal monitor strip (if paper being used) and on the paper or computer chart.

VITAL SIGN ASSESSMENT IN THE NEWBORN
RESPIRATIONS
1. Assess respirations when the infant is quiet or sleeping and before disturbing the infant for other assessments, if possible.
2. Observe, auscultate, and palpate the chest and abdomen.

3. Lift the infant's blanket and shirt to see the chest and abdomen. Observe the pattern of respirations before beginning to count.

4. If desired, place a hand lightly over the infant's chest or abdomen to feel the movement. Avoid covering the chest completely so that the chest excursions can be watched as well as palpated.

5. To auscultate respirations, move a stethoscope over the chest until the respirations are easily heard. This is often toward the right side of the infant's chest. After counting, move the stethoscope to listen to breath sounds in all areas.

6. Count for a full minute because respirations are normally irregular in the newborn.

7. If the infant is crying, allow the infant to suck on a pacifier or gloved finger. If crying continues, count the respirations and note on the chart that the infant was crying. Recheck later when the infant is quiet.

8. Expect the respiratory rate to be 30 to 60 breaths/minute when the infant is at rest. Observe and report signs of respiratory distress, including tachypnea, retractions, flaring, cyanosis, grunting, seesawing, apneic periods, and asymmetry of chest movements. Continue to watch infants whose respiratory rate is near the extremes of the normal range.

PULSE

1. Listen to the apical pulse while the infant is quiet and before disturbing the infant for other assessments, if possible.

2. Use a pediatric head on the stethoscope to listen to the apical pulse to hear the sounds more accurately.

3. If the infant is crying, insert a pacifier or a gloved finger into the infant's mouth.

4. If the infant cannot be quieted, increase concentration and time spent listening.

5. Listen briefly before beginning to count. Tapping a finger in rhythm with the beat may be helpful. Count for a full minute. Expect the heart rate to be 120 to 160 bpm at rest.

6. Move the stethoscope over the entire heart area. Assess for arrhythmias, murmurs, or other abnormal sounds. Refer any abnormalities.

TEMPERATURE
Axillary
1. Place the thermometer vertically along the chest wall with the tip of the thermometer against the skin in the center of the axillary space with the infant's arm held firmly against the body over the probe.
2. Read the thermometer at the proper time: electronic or digital, when the indicator sounds; other types according to manufacturer's direction. Normal range: 36.5° to 37.5° C (97.7°-99.5° F).

Rectal
NOTE: Taking rectal temperatures are not recommended under most circumstances.

1. Take a rectal temperature only when necessary and according to birth facility policy. Use the axillary method whenever possible to avoid the risk of perforation of the rectum.
2. Place the infant in a supine position and hold the ankles firmly in one hand. Bend the infant's knees against the abdomen and raise the legs to expose the anus. Or place the infant prone or on the side and separate the buttocks.
3. Lubricate the tip of the thermometer with water-soluble lubricant.
4. Insert the thermometer carefully and gently into the rectum.
5. Do not force the thermometer if it does not insert easily.
6. Hold the thermometer securely throughout the time it remains in the rectum.
7. Read the thermometer at the proper time: electronic when the indicator sounds; other types according to manufacturer's directions. Normal range: 36.5° to 37.6° C (97.7°-99.7° F).

WEIGHING AND MEASURING
THE NEWBORN
WEIGHT

1. Cover the scale with a blanket. Place a paper cover over the blanket if desired.
2. Balance or adjust the scale to zero after the covering is placed. Electronic scale: push the "on" button and check to see that the digital readout is at zero. The electronic scale is usually self adjusting. Balance scale: Adjust until the balance arm is horizontal.
3. Remove clothing and blankets from the infant and place it in supine position on the scale. Keep one hand just above the infant and watch carefully throughout the procedure to prevent the infant from sliding off the scale.
4. Wait until the infant is somewhat quiet. The electronic scale displays weight in pounds and ounces or in grams. Some electronic scales display an indicator when an accurate weight has been obtained. For a balance scale, move weights slowly until the arm is level.
5. Write the numbers down immediately. If the scale is covered with paper, the weight can be written on the paper and taken with the infant to the warmer. Write it on the nurses' notes when the infant is safely settled.
6. Compare weight with the normal range for term infants: 2500 to 4000 g (5 lb, 8 oz to 8 lb, 13 oz).

LENGTH
Ruler Printed on Scale or Crib

1. Place the infant in supine position with his or her head at the upper edge of the ruler.
2. While holding the infant with one hand so that the head does not move, use the other hand to fully extend the infant's leg along the ruler. Note the length at the bottom of the heel.

Tape Measure

1. Check that a paper tape has no partial tears in it so the measurement will be accurate.

2. Place the tape beside the infant, with the upper end at the top of the head. Tuck it beneath the shoulder, and extend it down to the feet.
3. Hold the tape straight alongside the infant's body while extending one leg full length. Be sure that the tape has not moved from the top of the head.
4. Another method is to mark the paper on which the infant is lying at the top of the head and the end of the extended leg. Then measure the distance between the two marks.
5. Compare with the normal range of 48 to 53 cm (19-21 inches).

HEAD AND CHEST CIRCUMFERENCE
1. Measure around the fullest part of the head with the tape placed around the occiput and just above the eyebrows.
2. Move the tape down to measure the chest at the level of the nipples. Be sure that the tape is even and taut.
3. Remove the tape by lifting or rolling the infant instead of pulling the tape to avoid injury to the infant's skin.
4. Compare measurements with the normal range. Head: 33 to 35.5 cm (13-14 inches). Chest: 30.5 to 33 cm (12-13 inches).

Section 7

Drug Guides

CONTENTS

BETAMETHASONE, DEXAMETHASONE
CLASSIFICATION
Corticosteroids

ACTION/INDICATIONS
Acceleration of fetal lung maturity to reduce the incidence
and severity of respiratory distress syndrome (RDS). Studies
suggest that antenatal steroids can also reduce the incidence
of intraventricular hemorrhage (IVH) and neonatal death
in the preterm infant. Greatest benefits accrue if at least
24 hours elapse between the initial dose and birth of the
preterm infant, but the drug is indicated if birth is not
imminent.

DOSAGE AND ROUTE
Betamethasone: 12 mg intramuscular (IM) for two doses, 24 hours apart
Dexamethasone: 6 mg IM every 12 hours for four doses

ABSORPTION
Rapid and complete after IM administration.

EXCRETION
Metabolized in the liver. Excreted in urine.

CONTRAINDICATIONS
Active infection, such as chorioamnionitis, is a relative contraindication, although further study is needed. The National Institutes of Health recommend use of corticosteroids for the woman who has preterm rupture of the membranes (24-32 weeks of gestation), but the American College of Obstetrics and Gynecology has not yet endorsed this recommendation.

PRECAUTIONS
Possible infection. Pregnancies complicated by diabetes.

ADVERSE REACTIONS
Few, owing to the short-term use of the drug. Pulmonary edema is possible secondary to sodium and fluid retention.

NURSING CONSIDERATIONS
Explain the potential benefits of corticosteroid administration to the preterm neonate. Explain that the drug cannot prevent or lessen the severity of all complications of prematurity. If the woman is diabetic, explain that more frequent blood glucose determinations are common because these levels are often elevated. Assess lung sounds. Report chest pain or heaviness or dyspnea.

BUTORPHANOL (STADOL)

CLASSIFICATION

Opioid analgesic

ACTION

Opioid analgesic with some agonist-antagonist effects; exact mechanism of action unknown; produces respiratory depression that does not increase markedly with larger doses.

INDICATIONS

Systemic pain relief during labor.

DOSAGE AND ROUTE

Intravenous: 1 mg every 3 to 4 hours; range 0.5 to 2 mg; may be given undiluted.

ABSORPTION

Onset of analgesia almost immediate with intravenous (IV) administration, peaks about 30 minutes, and lasts about 3 hours; faster onset and shorter duration of action than meperidine or morphine.

EXCRETION

Excreted in urine; crosses placental barrier; secreted in breast milk.

CONTRAINDICATIONS AND PRECAUTIONS

Contraindicated in persons who are hypersensitive; not used in opiate-dependent persons because antagonist activity of the drug may cause withdrawal symptoms in the woman or newborn; cautiously used during birth of preterm infant; drug actions potentiated (enhanced) by barbiturates, phenothiazines, cimetidine, and other tranquilizers.

ADVERSE REACTIONS

Respiratory depression or apnea (woman or newborn), anaphylaxis; dizziness, lightheadedness, sedation, lethargy, headache, euphoria, mental clouding, fainting, restlessness, excitement, tremors, delirium, insomnia; nausea, vomiting, constipation, increased biliary pressure, dry mouth, anorexia; flushing, altered heart rate and blood pressure, circulatory collapse; urinary retention; sensitivity to cold.

NURSING CONSIDERATIONS
Assess for allergies and opiate dependence. Observe vital signs and respiratory function in woman (12 per minute or more) and newborn (30 per minute or more). Have naloxone and resuscitation equipment available for respiratory depression in woman and neonate. Report nausea or vomiting to the birth attendant for a possible order for an antiemetic. Antiemetics or other central nervous system depressants may enhance the respiratory depressant effects of butorphanol.

CARBOPROST TROMETHAMINE (HEMABATE)
CLASSIFICATION
Prostaglandin, oxytocic

OTHER NAMES
Hemabate, Prostin/15M

ACTION
Stimulates contraction of the uterus.

INDICATIONS
Used for the treatment of postpartum hemorrhage caused by uterine atony. Also used for abortion.

DOSAGE AND ROUTE
Postpartum hemorrhage: 250 mcg IM. May repeat at 15- to 90-minute intervals for up to 8 doses.

ABSORPTION
Metabolized by the liver and by enzymes in the lungs.

EXCRETION
Primarily excreted in urine.

CONTRAINDICATIONS AND PRECAUTIONS
Contraindicated for women with hypersensitivity to carbo-prost or other prostaglandins; acute pelvic inflammatory disease; cardiac, pulmonary, renal, or hepatic disease. Use caution if the woman has a history of asthma, hypo-/hyper-tension, anemia, jaundice, diabetes, epilepsy.

ADVERSE REACTIONS/SIDE EFFECTS
Excessive dose may cause tetanic contraction and laceration or uterine rupture. May cause uterine hypertonus if used with oxytocin. Nausea, vomiting, diarrhea (frequent), fever, chills, facial flushing, headache, hyper-/hypotension.

NURSING CONSIDERATIONS
Should be refrigerated. Give via deep IM injection and aspi-rate carefully to avoid IV injection. Rotate sites if repeated. Monitor vital signs. Administer antiemetics and antidiar-rheals as ordered.

ERYTHROMYCIN OPHTHALMIC OINTMENT
CLASSIFICATION
Antibiotic

OTHER NAME
Ilotycin

ACTION
Inhibits protein synthesis in bacteria, bacteriostatic or bacte-ricidal (depending on organism).

INDICATIONS
Prophylaxis against the organisms *Neisseria gonorrhoeae* and *Chlamydia trachomatis;* helps prevent ophthalmia neona-torum in infants of mothers infected with gonorrhea and

conjunctivitis in infants of mothers infected with *Chlamydia;* prophylaxis against gonorrhea is required by law for all infants, whether or not the mother is known to be infected.

NEONATAL DOSAGE AND ROUTE
A "ribbon" of 0.5% erythromycin ointment, 1 to 2 cm (0.4-0.8 inch) long, is applied to the lower conjunctival sac of each eye within 1 hour after birth.

ADVERSE REACTION
Burning, itching. Irritation may result in chemical conjunctivitis, lasting 24 to 48 hours. Ointment may cause temporary blurred vision.

NURSING CONSIDERATIONS
Cleanse the infant's eyes before application, as needed. Hold the tube in a horizontal rather than a vertical position to prevent injury to the eye from sudden movement. Administer from the inner canthus to the outer canthus. Do not touch the tip of the tube to any part of the eye, because this may spread infectious material from one eye to the other. Do not rinse. Ointment may be wiped from outer eye after 1 minute. Observe for irritation. Use a new tube for each infant to prevent spread of infection. Other medications used for prevention of gonorrhea include tetracycline ointment, povidone-iodine, and silver nitrate solution.

HEPATITIS B IMMUNE GLOBULIN (HBIG)
CLASSIFICATION
Immune globulin

OTHER NAMES
BayHep B, Nabi-HB

ACTION
Provides antibodies and passive immunity to hepatitis B.

INDICATIONS
Prophylaxis for infants of hepatitis B surface antigen–positive mothers.

NEONATAL DOSAGE AND ROUTE
0.5 mL within 12 hours of birth intramuscularly in the anterolateral thigh; should not be given intravenously.

ABSORPTION
Absorbed slowly

EXCRETION
Unknown

CONTRAINDICATIONS
None known

ADVERSE REACTIONS
Pain and tenderness at the site, urticaria, anaphylaxis.

NURSING CONSIDERATIONS
Do not shake or give intravenously. Bathe infants before the injection to remove blood and prevent contamination of the injection site with maternal blood on the infant's skin. Hepatitis vaccine series should begin within 12 hours of birth. Give injections of vaccine and immune globulin at separate sites.

HEPATITIS B VACCINE
CLASSIFICATION
Vaccine

OTHER NAMES
Engerix-B, Recombivax HB

ACTION
Immunization against hepatitis B infection.

INDICATIONS
Prevention of hepatitis B in exposed and unexposed infants.

NEONATAL DOSAGE AND ROUTE
Recombivax HB: 5 mcg to infants of an infected mother, 2.5 mcg if the mother is not infected.
Engerix-B: 10 mcg (whether or not the mother is infected).

For infants of HBsAg-negative mothers the first dose of vaccine is given by 2 months. The second dose is given at least 4 weeks after the first dose. The third dose is given at least 16 weeks after the first dose and at least 8 weeks after the second dose but not before the infant is 24 weeks old.

For infants of HBsAg-positive mothers the vaccine is given within 12 hours of birth. HBIG is also given within 12 hours of birth at a different site than the vaccine. The second dose of vaccine is given at age 1 to 2 months and the last dose is not given before 24 weeks of age.

If the mother's HbsAg status is unknown, the infant receives the vaccine within 12 hours of birth and the mother is tested. If the HbsAg test is positive, the infant should receive HBIG as soon as possible and by 1 week of age. The second dose of vaccine is given at age 1 to 2 months and the last dose not before 24 weeks of age.

Give intramuscularly in the anterolateral thigh.

ABSORPTION
Absorbed slowly; not affected by maternal antibodies.

CONTRAINDICATIONS
Hypersensitivity to yeast.

ADVERSE REACTIONS
Pain or redness at the site, fever.

NURSING CONSIDERATIONS
If a vial is used, shake the solution well before preparing. Give vaccine within 12 hours of birth to infants of infected

mothers. Do not inject intravenously or intradermally. Bathe infants before the injection to prevent contamination of the injection site with maternal blood on the infant's skin. Obtain parental consent before administering.

HYDRALAZINE
CLASSIFICATION
Antihypertensive

ACTION
Relaxes arterial smooth muscle to reduce blood pressure.

INDICATIONS
Used in preeclampsia when blood pressure is elevated to a degree that might be associated with intracranial bleeding.

DOSAGE AND ROUTE
Obstetric uses in hypertensive disorders during pregnancy. Intravenous doses: 5 to 10 mg may be administered as often as every 15 to 20 minutes if necessary. Duration of action is 3 to 8 hours (ACOG, 2002; Roberts, 2004).

ABSORPTION
Widely distributed, crosses the placenta; enters breast milk in minimal concentrations.

EXCRETION
Metabolized and excreted by the liver.

CONTRAINDICATIONS AND PRECAUTIONS
Contraindicated in coronary artery disease, cerebrovascular disease, and hypersensitivity to hydralazine. Used cautiously in pregnancy; pregnancy category C.

ADVERSE REACTIONS
Headache, dizziness, drowsiness, hypotension that can interfere with uterine blood flow, epigastric pain, which may be confused with worsening preeclampsia.

NURSING CONSIDERATIONS

Obstetric clients are hospitalized before initiation of anti-hypertensive medications. Blood pressure and pulse must be monitored every 2 to 3 minutes for 30 minutes after initial dosage and periodically throughout the course of therapy. Therapy is repeated only when diastolic pressure exceeds limits set by physician or facility protocol, usually ≥105-110 mm Hg (ACOG, 2002; Roberts, 2004).

MAGNESIUM SULFATE

CLASSIFICATION

Miscellaneous anticonvulsant

ACTION

Decreases acetylcholine released by motor nerve impulses, thereby blocking neuromuscular transmission. Depresses the central nervous system (CNS) to act as an anticonvulsant; also decreases frequency and intensity of uterine contractions. Produces flushing and sweating due to decreased peripheral blood pressure.

INDICATIONS

Prevention and control of seizures in severe preeclampsia. Prevention of uterine contractions in preterm labor.

DOSAGE AND ROUTE

A common IV administration protocol for preeclampsia includes a loading dose and a continuous infusion using a controlled infusion pump. The loading dose is 4 to 6 g magnesium sulfate administered in 100 mL IV fluid over 15 to 20 minutes. The continuing infusion to maintain control is 2 g/hr. Doses are individualized as needed. Deep IM injection is acceptable but is painful. A primary IV infusion with no medication is maintained if the magnesium must be discontinued.

Magnesium sulfate may also be administered in a similar dose profile to stop preterm labor contractions.

ABSORPTION

Immediate onset following IV administration.

EXCRETION
Excreted by the kidneys.

CONTRAINDICATIONS AND PRECAUTIONS
Contraindicated in persons with myocardial damage, heart block, myasthenia gravis, or impaired renal function. Magnesium toxicity, possibly related to incomplete renal drug excretion, may be evidenced by thirst, mental confusion, or a decrease in reflexes.

ADVERSE REACTIONS
Result from magnesium overdose and include flushing, sweating, hypotension, depressed deep tendon reflexes, and CNS depression, including respiratory depression.

NURSING CONSIDERATIONS
Monitor blood pressure closely during administration. Assess for minimum respiratory rate of 12 breaths per minute, presence of deep tendon reflexes, and urinary output of at least 30 mL/hr before starting or continuing magnesium therapy. Place resuscitation equipment (suction, oxygen) in the room. Keep calcium gluconate, which acts as an antidote to magnesium, readily available.

METHYLERGONOVINE (METHERGINE)
CLASSIFICATION
Oxytocic

ACTION
Stimulates sustained contraction of the uterus and causes arterial vasoconstriction.

INDICATIONS
Used for the prevention and treatment of postpartum or post-abortion hemorrhage caused by uterine atony or subinvolution.

DOSAGE AND ROUTE
Usual dosage is 0.2 mg IM every 2 to 4 hours for a maximum of five doses. Change to the oral route 0.2 mg every 6 to

8 hours for a maximum of 7 days. IV use not recommended; use in life-threatening emergency only; may cause severe hypertension.

ABSORPTION
Well absorbed after the oral or IM route.

EXCRETION
Metabolized by the liver, excreted in the feces and urine.

CONTRAINDICATIONS AND PRECAUTIONS
Methylergonovine should never be used during pregnancy or to induce labor. Do not use IM if the mother is hypersensitive to ergot. Contraindicated for women with hypertension, severe hepatic or renal disease, coronary artery disease, peripheral vascular disease, hypocalcemia, sepsis, and before the fourth stage of labor.

ADVERSE REACTIONS
Nausea, vomiting, uterine cramping, hypertension, dizziness, headache, dyspnea, chest pain, palpitations, peripheral ischemia, and uterine and gastrointestinal cramping.

NURSING CONSIDERATIONS
Before administering the medication, assess the blood pressure (BP). Follow facility protocol if medication must be withheld (usually a reading of 136/90 or above). Caution the mother to avoid smoking because nicotine constricts blood vessels. Remind her to report any adverse reactions.

NALOXONE HYDROCHLORIDE (NARCAN)
CLASSIFICATION
Opioid antagonist

ACTION
Reverses central nervous system and respiratory depression caused by narcotics (opiates). Competes with narcotics at receptor sites.

INDICATIONS
Severe respiratory depression when the mother has received narcotics within 4 hours of delivery.

DOSAGE AND ROUTE
Available in 0.4 mg/mL, and 1 mg/mL. Dosage is 0.1 mg/kg. Given intravenously, intramuscularly, subcutaneously, or into an endotracheal tube. Intravenous and endotracheal routes are preferred during resuscitation.

ABSORPTION
Well absorbed by all routes. Onset of action is 1 to 2 minutes if given intravenously.

EXCRETION
Metabolized by the liver and excreted by kidneys.

CONTRAINDICATIONS AND PRECAUTIONS
Duration of effect is 45 to 60 minutes. The dose may need to be repeated because the opiate may have a longer half-life than naloxone. If given to an infant of a mother addicted to opiates, it will cause withdrawal and may cause seizures. Resuscitative measures should be used as necessary.

NURSING CONSIDERATIONS
Note the strength of the medication available when calculating the dose. Prepare the syringe before birth by drawing up more than is needed. After birth, the excess is removed from the syringe, and the amount is given according to the estimate of the infant's weight. Inject rapidly. Monitor for response, and be prepared to give repeated doses if necessary.

COMMON DOSAGES OF NALOXONE HYDROCHLORIDE (NARCAN)
Dosage must be calculated based on weight (0.1 mg/kg). The amount for various weights is given below for *two different drug concentrations.*

Infant's Weight	Total Dose	Drug Concentration 0.4 mg/mL	Drug Concentration 1 mg/mL
1 kg (2 lb, 3 oz)	0.1 mg	0.25 mL	0.1 mL
2 kg (4 lb, 7 oz)	0.2 mg	0.50 mL	0.2 mL
3 kg (6 lb, 10 oz)	0.3 mg	0.75 mL	0.3 mL
4 kg (8 lb, 13 oz)	0.4 mg	1 mL	0.4 mL

OXYTOCIN (PITOCIN)
CLASSIFICATION
Oxytocic

ACTION
Synthetic compound identical to the natural hormone from the posterior pituitary. Stimulates uterine smooth muscle, resulting in increased strength, duration, and frequency of uterine contractions. Uterine sensitivity to oxytocin increases gradually during gestation. Oxytocin has vasoactive and antidiuretic properties.

INDICATIONS
Induction or augmentation of labor at or near term. Maintenance of firm uterine contraction after birth to control postpartum bleeding. Management of inevitable or incomplete abortion.

DOSAGE AND ROUTE
Induction or Augmentation of Labor
1. Intravenous infusion via a secondary (piggyback) line. Oxytocin infusion is controlled with a pump. Various dilutions of oxytocin and balanced electrolyte solution may be used. Mixtures having 60 mU/mL are convenient because the mL/hr setting on the infusion pump is the same number as the mU/min infused, reducing the chance for errors. Common mixtures that provide 60 mU/mL of oxytocin include (1) 15 units of oxytocin (1.5 mL) plus 250 mL of solution; (2) 30 units (3 mL) of oxytocin plus

500 mL solution; (3) 60 units (6 mL) of oxytocin plus 1000 mL solution. Lower concentrations, such as 10 to 20 units of oxytocin plus 1000 mL of solution may also be used. The drug may be given in 10-minute pulsed infusions rather than continuously.

2. Guidelines for oxytocin administration from the American College of Obstetricians and Gynecologists* provide examples of low- and high-dose oxytocin labor induction protocols. Depending on the protocol followed, the following recommendations are provided: (1) starting dosages of 0.5 to 6 mU/min, and (2) increasing dosage by 1- to 2-mU/min increments every 15 to 40 minutes. High-dose protocols may increase the dose in increments of up to 6 mU/min. The actual oxytocin dose is based on uterine response and absence of adverse effects. Higher starting doses, higher dose increases, and shorter intervals between dose increases are most likely to result in uterine hyperstimulation. A lower starting dose and lower rate increase increments are usually required to augment labor.

3. After an adequate contraction pattern is established and the cervix is dilated 5 to 6 cm, the oxytocin may be reduced by similar increments.

Control of Postpartum Bleeding
Intravenous infusion: Dilute 10 to 40 units in 1000 mL of intravenous solution. The rate of infusion must control uterine atony. Begin at a rate of 20 to 40 mU/min, increasing or decreasing the rate according to uterine response and the rate of postpartum bleeding. Correcting any identifiable cause of the hemorrhage should also be done. *Intramuscular injection:* Inject 10 units after delivery of the placenta.

Inevitable or Incomplete Abortion
Dilute 10 units in 500 mL of intravenous solution and infuse at a rate of 10 to 20 mU/min. Other dilutions are acceptable.

*American College of Obstetricians and Gynecologists. (1999). *Induction of labor* (ACOG Practice Bulletin No. 10). Washington, DC: Author.

ABSORPTION
Intravenous, immediate; intramuscular, 3 to 5 minutes.

EXCRETION
Liver and urine.

CONTRAINDICATIONS AND PRECAUTIONS
Include, but are not limited to, placenta previa, vasa previa, nonreassuring fetal heart rate patterns, abnormal fetal presentation, prolapsed umbilical cord, presenting part above the pelvic inlet, previous classic or other fundal uterine incision, active genital herpes infection, pelvic structural deformities, invasive cervical carcinoma.

ADVERSE REACTIONS
Most result from hypersensitivity to drug or excessive dosage. Adverse reactions include hypertonic uterine activity, impaired uterine blood flow, uterine rupture, and abruptio placentae. Uterine hypertonicity may result in fetal bradycardia, tachycardia, reduced fetal heart rate variability, and late decelerations. Fetal asphyxia may occur with diminished uterine blood flow. Fetal or maternal trauma, or both, may occur from rapid birth. Prolonged administration may cause maternal fluid retention, leading to water intoxication. Hypotension (seen with rapid intravenous injection), tachycardia, cardiac dysrhythmias, and subarachnoid hemorrhage are rare adverse reactions.

Drug interactions include vasopressors and the herb ephedra, causing hypertension.

NURSING CONSIDERATIONS
Intrapartum: Assess the fetal heart rate for at least 20 minutes before induction to identify reassuring or nonreassuring patterns. Perform Leopold's maneuvers, a vaginal examination, or both to verify a cephalic fetal presentation. If nonreassuring fetal heart rate patterns are identified or if fetal presentation is other than cephalic, notify the physician and do not begin induction until an ultrasound is done to determine fetal presentation.

Observe uterine activity for establishment of effective labor pattern: contraction frequency every 2 to 3 minutes, duration of 40 to 90 seconds, intensity of 50 to 80 mm Hg (if measured with an intrauterine pressure catheter). Observe for hypertonic uterine activity: contractions less than 2 minutes apart, rest interval shorter than 30 seconds, duration longer than 90-120 seconds, or an elevated resting tone greater than 20 mm Hg (if measured with an intrauterine pressure catheter).

Observe fetal heart rate for nonreassuring patterns such as tachycardia, bradycardia, decreased variability, and late decelerations.

If uterine hypertonicity or a nonreassuring fetal heart rate pattern occurs, intervene to reduce uterine activity and increase fetal oxygenation: stop the oxytocin infusion; increase the rate of nonadditive solution; position the woman in a side-lying position; and administer oxygen by snug facemask at 8 to 10 L/min. Notify the physician of adverse reactions, nursing interventions, and response to interventions. Record the maternal blood pressure, pulse, and respirations every 30 to 60 minutes or with each dosage increase. Record intake and output.

Postpartum: Observe uterus for firmness, height, and deviation. Massage until firm if uterus is soft ("boggy"). Observe lochia for color, quantity, and presence of clots. Notify birth attendant if uterus fails to remain contracted or if lochia is bright red or contains large clots. Assess for cramping. Assess vital signs every 15 minutes or according to protocol. Monitor intake and output and breath sounds to identify fluid retention or bladder distention.

Inevitable or incomplete abortion: Observe for cramping, vaginal bleeding, clots, and passage of products of conception. Observe maternal vital signs, intake, and output as noted under postpartum nursing implications.

RH$_0$(D) IMMUNE GLOBULIN
CLASSIFICATION
Concentrated immunoglobulins directed toward the red blood cell antigen Rh$_0$(D).

ACTION

Prevents production of anti-Rh_o(D) antibodies in Rh-negative women who have been exposed to Rh-positive blood by suppressing the immune reaction of the Rh-negative woman to the antigen in Rh-positive blood; prevents antibody response and thus prevents hemolytic disease of the newborn in future Rh-positive pregnancies. Used for both males and females who are Rh-negative but exposed to Rh-positive blood or for immune thrombocytopenic purpura (ITP).

INDICATIONS (PREGNANCY RELATED)

Administered to Rh-negative women who have been exposed to Rh-positive blood by:

1. Delivering an Rh-positive infant.
2. Aborting an Rh-positive fetus.
3. Having chorionic villus sampling, amniocentesis, or intraabdominal trauma while carrying an Rh-positive fetus.
4. Receiving inadvertent transfusion of Rh-positive blood.

DOSAGE AND ROUTE

One *standard* dose (300 mcg) administered intramuscularly:

1. At 28 weeks of pregnancy and within 72 hours of delivery.
2. Within 72 hours following termination of a pregnancy of 13 weeks or more of gestation.

One *microdose* (50 mcg) within 72 hours after the termination of a pregnancy of less than 13 weeks of gestation.

Dose is calculated based on the volume of fetal-maternal hemorrhage or Rh-positive blood administered in transfusion accidents. A standard dose will protect against 30 mL of Rh-positive whole blood or 15 mL of packed red blood cells (RBCs) (Weiner & Buhimschi, 2004).

ABSORPTION

Well absorbed from intramuscular sites.

EXCRETION
Metabolism and excretion unknown.

CONTRAINDICATIONS AND PRECAUTIONS
Women who are Rh-positive or women previously sensitized to $Rh_o(D)$ should not receive $Rh_o(D)$ immune globulin. It is used cautiously for women with previous hypersensitivity reactions to immune globulins.

ADVERSE REACTIONS
Local pain at intramuscular site, fever, or both.

NURSING CONSIDERATIONS
Type and antibody screen of the mother's blood and cord blood type of the newborn must be performed to determine the need for the medication. The mother must be Rh-negative and negative for Rh antibodies. The newborn must be Rh-positive. If the fetal blood type after termination of pregnancy is uncertain, the medication should be administered. The newborn may have a weakly positive antibody test if the woman received $Rh_o(D)$ immune globulin during pregnancy. The drug is administered to the mother, not the infant. The deltoid muscle is recommended for intramuscular administration.

RUBELLA VACCINE
CLASSIFICATION
Attenuated live virus vaccine

ACTION
Vaccination produces a modified rubella infection that is not communicable, causing the formation of antibodies against rubella virus.

INDICATIONS
The vaccine is administered after childbirth or abortion to women whose antibody screen shows they are not immune to rubella (German measles). This prevents rubella infection

and possible severe congenital defects in the fetus during a subsequent pregnancy.

DOSAGE AND ROUTE
The entire reconstituted volume of a single dose vial or 0.5 mL from a multiple dose vial. Inject subcutaneously in the outer aspect of the upper arm.

ABSORPTION
Well absorbed

CONTRAINDICATIONS AND PRECAUTIONS
The vaccine is contraindicated in women who have a respiratory or febrile infection, active untreated tuberculosis, or conditions that affect the bone marrow or lymphatic systems or are immunosuppressed, pregnant, or sensitive to neomycin or eggs. The attenuated virus may appear in breast milk and some infants develop a rash, but this is not a contraindication to vaccination of lactating women. It should be deferred for 3 months in clients receiving immune globulin or blood transfusions. Although it can be given after $Rh_o(D)$ immune globulin, women receiving the vaccine should be tested for immune status at 6 to 8 weeks to be sure they are immune (Centers for Disease Control and Prevention [CDC], 2003).

ADVERSE REACTIONS
Transient stinging at site, fever, lymphadenopathy, arthralgia, and transient arthritis are the most common adverse reactions.

NURSING CONSIDERATIONS
Previously, the woman and her partner were warned to avoid pregnancy for at least 3 months after vaccination because of the possibility that a fetus might be affected by the live virus in the vaccine. The CDC has changed this period to 4 weeks. Signed informed consent is usually required.

Vials should be refrigerated. Reconstitute only with diluent supplied with the vial. Use immediately after reconstitution and discard if not used within 8 hours. Protect from light. Do not give at the same time as immune globulin.

TERBUTALINE
CLASSIFICATION
Beta-adrenergic agent

ACTION
Stimulates beta-adrenergic receptors of the sympathetic nervous system. Action results primarily in bronchodilation and inhibition of uterine muscle activity. Increases pulse rate and widens pulse pressure.

INDICATIONS
Stop preterm labor. Reduce or stop hypertonic labor contractions, whether natural or stimulated. Tolerance and loss of tocolytic effect occur with prolonged use.

DOSAGE AND ROUTE
1. *IV infusion:* Begin at the ordered rate of approximately 0.01 to 0.05 mg/min. Increase rate if needed to stop contractions by 0.01 mg/min at 10- to 30-minute intervals until contractions stop (maximum of 0.08 mg/min). The infusion rate is not increased or may be decreased if the maternal pulse rate remains greater than 120 bpm or systolic blood pressure falls below 80-90 mm Hg. Maintain this dose for at least 1 hour; then reduce the rate at 20-minute intervals to reach minimum maintenance dose. Continue maintenance dose for 12 hours or as ordered after contractions stop.
2. *Subcutaneous (subQ)* (most common parenteral route): Intermittent injections, 0.25 mg, every 3 to 4 hours. A subcutaneous programmed infusion pump may be used for low-dose continuous (baseline) drug infusion plus intermittent bolus doses of approximately 0.25 mg at times of greatest uterine activity. The subcutaneous pump is typically placed and its programming for continuous and

bolus doses verified before removing the intermittent IV
terbutaline line or *magnesium sulfate infusion.*
3. *Oral:* 2.5 to 5 mg every 2 to 4 hours.

When changing from IV to oral therapy, give oral dose
30 minutes before discontinuing IV infusion.

ABSORPTION
1. *IV:* Prompt; duration about 2 hours.
2. *subQ:* 6 to 15 minutes; duration 1½ to 4 hours.
3. *Oral:* 1 to 2 hours; duration 4 to 8 hours.

EXCRETION

Metabolized in the liver. Excreted in urine.

CONTRAINDICATIONS
Hypersensitivity. Contraindicated before 20 weeks of gestation and if continuing the pregnancy is hazardous to the
mother or fetus, as in fetal distress, premature rupture of
membranes, hemorrhage, chorioamnionitis, and intrauterine
fetal death. Contraindicated in conditions that may be adversely
affected by beta-adrenergic agents (uncontrolled diabetes,
hyperthyroidism, bronchial asthma treated with other
beta-adrenergic agents or steroids, cardiac dysrhythmias,
hypovolemia, uncontrolled hypertension).

PRECAUTIONS
Terbutaline is not approved by the U.S. Food and Drug
Administration (FDA) for inhibiting uterine activity, although
it is widely used for this purpose. Research has been mixed
regarding the drug effects of terbutaline for this purpose,
but its lower risk for adverse side effects combined with some
efficacy has maintained terbutaline's use as a tocolytic.

ADVERSE REACTIONS
1. *Cardiovascular:* Maternal and fetal tachycardia, palpitations,
cardiac dysrhythmias, chest pain, wide pulse pressure

2. *Respiratory:* Dyspnea, chest discomfort
3. *Central nervous system:* Tremors, restlessness, weakness, dizziness, headache
4. *Metabolic:* Hypokalemia, hyperglycemia
5. *Gastrointestinal:* Nausea, vomiting, reduced bowel motility
6. *Skin:* Flushing, diaphoresis

NURSING CONSIDERATIONS

Diagnostic studies that may be ordered related to terbutaline therapy: electrocardiogram, blood glucose, electrolytes, urinalysis. Explain common side effects that are usually well tolerated, such as palpitations, tremors, restlessness, weakness, headache. Assess fetal heart rate (FHR), usually with continuous electronic fetal monitoring when the drug is initiated, recording rate and patterns at recommended intervals and with IV dose increases. Assess maternal pulse, respirations, and blood pressure by same schedule as for FHR. Maintain adequate IV or oral hydration. Encourage the woman to empty her bladder every 2 hours. Notify the physician for significant or unacceptable side effects (maternal heart rate >120 bpm, respirations >24/minute, dyspnea, pulmonary edema, systolic blood pressure <80-90 mm Hg, FHR >160 bpm, chest pain). Report continuing or recurrent uterine activity. Teach signs and symptoms of recurrent preterm labor and follow-up medical care after discharge.

VITAMIN K₁ (PHYTONADIONE)
CLASSIFICATION

Fat-soluble vitamin, antihemorrhagic

OTHER NAMES

AquaMEPHYTON, Mephyton, Konakion

ACTION

Promotes the formation of factors II (prothrombin), VII, IX, and X by the liver for clotting; provides vitamin K, which is not synthesized in the intestines for the first 5 to 8 days after birth because the newborn lacks intestinal flora necessary for vitamin K production.

INDICATION
Prevention or treatment of vitamin K–dependent bleeding (hemorrhagic disease of the newborn).

NEONATAL DOSAGE AND ROUTE
0.5 to 1 mg (0.25-0.5 mL of solution containing 2 mg/mL) given once intramuscularly within 1 hour of birth for prophylaxis (lower dose is given to infants weighing <2500 g); higher doses or repeated doses may be used if the mother took anticonvulsants during pregnancy or if the infant shows bleeding tendencies.

ABSORPTION
Readily absorbed after intramuscular injection; effective within 1 to 2 hours; metabolized in the liver.

ADVERSE REACTIONS
Erythema, pain, and edema at site of administration; anaphylaxis, hemolysis or hyperbilirubinemia, especially in a preterm infant or when large doses are used.

NURSING CONSIDERATIONS
Protect the drug from light until just before administration because it decomposes and loses potency on exposure to light. Observe all infants for signs of vitamin K deficiency: ecchymoses or bleeding from any site. Check that the newborn has had vitamin K before a circumcision is performed.

Table 7-1	Drugs Commonly Used for Intrapartum Pain Management
Drug/Dose	**Comments**
Opioid Analgesics	
Meperidine (Demerol) 12.5-50 mg every 2-4 hr IV; may be given by PCA	Respiratory depression (primarily in the neonate) is the main side effect.
Fentanyl (Sublimaze) 50-100 mcg; may be repeated every hour; may be given by PCA Adjunct to epidural analgesia during labor (dose individualized)	Onset is quick (5 min for IV administration), but duration of action is short. Less nausea, vomiting, and respiratory depression occurs than with meperidine. Epidural use may cause pruritus.
Butorphanol (Stadol) 1 mg every 3-4 hr; range 0.5-2 mg IV; may be given by PCA	Has some narcotic antagonist effects; should not be given to the opiate-dependent woman (may precipitate withdrawal) or after other narcotics such as meperidine (may reverse their analgesic effects); also a respiratory depressant.
Nalbuphine (Nubain) 10 mg every 3-6 hr IV; may be given by PCA	Same as butorphanol. 5-10 mg may be given to relieve pruritus associated with epidural narcotics.

IV, Intravenously; *PCA*, patient-controlled analgesia; *IM*, intramuscularly; *PO*, orally.

Continued

Table 7-1	Drugs Commonly Used for Intrapartum Pain Management—cont'd
Drug/Dose	**Comments**
Adjunctive Drugs	
Promethazine (Phenergan) 6.25-25 mg every 4-6 hr IV	Given for nausea and vomiting in labor. Duration of action is longer than most narcotics; may enhance respiratory depressant effects of narcotics.
Diphenhydramine (Benadryl) 10-50 mg every 4-6 hr IV	Given to relieve pruritus from epidural narcotics.
Hydroxyzine (Atarax, Vistaril) 25-100 mg IM Z-track only	See promethazine.
Narcotic Antagonists	
Naloxone (Narcan) Adult: To reduce respiratory depression induced by opioids: 0.4-2 mg IV To reverse pruritus from epidural opioids: 0.04-0.2 mg IV or IV infusion 5-10 mcg/kg/hr Neonatal resuscitation: 0.1 mg/kg IV (umbilical vein) or intratracheal	Action shorter than most narcotics it reverses; must observe for recurrent respiratory depression and be prepared to give additional doses. Small doses (0.04-0.08 mg) may be given to reduce pruritus from epidural opioids. Resuscitation in Newborns (see p. 439).
Naltrexone (Trexan) 3-6 mg PO × 1 dose	Long-acting drug to relieve pruritus from epidural narcotics. May reduce some analgesic effect when given for pruritus.

IV, Intravenously; *PCA,* patient-controlled analgesia; *IM,* intramuscularly; *PO,* orally.

Appendix A

Laboratory Values in Pregnant and Nonpregnant Women

Appendix A	Laboratory Values in Pregnant and Nonpregnant Women	
Value	**Nonpregnancy**	**Pregnancy**
Blood volume, total (mL/kg)	55-80	Increases 40%-50%
Plasma volume (mL/kg)	30-45	Increases 50% (1200-1300 mL above nonpregnant levels)
Red blood cell volume (mL/kg)	20-35	Increases 25%-33% (average total increase of 250-450 mL)
Red blood cell count (1,000,000/mm³)	4.2-5.4	Decreases slightly because of hemodilution
Hemoglobin (g/dL)	12-16	At least 11 g/dL during first and third trimesters and at least 10.5 g/dL during second trimester
Hematocrit, packed cell volume (%)	37-47	>33
White blood cell count (1000/mm³)	5-10	5-12 Rises during labor and early postpartum

Continued

Appendix A	**Laboratory Values in Pregnant and Nonpregnant Women—cont'd**	
Value	**Nonpregnancy**	**Pregnancy**
Platelets (1000/mm^3)	150-400	150-400 or slightly decreased
Prothrombin time (sec)	11-12.5	Slight decrease but remains within normal limits
Activated partial thromboplastin time (sec)	21-35	Slight decrease but remains within normal limits
D dimer	Negative	Negative
Glucose, blood		
Fasting (mg/dL)	70-105	95 or lower
Postprandial (mg/dL)	<140	<140
Creatinine, serum (mg/dL)	0.5-1.1	0.5
Creatinine clearance, urine (mL/min)	87-107	110-180
Fibrinogen (mg/dL)	200-400	300-600

Data from Blackburn, S.T. (2003). *Maternal, fetal, and neonatal physiology: A clinical perspective* (2nd ed.). St. Louis: Saunders; Cunningham, F.G., Leveno, K.J., Bloom, S.L., Hauth, J.C., Gilstrap, L., & Wenstrom, K.D. (2005). *Williams obstetrics* (22nd ed.). New York: McGraw-Hill; Fischbach, F.T. & Dunning, M.B. (2004). *A manual of laboratory and diagnostic tests* (7th ed.). Philadelphia: Lippincott Williams & Wilkins; Gordon, M.C. (2002). Maternal physiology in pregnancy. In S.G. Gabbe, J.R. Niebyl, & J.L. Simpson (Eds.), *Obstetrics: Normal and problem pregnancies* (4th ed.). Philadelphia: Churchill Livingstone; Moore, T.R. (2004). Diabetes in pregnancy. In R.K. Creasy, R. Resnik, & J.D. Iams (Eds.), *Maternal-fetal medicine: Principles and practice* (5th ed.). Philadelphia: Saunders; and Pagana, K.D. & Pagana, T.J. (2005). *Mosby's diagnostic and laboratory test reference* (7th ed.). St. Louis: Mosby.

Appendix B

Laboratory Values in the Newborn

Appendix B	Laboratory Values in the Newborn

Test, Specimen, and Unit of Measurement	Age	Normal Range
Red blood cell count, whole blood (1,000,000/mm³)	Cord	3.9-5.5
	1-3 days	4-6.6
	1 wk	3.9-6.3
	1 mo	3-5.4
Hemoglobin, whole blood (g/dL)	1-3 days (capillary)	14.5-22.5
	2 mo	9-14
Hematocrit, whole blood (%)	1 day (capillary)	48-69
	2 days	48-75
	3 days	44-72
	2 mo	28-42
White blood cell count, whole blood (1000/mm³)	Birth	9-30
	24 hr	9.4-34
	1 mo	5-19.5
White blood cell differential count, whole blood		
Myelocytes (%)		0
Neutrophils ("bands") (%)		3-5
Neutrophils ("segs") (%)		54-62
Lymphocytes (%)		25-33
Monocytes (%)		3-7
Eosinophils (%)		1-3
Basophils (%)		0-0.75

Adapted from Nicholson, J.F. & Pesce, M.A. (2004). Reference ranges for laboratory tests and procedures. In R.E. Behrman, R.M. Kliegman, & H.B. Jenson (Eds.), *Nelson textbook of pediatrics* (17th ed., pp. 2396-2427). Philadelphia: Saunders.

Continued

Appendix B	**Laboratory Values in the Newborn—cont'd**

Test, Specimen, and Unit of Measurement	Age	Normal Range
Platelet count, whole blood (1000/mm³)	Newborn, >1 wk	84-478 150-400
Glucose, serum (mg/dL)	Cord	45-96
	1 day	40-60
	Newborn, >1 day	50-90
Calcium, serum (mg/dL)	Cord	9-11.5
	Newborn, 3-24 hr	9-10.6
	24-48 hr	7-12
	4-7 days	9-10.9
Magnesium, plasma (mg/dL)	Newborn, 0-6 days	1.2-2.6

		Normal Range	
		Preterm	**Full-Term**
Bilirubin, total serum (mg/dL)	Cord	<2	<2
	0-1 day	<8	<6
	1-2 days	<12	<8
	2-5 days	<16	<12
	>5 days	<20	<10
Bilirubin, direct (conjugated) serum (mg/dL)		0-0.2	0-0.2

Appendix C

Use of Drugs and Botanical (Herbal) Preparations during Pregnancy, Breastfeeding, and Women's Health

FDA PREGNANCY RISK CATEGORIES

The U.S. Food and Drug Administration (FDA) has assigned pregnancy risk categories to many drugs on the basis of their known relative safety or danger to the fetus and whether safer alternative drugs exist. Depending on fetal effects or nearness of birth, drugs may carry different risk categories at different points during pregnancy. For many drugs, little is known about the fetal risk. FDA categories are as follows:

A: No evidence of risk to the fetus exists.

B: Animal reproduction studies have not demonstrated a risk to the fetus. No adequate and well-controlled studies have been done in pregnant women.

C: Animal reproduction studies have shown an adverse effect on the fetus, but no adequate, well-controlled studies have been done in humans. Potential benefits may warrant use of the drug in pregnant women despite fetal risks. Or, animal studies show adverse effect on fetus, but human studies with pregnant women have not demonstrated a risk to the fetus in any trimester of pregnancy.

D: There is positive evidence of human fetal risk based on adverse reaction data, but potential benefits may warrant use of the drug in pregnant women despite fetal risks. Essentially, no safer alternatives to the drug are available.

X: There is positive evidence of human fetal risk based on animal or human studies and/or adverse reaction data. The risks of using the drug in pregnant women clearly outweigh potential benefits. Safer alternatives to these drugs may be available.

DRUG USE DURING LACTATION

The effects of many drugs when used during lactation have not been studied. In general, if a drug is safe for use in infants, it is probably safe for the lactating woman to take. Other drugs are known not to be excreted in breast milk or are excreted in an inactive form or very low concentrations. Modifying the time of maternal ingestion may reduce transfer of the drug to the infant. Some drugs are undesirable because they suppress lactation, which is a problem primarily in the earliest stages of breastfeeding.

Use of Drugs and Botanical (Herbal) Preparations during Pregnancy, Breastfeeding, and Women's Health		
Drug	**Use during Pregnancy**	**Use during Breastfeeding**
Amebicides		
Metronidazole (Flagyl)	*Risk category B.* Previous concern about teratogenic effects on the fetus have not been supported (CDC, 2002). Treatment of choice for trichomoniasis but may also be chosen as part of drug regimen for inflammatory bowel disease or postpartum endometritis.	Breastfeeding may be discontinued for 12-24 hr during single-dose treatment of mother. However, few known adverse infant effects.
Analgesics		
Aspirin	*Risk category C (D in third trimester).* Has been linked to fetal gastroschisis and small intestine atresia.	Single doses not associated with risk to breastfeeding infant. Greater potential risk if mother requires higher doses for a disorder such as arthritis.
Acetaminophen (Tylenol, Datril, Tempra)	*Risk category B.* Problems have not been documented, but drug crosses	Safe. Very small amounts secreted into breast milk.

Continued

Use of Drugs and Botanical (Herbal) Preparations during Pregnancy, Breastfeeding, and Women's Health—cont'd

Drug	Use during Pregnancy	Use during Breastfeeding
	placenta in low concentrations. Maximum dose 4 g/day. Drug often combined with other medications and should be considered when determining the maximum daily dose received.	
Opiate analgesics: butorphanol [Stadol], fentanyl [Sublimaze], hydrocodone [Duocet, Lortab, Norco, Vicodin, Zydone], hydromorphone [Dilaudid], meperidine [Demerol], morphine, nalbuphine [Nubain], oxycodone [Percocet, Tylox, Percodan]	*Most are risk category B or C.* Neonatal respiratory depression is the most significant adverse effect when large amounts of opiates are used during labor, making them category D drugs at this time. Neonatal withdrawal may occur if the woman is addicted to an opiate drug.	Most narcotics given briefly and in therapeutic doses are compatible with breastfeeding, including intrathecal (before epidural catheter removal) morphine given postoperatively. Prolonged infant sedation during the early postpartum period may occur with maternal meperidine analgesia.
Nonsteroidal antiinflammatory drugs (NSAIDs): fenoprofen [Nalfon], flurbiprofen [Ansaid], ibuprofen [Advil, Motrin,	*Risk category B or C; category D in third trimester.* May prolong pregnancy or labor because of antiprostaglandin effects. Indomethacin	Ibuprofen, indomethacin, and naproxen are AAP approved. All should be used cautiously owing to potential for infant bleeding. Indomethacin has been used

Nuprin], indomethacin [Indocin], ketoprofen [Actron, Orudis], naproxen [Aleve, Anaprox]	associated with premature closure of ductus arteriosus or oligohydramnios in fetus but may be given in limited doses to stop preterm labor or reduce excess amniotic fluid in hydramnios.	for treatment of neonatal patent ductus arteriosus.
COX-2 inhibitors: celecoxib [Celebrex]	Risk category C. Associated with oligohydramnios and constriction of the ductus arteriosus. Greater risk of adverse cardiovascular effects has caused two related COX-2 inhibitors (rofecoxib [Vioxx], valdecoxib [Bextra]) to be withdrawn from the market. See www.fda.gov for latest information on COX-2 inhibitors and other drugs.	No adverse effects via milk reported. Observe for infant gastrointestinal (GI) cramping, diarrhea, effects similar to those reported in adults.
Migraine agents: almotriptan [Axert], frovatriptan [Frova], naratriptan [Amerge], rizatriptan [Maxalt], sumatriptan [Imitrex]	Risk category C. Minimal well-controlled studies about fetal safety during pregnancy.	No identified pediatric concerns regarding breast milk, but caution recommended. Pumping and discarding milk for 24 hr after medication administration prevents transfer to infant.

Continued

Use of Drugs and Botanical (Herbal) Preparations during Pregnancy, Breastfeeding, and Women's Health—cont'd

Drug	Use during Pregnancy	Use during Breastfeeding
Antiallergics		
Antihistamines (see middle column for drugs)	*Risk category B:* chlorpheniramine (Chlor-Trimeton), clemastine (Contac, Tavist), diphenhydramine (Benadryl), loratadine (Claritin), meclizine (Antivert, Dramamine). *Risk category C:* astemizole (Hismanal), brompheniramine (Dimetane), phenylephrine (Neo-Synephrine), terfenadine (Seldane), triprolidine (Alleract).	All should be used with caution. Most are safe but may cause infant drowsiness. If these adverse effects occur, a different drug may be tried. Clemastine noted by AAP to be given with caution because of one case of infant irritability, refusal to feed, neurologic symptoms, seizures, and a high-pitched cry.
Antiasthmatics (See also Decongestants, Hormones, Corticosteroids Other Than Inhalers)		
Corticosteroid inhalers: beclomethasone [Beclovent, Vanceril], triamcinolone [Aristocort, Azmacort, Nasacort]	*Risk category C.*	Safety in lactation not fully known, but no reported problems following breast milk ingestion.

Continued

NSAID asthma medications: cromolyn [Intal, NasalCrom, Opticrom], nedocromil [Alocril, Miraze]	*Risk category B.*	Minimal oral absorption. No reported adverse effects via milk.
Epinephrine: Adrenalin, Sus-Phrine, Primatene	*Risk category C.* To treat bronchospasm in acute asthma attack.	Observe for brief infant stimulation after maternal drug use.
Leukotriene pathway modulators: montelukast [Singulair], zafirlukast [Accolate], zyleuton [Zyflo]	*Risk category B:* (zafirlukast, montelukast) and C (zyleuton).	No reported problems via breast milk; little published experience.
Bronchodilators: albuterol [Proventil, Ventolin], metaproterenol [Alupent]	*Risk category C.* May inhibit uterine contractions.	Unknown if secreted in milk; use cautiously.

Anticoagulants

Enoxaparin (Lovenox)	*Risk category B.* Not interchangeable with heparin.	Unlikely to produce clinically relevant levels in breast milk because of molecular size.
Heparir.	*Risk category C.*	Not excreted in breast milk.
Warfarin (Coumadin)	*Risk category X.* Known teratogen that should be used during pregnancy only if the benefits outweigh risks. Associated with CNS and facial malformations, mental retardation, prenatal growth deficiency, and other fetal defects.	Small amounts secreted in milk. Infant bleeding abnormalities may result. Avoidance of breastfeeding during therapy may be recommended.

Use of Drugs and Botanical (Herbal) Preparations during Pregnancy, Breastfeeding, and Women's Health—cont'd

Drug	Use during Pregnancy	Use during Breastfeeding
Anticonvulsants		
Carbamazepine (Tegretol); oxcarbazepine (Trileptal)	*Risk category C.* Associated with craniofacial abnormalities, underdeveloped fingernails, neural tube defects, and developmental delay.	Small amounts secreted in breast milk; accumulation does not seem to occur. Observe infant for sedation.
Clonazepam (Klonopin)	*Risk category D.* No firm evidence that clonazepam is teratogenic. Infant after birth may display mild sedation, hypotonia, poor sucking.	Enters breast milk in a possibly relevant quantity.
Magnesium sulfate	*Risk category A* during early pregnancy. Infants exposed to magnesium sulfate 2 hr before birth may exhibit respiratory depression, hypotonic muscle tone, depressed reflexes, hypocalcemia, or cardiac dysrhythmias. Although infant risks	Level in milk return to normal about 24 hr after drug is stopped.

Drug		
Phenobarbital	exist when drug used during labor, complications of preeclampsia and eclampsia are greater. *Risk category D.* Fetal addiction with subsequent withdrawal is possible but rare at dose levels used for seizure control. Abnormalities similar to those seen in infants exposed to carbamazepine, phenytoin, and valproic acid have been reported.	Infant serum levels approximately one third of adult levels. Psychomotor delay and sedation possible.
Fosphenytoin (Cerebyx); phenytoin (Dilantin)	*Risk category D.* Few studies of fosphenytoin. Risk for fetal malformations with phenytoin, specifically congenital heart defects and cleft palate, is double that in the general population.	Methemoglobinemia, drowsiness, and poor sucking have been reported. Most studies do not suggest problems.
Primidone (Mysoline)	*Risk category D.*	Drug and its metabolites are secreted into breast milk. Has been associated with neonatal sedation.
Topiramate (Topamax)	*Risk category C.*	No studies available. Use with caution.

Continued

Use of Drugs and Botanical (Herbal) Preparations during Pregnancy, Breastfeeding, and Women's Health—cont'd

Drug	Use during Pregnancy	Use during Breastfeeding
Valproic acid (Depakene)	*Risk category D.* Associated with neural tube defects and craniofacial, cardiac, and hand abnormalities.	Secreted in small amounts. May cause drowsiness. Used for treatment of infant seizures.
Antidiabetics		
Insulin	*Risk category B.* Insulin is the drug of choice during pregnancy because it does not cross placenta.	Orally ingested insulin would be destroyed in infant's GI tract.
Oral hypoglycemic agents: metformin [Glucophage], nateglinide [Starlix], pioglitazone [Actos], repaglinide [Prandin], rosiglitazone [Avandia]	*Risk category B:* Metformin. *Risk category C:* Remaining drugs.	Safety not established for most oral hypoglycemics. Observe for infant hypoglycemia if used.
Antifungals		
Fluconazole (Diflucan), miconazole (Monistat),	*Risk category C.*	Fluconazole excreted in breast milk at levels similar to the mother's

nystatin (Mycostatin), terconazole (Terazol)

plasma level. Most considered safe if ingested in breast milk.

Antihypertensives (see also Diuretics)

ACE inhibitors: benazepril [Lotensin], captopril [Capoten], enalapril [Vasotec], fosinopril [Monopril], lisinopril [Prinivil, Zestril], quinapril [Accupril], ramipril [Altace], trandolapril [Mavik]

Risk category D (primarily second and third trimesters). Renal dysplasia leading to oligohydramnios may result in pulmonary hypotension and death after birth.

Observe for infant hypotension. Fewer safety data available for newer agents.

Beta-adrenergic blockers: acebutolol [Monitan, Sectral], atenolol [Tenormin], betaxolol [Kerlone], labetalol [Normodyne], metoprolol [Lopressor, Toprol], nadolol [Corgard], penbutolol [Levatol], pindolol [Viskin], propranolol [Inderal]

Risk category B (pindolol). Possible fetal or neonatal effects include intrauterine growth restriction, neonatal hypotension, bradycardia, transient tachypnea, respiratory depression, and hypoglycemia.
Risk category C (labetalol, metoprolol, nadolol, penbutolol, propranolol).
Risk category D (acebutolol, atenolol).

Acebutalol, labetalol, metoprolol, nadolol, and propranolol considered safe. Less known about other drugs. Observe infant for possible effects listed under Use during Pregnancy.

Continued

Use of Drugs and Botanical (Herbal) Preparations during Pregnancy, Breastfeeding, and Women's Health—cont'd

Drug	Use during Pregnancy	Use during Breastfeeding
Calcium channel blockers: amlodipine [Norvasc], diltiazem [Cardizem], nicardipine [Cardene], nifedipine [Adalat, Procardia], verapamil [Calan, Isoptin]	*Risk category C.* May benefit fetus by reducing resistance to placental blood flow. Nifedipine and verapamil may be given to reduce preterm contractions, prolonging pregnancy.	Diltiazem, nifedipine, verapamil generally considered safe, although diltiazem levels in breast milk may reach maternal serum levels. Less known about other drugs listed.
Centrally acting antihypertensives: clonidine [Catapres], guanabenz [Wytensin], guanadrel [Hylorel], guanfacine [Tenex], methyldopa [Aldomet]	*Risk category B* (guanadrel, guanfacine, methyldopa). *Risk category C* (clonidine, guanabenz). Methyldopa is an accepted antihypertensive drug during first trimester of pregnancy.	Methyldopa is considered safe. Little information about effects of the other centrally acting antihypertensive drugs on lactation. Observe infant for hypotension.
Vasodilators: eprosartan [Teveten], hydralazine [Apresoline], minoxidil [Loniten], nitroprusside [Nipride, Nitropress]	*Risk category C; risk category D in second and third trimesters for* eprosartan. Hydralazine is drug of choice for hypertension during pregnancy. Nitroprusside given in carefully titrated doses to control severe hypertension during pregnancy.	Hydralazine considered safe, but less is known about minoxidil use. Nitroprusside is a concern because of drug's conversion to potentially toxic thiocyanate metabolite.

Antimicrobials

Aminoglycosides: gentamicin [Garamycin], streptomycin, tobramycin [Tobrex, Nebcin]	*Risk categories C and D.* Associated with hearing loss and renal toxicity. Monitoring of blood levels reduces risk of adverse effects.	Most drugs in this class are considered safe because minimal amounts are secreted in breast milk and drugs are poorly absorbed if orally ingested. Observe for changes in GI flora.
Macrolides: azithromycin [Zithromax], clarithromycin [Biaxin], erythromycin [EES, Erythrocin, Ilotycin]	*Risk category B.*	Appear to be safe. Drugs available in pediatric preparations.
Cephalosporins first- through fourth-generation drugs	*Risk category B.*	Most are considered safe for breastfeeding.
Chloramphenicol (Chloromycetin)	*Risk category D.* Not recommended for use near term because it is associated with neonatal "gray baby syndrome" (rapid respiration, ashen and pale color, poor feeding, abdominal distention, vasomotor collapse, death).	Generally unsafe in breastfeeding mothers because of potential toxicity and "gray baby syndrome" risk for newborns.
Fluoroquinolones: ciprofloxacin [Cipro], levofloxacin [Levaquin], norfloxacin [Chibroxin], ofloxacin [Floxin]	*Risk category C.* Animal studies have shown skeletal abnormalities.	Potentially hazardous. Ofloxacin and ciprofloxacin reach breast milk concentrations similar to or higher than maternal plasma. Less is known about other drugs. Observe infant for diarrhea.

Continued

Use of Drugs and Botanical (Herbal) Preparations during Pregnancy, Breastfeeding, and Women's Health—cont'd

Drug	Use during Pregnancy	Use during Breastfeeding
Nitrofurantoin (Furadantin, Macrodantin)	*Risk category B.* Crosses placenta. Animal studies reassuring, and no evidence suggests drug is teratogenic.	Should avoid if infant is younger than 1 mo. Risk for hemolytic anemia if infant has an enzyme (G-6-PD) deficiency.
Penicillins: amoxicillin [Amoxil], ampicillin [Omnipen, Polycillin], penicillin G	*Risk category B.* No reported adverse fetal effects. Penicillins combined with beta-lactamase inhibitors (amoxicillin and clavulanate [Augmentin], ticarcillin and clavulanate [Timentin], and ampicillin and subbactam [Unasyn]) also are risk category B.	Low concentrations of penicillins in breast milk, including those combined with beta-lactamase inhibitors. Observe for infant diarrhea or candidiasis.
Sulfonamides: sulfadiazine [Coptin], sulfamethoxazole [Gantanol], sulfisoxazole [Gantrisin]	*Risk category C.*	AAP recommends caution in use of breast milk if infant has jaundice or G-6-PD deficiency and in the ill or preterm infant.
Tetracycline	*Risk category D.* Can interfere with tooth enamel formation and cause discolored teeth. Prenatal exposure does not affect permanent teeth.	Thought to be compatible with breastfeeding. Oral ingestion appears to be safe, although few well-controlled studies exist.

Vancomycin (Vancocin)	*Risk category B.* Used for maternal methicillin-resistant *Staphylococcus aureus* infections and prophylaxis to prevent endocarditis.	Thought to be safe because oral absorption by breastfeeding infant is minimal.

Antiretrovirals

Nucleoside reverse transcriptase inhibitors (NRTIs): abacavir [ABC, Ziagen], didanosine [ddI, Videx], lamivudine [3TC, Epivir], stavudine [d4T, Zerit], tenofovir DF [Viread, TDF], zalcitabine [ddC, Hivid], zidovudine [ZDV, Retrovir]	*Risk category B* (didanosine). *Risk category C* (abacavir, lamivudine, stavudine, tenofovir DF, zalcitabine, zidovudine). Zidovudine is recommended for HIV-seropositive women to reduce risk for perinatal transmission of the virus.	Breastfeeding not recommended because of possibility of HIV transmission to infant.
Nonnucleotide reverse transcriptase inhibitors (NNRTIs): delavirdine [DLV, Rescriptor], efavirenz [Sustiva, EFV], nevirapine [NVP, Viramune]	*Risk category C.* Efavirenz category C first trimester, category D second and third trimesters.	Breastfeeding not recommended because of possibility of HIV transmission to infant.
Fusion inhibitors: enfuvirtide [Fuzeon, T-20]	*Risk category B.*	Breastfeeding not recommended because of possibility of HIV transmission to infant.

Continued

Use of Drugs and Botanical (Herbal) Preparations during Pregnancy, Breastfeeding, and Women's Health—cont'd

Drug	Use during Pregnancy	Use during Breastfeeding
Protease inhibitors (PIs): amprenavir [Agenerase], indinavir [Crixivan], nelfinavir [Viracept], ritonavir [Norvir], saquinavir [Invirase]	*Risk category B:* nelfinavir, ritonavir, saquinavir. *Risk category C:* amprenavir, indinavir.	Breastfeeding not recommended because of possibility of HIV transmission to infant.
Antituberculosis Agents (see also *Antimicrobials*)		
Ethambutol (Myambutol)	*Risk category B.* No evidence of increased abnormalities.	Small amounts of ethambutol are excreted into breast milk.
Isoniazid (INH)	*Risk category C.*	Scant drug levels found in breast milk. Observe infant for hepatitis, vision changes.
Pyrazinamide	*Risk category C.* No adverse experience with this widely prescribed agent.	None reported in breast milk.
Rifampin (Rifadin)	*Risk category C.*	Trace amounts excreted in breast milk.

Antitussives and Expectorants

Dextromethorphan (Robitussin-DM)	*Risk category C.* No reported adverse effects.
Guaifenesin (Robitussin)	*Risk category C.* Usefulness as an expectorant is questionable. No reported adverse effects.

Antiviral Agents

Genital herpes infection therapy: acyclovir [Avirax, Zovirax], foscarnet [Foscavir], valacyclovir [Valtrex]	*Risk category B* (acyclovir). *Risk category C* (foscarnet, valacyclovir). Few reported toxicities except foscarnet associated with higher milk levels than other drugs. Wash topical drug from area before nursing, and consult with physician about breastfeeding safety if lesion is present on nipple.
Ribavirin (Virazole)	*Risk category X.* Administered by aerosol, usually to young children only. Women who are pregnant or may become pregnant should avoid exposure. Drug is most often given to young children hospitalized with respiratory syncytial virus (RSV), so transfer to breast milk is not likely.

Cardiac Medications

Antiarrhythmics for serious arrhythmias: amiodarone [Cordarone, Pacerone], bretylium [Bretylol]	*Risk category C* (bretylium). *Risk categories D* (amiodarone). May reduce uterine blood flow. Possible neurotoxic effects of amiodarone. Used for life-threatening arrhythmias; woman unlikely to be nursing.

Continued

Use of Drugs and Botanical (Herbal) Preparations during Pregnancy, Breastfeeding, and Women's Health—cont'd

Drug	Use during Pregnancy	Use during Breastfeeding
Digitoxin (Crystodigin), digoxin (Lanoxin)	*Risk category C.* Has been used to treat fetal cardiac arrhythmias.	Digitoxin considered safe, but less known about digitoxin safety.
Lidocaine (used as antiarrhythmic) (Xylocaine)	*Risk category B.*	Lidocaine considered safe for breastfeeding.
Decongestants		
Ephedrine, epinephrine (EpiPen, Sus-Phrine)	*Risk category C.* Ephedrine is also used to support blood pressure during epidural or subarachnoid block during intrapartum period.	Acute, one-time use of ephedrine or epinephrine is likely to be safe. Breastfeeding not recommended if drug regularly used by mother.
Nasal sprays: oxymetazoline [Afrin, Coricidin, Dristan], phenylephrine [Neo-Synephrine], phenylpropanolamine [Kleer, Propan], fluticasone [Flonase, Flovent]	*Risk category C.* Avoid during third trimester.	Minimal amounts secreted in milk (oxymetazoline and phenylephrine). Less information available about fluticasone and phenylpropanolamine in milk secretion.
Pseudoephedrine (Sufedrine, Sudafed)	*Risk category C.* Avoid during first trimester because fetus may	Generally considered safe for breastfeeding if used

Diuretics

		occasionally rather than chronically.
Carbonic anhydrase inhibitors: acetazolamide [Diamox], methazolamide [Neptazane]	*Risk category C.*	Acetazolamide is considered safe. Safety of methazolamide unknown.
Loop diuretics: ethacrynic acid [Edecrin], furosemide [Lasix], torsemide [Demadex]	*Risk category B* (ethacrynic acid). *Risk category C* (furosemide, torsemide).	Few well-controlled studies; effects probably minimal. Maternal use could suppress lactation.
Potassium-sparing diuretics: amiloride [Midamor], spironolactone [Aldactone], triamterene [Dyrenium]	*Risk category B* (amiloride, triamterene). *Risk category D* (spironolactone).	Amiloride concentrated in breast milk. Few studies of triamterene. Spironolactone considered safe by AAP.
Thiazide diuretics: chlorothiazide [Diuril], hydrochlorothiazide [HydroDIURIL]	*Risk category D.* Decreased intravascular volume may reduce uteroplacental perfusion and result in growth retardation. Metabolic disturbances and thrombocytopenia may occur in mother and fetus. *Risk category B.*	Considered safe during lactation.
Thiazide-like diuretics: chlorthalidone [Hygroton], indapamide [Lozide, Lozol], metolazone [Mykrox, Zaroxolyn]		Chlorthalidone considered by AAP to be safe during lactation but may reduce milk supply.

Continued

Use of Drugs and Botanical (Herbal) Preparations during Pregnancy, Breastfeeding, and Women's Health—cont'd

Drug	Use during Pregnancy	Use during Breastfeeding
Hormones		
Corticosteroids: beclomethasone [Vanceril, Beclovent], betamethasone [Celestone], cortisone [Cortone], dexamethasone [Decadron], prednisolone [Delta-Cortef, Prelone], prednisone [Deltasone]	*Risk category C.* Prednisone or prednisolone (category B) is common for asthmatic woman who needs steroids. Betamethasone and dexamethasone are used to accelerate maturation of fetal lungs if preterm delivery is likely.	Prednisone and prednisolone compatible with breastfeeding. Delay nursing 4 hr after dose to reduce transfer to infant. Remove from nipples before nursing if applied topically.
Clomiphene citrate (Clomid)	*Risk category X.* Questionable association with neural tube defects. Drug is discontinued after pregnancy is achieved.	Unlikely to be given during lactation because the drug is for infertility treatment.
Danazol (Danocrine)	*Risk category X.* May cause virilization of female fetus.	Breastfeeding not advised.
Estrogens (Azumon, Conjugen, Ovest, Premarin)	*Risk category X.* No indication for estrogens during pregnancy.	Try to delay drug until breastfeeding is firmly established.

Estradiol (Alora, Climara, Estrace, Estraderm, Estring, FemPatch, Vivelle)

Risk category X. Contraceptives; not indicated during pregnancy.

Safe during lactation. Early use sometimes reduces milk volume secreted.

Estrogen-progestin combinations

Risk category X. Risks and benefits must be individually evaluated because a higher risk for cardiovascular disease was found in women who take the combination for menopausal symptoms. Doses much higher than those for oral contraceptives and are associated with masculinization of the female fetus's genitalia.

Ideally, avoid until lactation is well established for best quantity and quality of breast milk.

Progesterone (Gesterol 50, Lutolin-S, Progestagect-50, Prometrium, Crinone)

Risk category D. Most often given for amenorrhea, hormone replacement therapy, infertility (luteal phase support only during pregnancy).

Generally considered safe for use when breastfeeding.

Psychoactive Drugs

Benzodiazepines: alprazolam [Xanax], chlordiazepoxide [Librium, Libritabs], clonazepam [Klonopin], diazepam [Valium], flurazepam [Dalmane], lorazepam [Ativan],

Most are risk category D. Some reports of mild facial abnormalities and developmental delay, but no conclusive studies. Use during the third trimester may slow the infant's neurologic development and result in sedation

Potentially hazardous because of the long half-lives of many drugs in this class and the potential development of dependence. Few reported adverse effects, but observe infant for sedation, poor feeding.

Continued

Use of Drugs and Botanical (Herbal) Preparations during Pregnancy, Breastfeeding, and Women's Health—cont'd

Drug	Use during Pregnancy	Use during Breastfeeding
midazolam [Versed], oxazepam [Serax], temazepam [Restoril], triazolam [Halcion]	after birth. Midazolam is primarily used as a brief maternal perioperative sedative. The following sedative-hypnotic drugs in this class are *risk category X*: flurazepam, temazepam, and triazolam.	
Anxiolytic: meprobamate [Equanil, Miltown]	*Risk category D.* Has been associated with cardiac malformations.	Concentrations in milk are higher than in maternal serum. Observe for infant sedation.
Antipsychotic: lithium [Eskalith, Lithobid]	*Risk category D.* Slightly increased risk for cardiac abnormalities.	Infant blood concentration of lithium reaches $1/2$ to $1/3$ of the mother's concentration. Infant drug levels should be evaluated. T-wave abnormalities and decreased muscle tone have been noted.
Atypical antidepressants: bupropion [Wellbutrin], mirtazapine [Remeron], nefazodone [Serzone],	*Risk category B* (bupropion). *Risk category C* (mirtazapine, nefazodone, trazodone, venlafaxine).	Trazodone minimally excreted in breast milk. Unknown if other atypical antidepressants are excreted in breast milk.

trazodone [Desyrel], venlafaxine [Effexor]

Phenothiazines: chlorpromazine [Thorazine], prochlorperazine [Compazine], thioridazine [Mellaril]

Risk category C. Risk of malformations is uncertain, but these are probably safe for use in humans. Alcohol may increase CNS depression. Taking other drugs with phenothiazines may alter serum levels of one or more of the drugs taken.

Neonatal hypoglycemia has been reported with chlorpromazine. Less known about breastfeeding effects of maternal prochlorperazine and thioridazine.

Monoamine oxidase inhibitors (MAOIs): phenelzine [Nardil], tranylcypromine [Parnate]

Risk category C. Documented interactions between opioids and MAOIs. Potential risks if taken near the time other drugs were taken. Consult a detailed drug guide. Little documentation of fetal effects.

Few published reports related to entry of these MAOI drugs into breast milk.

Tricyclic antidepressants: amitriptyline [Elavil], amoxapine [Asendin], clomipramine [Anafranil], desipramine [Norpramin], doxepin [Adepin, Sinequan], imipramine [Tofranil], nortriptyline [Aventyl, Pamelor], protriptyline [Vivactil]

Risk category C for most tricyclics. *Risk category D* for imipramine and nortriptyline, however. Several studies have shown that tricyclic antidepressant use during pregnancy is most likely not teratogenic.

Few contraindications for most tricyclic antidepressants. Infant apnea and drowsiness with maternal doxepin intake have been described.

Continued

Use of Drugs and Botanical (Herbal) Preparations during Pregnancy, Breastfeeding, and Women's Health—cont'd

Drug	Use during Pregnancy	Use during Breastfeeding
Selective serotonin reuptake inhibitors (SSRIs): citalopram [Celexa], escitalopram [Lexapro], fluoxetine [Prozac], fluvoxamine [Luvox], paroxetine [Paxil], sertraline [Zoloft]	*Risk category C except for sertraline (risk category B).*	Most considered safe for breastfeeding infant. Citalopram and escitalopram have been associated with excessive somnolence, decreased intake, and infant weight loss.
Other psychoactive drugs: bupropion [Wellbutrin], mirtazapine [Remeron], nefazodone [Serzone], trazodone [Desyrel], venlafaxine [Effexor]	*Risk category C except for bupropion (risk category B).*	Few reports on breast milk safety for infants for most drugs. No AAP contraindications for bupropion or trazodone. Observe infant for sedation.
Thyroid Drugs		
Antithyroids: methimazole [Tapazole], propylthiouracil [PTU]	*Risk category D.* May result in neonatal goiter or hypothyroidism, although uncommon at usual	Approved by AAP. Neonatal thyroid function apparently unaffected by maternal treatment.

Potassium iodide (SSKI, Thyro-Block)	therapeutic doses. Methimazole has possible association with scalp defects. PTU is drug of choice during pregnancy.	
	Risk category D. Long-term exposure may produce fetal thyroid enlargement or hypothyroidism.	May cause rash or suppress infant's thyroid function. Dose should not be higher than RDA (recommended daily allowance).
Thyroid replacement hormone: levothyroxine [Levoxyl, Synthroid]	*Risk category A.* Crosses placenta only to limited extent.	Apparently safe during breastfeeding.

Vitamins and Retinoids

Retinoids: isotretinoin [Accutane]	*Risk category X.* Related to vitamin A. Associated with severe fetal malformations (microcephaly, ear abnormalities, cardiac defects, central nervous system abnormalities).	Contraindicated for use during breastfeeding because of severe fetal effects.
Vitamin A	*Risk category A* at doses no higher than 6000 USP units/day (risk category X at doses higher than RDA limits). Excess intake may lead to abnormalities noted for isotretinoin.	Breast milk usually supplies sufficient vitamin A to infant. Mother should not take more than 6000 international units per day.

Continued

Use of Drugs and Botanical (Herbal) Preparations during Pregnancy, Breastfeeding, and Women's Health—cont'd

Drug	Use during Pregnancy	Use during Breastfeeding
Vitamin D	*Risk category A* (risk category D at doses above RDA). Excess intake associated with malformations, including aortic stenosis, facial abnormalities, and mental retardation.	AAP approved. Infant serum level assessment recommended if mother taking a therapeutic dose.
Miscellaneous Drugs		
Nicotine gum; nicotine transdermal patch	*Risk category C* (nicotine gum). *Risk category D* (transdermal nicotine). Risk category X if used in overdose. Stopping nicotine intake by ceasing smoking lowers complications such as preterm birth.	Lactation safe, although drug is passed into breast milk. Infant exposure to passive environmental nicotine smoke is not considered safe, however.

Herbal and Botanical Preparations

Botanical Preparation	Uses	Risks for Use during Pregnancy and Lactation
Black cohosh (baneberry, black snakeroot, bugbane, squaw root, rattle root)	Phytoestrogen effects to reduce symptoms during menopause.	Pregnancy risk category X because of uterine stimulant effects. Unknown lactation effects but may reduce milk production with estrogenic effects.
Blue cohosh (blue ginseng, squaw root, papoose root, yellow ginseng)	Uterine stimulant. Similar to nicotine, resulting in hypertension, gastric stimulation, and coronary vasoconstriction.	Pregnancy risk category X. Has been used short term to stimulate delivery. No data for lactation safety but considered a high-risk herbal supplement.
Capsaicin (Zostrix, Axsain, Capsin, Capzasin-P, No-Pain, Absorbine Jr. Arthritis, Arthricare)	Topical application for pain associated with osteoarthritis, fibromyalgia, peripheral neuropathy, shingles. Avoid contact with eyes.	Pregnancy risk category C; little data on risk during lactation. Considered safe for children >2 yr of age.
Chamomile (German chamomile, Hungarian chamomile, pinheads, wild chamomile)	Antiinflammatory, antispasmodic, sedative. Treatment of nausea, GI spasms, diarrhea, insomnia. Topical treatment of hemorrhoids. Caution required in those with asthma or allergic to ragweed.	Uterotonic effects with unknown risk. Should be avoided in pregnancy and lactation.

Continued

Herbal and Botanical Preparations—cont'd

Botanical Preparation	Uses	Risks for Use during Pregnancy and Lactation
Echinacea (black Susan, snakeroot, comb flower, red sunflower, scurvy root)	Antiviral, antibiotic effects to reduce cold and flu symptoms, stimulate wound healing. Long-term daily doses may suppress rather than stimulate immune response. Should not be taken by those with autoimmune disease.	Contraindicated in pregnancy. Pregnancy risk category C because of possible immune suppression. No data on lactation effects.
Evening primrose oil	Treatment of premenstrual syndrome (PMS), menopausal symptoms. Seizure risk increased if combined with antipsychotics.	No pregnancy risk category assigned. Appears to be safe for use in pregnancy and lactation.
Feverfew (bachelor button, featherfew, midsummer daisy, Santa Maria)	Prevention of migraines. Should not be used with prescription headache drugs. May cause uterine contraction or abortion.	Contraindicated in pregnancy and lactation.
Glucosamine	Treatment of osteoarthritis to reduce pain and improve movement.	Increases blood glucose levels. Avoid use in pregnancy and lactation.

Goldenseal	Antibiotic, antiseptic, antiinflammatory effects. Uses include wound healing, treatment of upper respiratory infections, uterine bleeding, and enhancement of insulin.	Contraindicated in pregnancy and lactation. May cause premature contractions. Short-term use only because product may cause inflammation of mucosa.
Kava (also known as kava-kava) (Awa, Kew, Tonga)	Treatment of anxiety, stress, restlessness; sedation or sleep enhancement. Effects similar to alcohol. Mixing with alcohol increases toxicity.	Contraindicated in pregnancy and lactation.
St. John's wort	Treatment of mild to moderate depression. Possible interaction with therapeutic drugs and other herbal preparations: cyclosporine, digoxin, ACE inhibitors, indinavir, ginseng, chamomile, goldenseal, kava, valerian.	Contraindicated in pregnancy and lactation. May cause increased muscle tone of uterus. Pregnancy risk category C. Infant effects may include colic, drowsiness, lethargy.
Valerian (valerian root)	Sedative for insomnia, sleeping disorders associated with anxiety, restlessness.	Inadequate data to determine effects during pregnancy. Sedative effects discourage use in lactating woman.

REFERENCES & READINGS

American Academy of Pediatrics (AAP) and American College of Obstetricians and Gynecologists (ACOG). (2002). *Guidelines for perinatal care* (5th ed.). Elk Grove Village, IL, and Washington, DC: Authors.

American Academy of Pediatrics Committee on Drugs. (2001). Transfer of drugs and other chemicals into human milk. *Pediatrics, 108*(3), 776-789.

American Academy of Pediatrics Committee on Drugs. (2000). Use of psychoactive medications during pregnancy and possible effects on the fetus and newborn (RE9866). *Pediatrics, 105*(4), 880-887.

Andrade, S.E., Gurwitz, J.H., Davis, R.L., Chan, K.A., Finkelstein, J.A., Fortman, K., et al. (2004). Prescription drug use in pregnancy. *American Journal of Obstetrics & Gynecology, 191*(2), 398-407.

Andres, R.L. (2004). Effects of therapeutic, diagnostic, and environmental agents and exposure to social and illicit drugs. In R.K. Creasy, R. Resnik, & J.D. Iams (Eds.), *Maternal-fetal medicine: Principles and practice* (5th ed., pp. 281-314). Philadelphia: Saunders.

Blanchard, D.G., & Shabetai, R. (2004). Cardiac diseases. In R.K. Creasy, R. Resnik, & J.D. Iams (Eds.), *Maternal-fetal medicine: Principles and practice* (5th ed., pp. 815-843). Philadelphia: Saunders.

Centers for Disease Control and Prevention. (2002). Sexually transmitted diseases treatment guidelines. *MMWR Morbidity and Mortality Weekly Report, 51*(RR-6). www.cdc.gov/STD/treatment/rr5106.pdf

Cunningham, F.G., Leveno, K.J., Bloom, S.L., Hauth, J.C., Gilstrap, L.C., & Wenstrom, K.D. (2005). *Williams obstetrics* (22nd ed.). New York: McGraw-Hill.

Fontaine, K.L. (2005). *Complementary and alternative therapies for nursing practice* (2nd ed.). Upper Saddle River, NJ: Prentice-Hall.

Gahart, B.L., & Nazareno, A.R. (2005). *2005 intravenous medications* (21st ed.). St. Louis: Mosby.

Gal, P., & Reed, M.D. (2004). Medications. In R.E. Behrman, R.M. Kliegman, & H.B. Jenson (Eds.), *Nelson textbook of pediatrics* (17th ed., pp. 2432-2501). Philadelphia: Saunders.

Gibbs, R.S., Sweet, R.L., & Duff, W.P. (2004). Maternal and fetal infectious disorders. In R.K. Creasy, R. Resnik, & J.D. Iams (Eds.), *Maternal-fetal medicine: Principles and practice* (5th ed., pp. 741-801). Philadelphia: Saunders.

Hale, T.W. (2004). *Medications and mothers' milk* (11th ed.). Amarillo, TX: Pharmasoft Medical Publishing.

Harkness, R., & Bratman, S. (2003). *Mosby's handbook of drug-herb and drug-supplement interactions.* St. Louis: Mosby.

Hodgson, B.B. (2005). *Nursing drug handbook 2005.* Philadelphia: Saunders.

Kemper, K.J., & Gardiner, P. (2004). Herbal medicines. In R.E. Behrman, R.M. Kliegman, & H.B. Jenson (Eds.), *Nelson textbook of pediatrics* (17th ed., pp. 2502-2505). Philadelphia: Saunders.

Lawrence, R.M., & Lawrence, R.A. (2004). The breast and the physiology of lactation. In R.K. Creasy, R. Resnik, & J.D. Iams (Eds.), *Maternal-fetal medicine: Principles and practice* (5th ed., pp. 135-153). Philadelphia: Saunders.

Lawrence, R.M., & Lawrence, R.A. (2005). *Breastfeeding: A guide for the medical profession* (6th ed.). St. Louis: Mosby.

Minkoff, H.L. (2004). Human immunodeficiency virus. In R.K. Creasy, R. Resnik, & J.D. Iams (Eds.), *Maternal-fetal medicine: Principles and practice* (5th ed., pp. 803-814). Philadelphia: Saunders.

Public Health Service Task Force. (2005). *Recommendations for using anti-retroviral drugs in pregnant HIV-1 infected women for maternal health and interventions to reduce perinatal HIV-1 transmission in the United States.* Retrieved April 13, 2005, from http://AIDSinfo.nih.gov.

Public Health Service Task Force. (2005). *Safety and toxicity of individual antiretroviral agents in pregnancy.* Retrieved April 13, 2005, from http://AIDSinfo.nih.gov.

Skidmore-Roth, L. (2004). *Mosby's handbook of herbs and natural supplements* (2nd ed.). St. Louis: Mosby.

Skidmore-Roth, L. (2005). *Mosby's nursing drug reference.* St. Louis: Mosby.

Spencer, J.W. & Jacobs, J.J. (2004). *Complementary and alternative medicine: An evidence-based approach* (2nd ed.). St. Louis: Mosby.

U.S. Department of Health and Human Services. (2004). AIDS info: Approved medications to treat HIV infection. Retrieved April 1, 2004, from www.AIDSinfo.nih.gov.

Weiner, C.P., & Buhimschi, C. (2004). *Drugs for pregnant and lactating women.* New York: Churchill Livingstone.

Bibliography

American Academy of Pediatrics (AAP) and American College of Obstetricians and Gynecologists (ACOG). (2002). *Guidelines for perinatal care* (5th ed.). Elk Grove Village, IL: Authors.

American Academy of Pediatrics Committee on Drugs (2001). Transfer of drugs and other chemicals into human milk. *Pediatrics, 108*(3), 776-789.

American Academy of Pediatrics Committee on Drugs (2000). Use of psychoactive medications during pregnancy and possible effects on the fetus and newborn (RE9866). *Pediatrics, 105*(4), 880-887.

American Cancer Society. (2004). *Detailed guide: Breast cancer: What are the risk factors for breast cancer?* Retrieved March 22, 2005, from www.cancer.org/docroot/home/index.asp.

American College of Obstetricians and Gynecologists (ACOG). (2003a). *Breast cancer screening: ACOG Practice Bulletin No. 42.* Washington, DC: Author.

American College of Obstetricians and Gynecologists (ACOG). (2002). *Diagnosis and management of preeclampsia and eclampsia: ACOG Practice Bulletin No. 33.* Washington, DC: Author.

American College of Obstetricians and Gynecologists (ACOG). (2001). *Chronic hypertension in pregnancy: ACOG Practice Bulletin No. 29.* Washington, DC: Author.

American College of Obstetricians and Gynecologists (ACOG). (2001). *Use of botanicals for management of menopausal symptoms: ACOG Practice Bulletin No. 28.* Washington, DC: Author.

Andrade, S.E., Gurwitz, J.H., Davis, R.L., Chan, K.A., Finkelstein, J.A., Fortman, K., et al (2004). Prescription drug use in pregnancy. *American Journal of Obstetrics & Gynecology, 191*(2), 398-407.

Andres, R.L. (2004). Effects of therapeutic, diagnostic, and environmental agents and exposure to social and illicit drugs. In R.K. Creasy, R. Resnik, & J.D. Iams (Eds.), *Maternal-fetal medicine: Principles and practice* (5th ed., pp. 281-314). Philadelphia: Saunders.

Biancuzzo, M. (2003). *Breastfeeding the newborn: Clinical strategies for nurses* (2nd ed.). St. Louis: Mosby.

Blackburn, S.T. (2003). *Maternal, fetal, and neonatal physiology: A clinical perspective* (2nd ed.). St. Louis: Saunders.

Blanchard, D.G., & Shabetai, R. (2004). Cardiac diseases. In R.K. Creasy, R. Resnik, & J.D. Iams (Eds.), *Maternal-fetal medicine: Principles and practice* (5th ed., pp. 815-843). Philadelphia: Saunders.

Bond, L. (2004). Physiology of pregnancy. In S. Mattson & J.E. Smith (Eds.), *Core curriculum for maternal-newborn nursing* (3rd ed., pp. 96-123). St. Louis: Saunders.

Burrow, G.N., Duffy, T.P., & Copel J.A. (2004), *Medical complications during pregnancy* (6th ed.). Philadelphia: Saunders.

Centers for Disease Control and Prevention. (2002). Sexually transmitted diseases treatment guidelines, 2002. *MMWR Morbidity and mortality weekly report, 51* (RR6). Retrieved February 12, 2005, from www.cdc.gov/STD/treatment/rr5106.pdf.

Cheffer, N.D., & Rannalli, D.A. (2004). Newborn biologic/behavioral characteristics and psychosocial adaptations. In S. Mattson & J.E. Smith (Eds.), *Core curriculum for maternal-newborn nursing* (3rd ed., pp. 437-484). St. Louis: Saunders.

Coverston, C. R. (2004). Psychology of pregnancy. In S. Mattson & J.E. Smith (Eds.), *Core curriculum for maternal-newborn nursing* (3rd ed., pp. 124-143). St. Louis: Saunders.

Creasy, R.K., Resnik, R., & Iams, J.D. (Eds.), *Maternal-fetal medicine: Principles and practice* (5th ed.). Philadelphia: Saunders.

Cunningham, F.G., Leveno, K.J., Bloom, S.L., Hauth, J.C., Gilstrap, L.C., & Wenstrom, K.D. (2005). *Williams obstetrics* (22nd ed.). New York: McGraw-Hill.

Feinstein, N.F., Torgersen, K.L., & Atterbury, J. (Eds.). (2003). *AWHONN's fetal heart monitoring: Principles and practices* (3rd ed.). Dubuque, IA: Kendall/Hunt.

Feinstein, N.F., Sprague, A., & Trépanier, M.J. (2000). *Fetal heart rate auscultation.* Washington, DC: Association of Women's Health Obstetric, and Neonatal Nurses.

Fischbach, F. (2000). *A manual of laboratory and diagnostic tests* (6th ed.). Philadelphia: Lippincott.

Fontaine, K.L. (2005). *Complementary & alternative therapies for nursing practice* (2nd ed.). Upper Saddle River, NJ: Pearson Prentice Hall.

Gahart, B.L., & Nazareno, A.R. (2005). *2005 intravenous medications* (21st ed.). St. Louis: Mosby.

Gal, P., & Reed, M.D. (2004). Medications. In R.E. Behrman, R.M. Kliegman, & H.B. Jenson (Eds.), *Nelson textbook of pediatrics* (17th ed., pp. 2432-2501). Philadelphia: Saunders.

Gibbs, R.S., Sweet, R.L., & Duff, W.P. (2004). Maternal and fetal infectious disorders. In R.K. Creasy, R. Resnik, & J.D. Iams (Eds.), *Maternal-fetal medicine: Principles and practice* (5th ed., pp. 741-801). Philadelphia: Saunders.

Gilbert, E.S., & Harmon, J.S. (2003). *Manual of high risk pregnancy and delivery* (3rd ed.). St. Louis: Mosby.

Gordon, M.C. (2002).Maternal physiology in pregnancy. In S.G. Gabbe, J.R. Niebyl, & J.L. Simpson (Eds.), *Obstetrics: Normal and problem pregnancies* (4th ed.). New York: Churchill Livingstone.

Grodner, M., Long, S., & DeYoung, S. (2004). *Foundations and clinical applications of nutrition, a nursing approach* (3rd ed.). St. Louis: Mosby.

Hale, T.W. (2004). *Medications and mothers' milk* (11th ed.). Amarillo, TX: Pharmasoft Medical Publishing.

Harkness, R., & Bratman, S. (2003). *Mosby's handbook of drug-herb and drug-supplement interactions*. St. Louis: Mosby.

Hatcher, R.A., Trussell, J., Stewart, F., Nelson, A.L., Cates, W., Guest, F., & Kowal, D. *Contraceptive technology* (18th ed., pp. 495-530). New York: Ardent Media.

Hodgson, B.B. (2005). *Nursing drug handbook 2005*. Philadelphia: Saunders.

Kemper, K.J., & Gardiner, P. (2004). Herbal medicines. In R.E. Behrman, R.M. Kliegman, & H.B. Jenson (Eds.), *Nelson textbook of pediatrics* (17th ed., pp. 2502-2505). Philadelphia: Saunders.

Kilpatrick, S.J., & Laros, R.K. (2004). Maternal hematologic disorders. In R.K. Creasy, R. Resnik, & J.D. Iams (Eds.), *Maternal-fetal medicine: Principles and practice* (5th ed., pp. 975-1004). Philadelphia: Saunders.

Laros, R.K. (2004). Thromboembolic disease. In R.K. Creasy, R. Resnik, & J.D. Iams (Eds.), *Maternal-fetal medicine: Principles and practice* (5th ed., pp. 845-857). Philadelphia: Saunders.

Lawrence, R.M., & Lawrence, R.A. (2004). The breast and the physiology of lactation. In R.K. Creasy, R. Resnik, & J.D. Iams (Eds.), *Maternal-fetal medicine: Principles and practice* (5th ed., pp. 135-153). Philadelphia: Saunders.

Lawrence, R.M., & Lawrence, R.A. (2005). *Breastfeeding: A guide for the medical profession* (6th ed.). St. Louis: Mosby.

Leibowitz, D., & Hoffman, J. (2000). Fertility drug therapies: Past, present, and future. *Journal of Obstetric, Gynecologic, and Neonatal Nursing, 29*(2), 201-210.

Martin, J.A., Hamilton, B.E., Sutton, P.D., Ventura, S.J., Menacker, F., & Munson, M.L. (2003). Births: Final data for 2002. *National Vital Statistics Reports, 52*(10), 1-113.

Minkoff, H.L. (2004). Human immunodeficiency virus. In R.K. Creasy, R. Resnik, & J.D. Iams (Eds.), *Maternal-fetal medicine: Principles and practice* (5th ed., pp. 803-814). Philadelphia: Saunders.

Moore, M.L., & Moos, M. (2003). *Cultural competence in the care of childbearing families*. White Plains, NY: March of Dimes.

Moore, T.R. (2004). Diabetes in pregnancy. In R.K. Creasy, R. Resnik, J.D. Iams (Eds.), *Maternal-fetal medicine: Principles and practice* (5th ed.). Philadelphia: Saunders.

National High Blood Pressure Education Program Working Group on High Blood Pressure in Pregnancy (2000). Report of the National high blood pressure program working group on high blood pressure in pregnancy. *American Journal of Obstetrics and Gynecology, 183*(1), S1-S22.

Nicholson, J.F., & Pesce, M.A. (2004). Reference ranges for laboratory tests and procedures. In R.E. Behrman, R.M. Kliegman, & H.B. Jenson (Eds.),

Nelson textbook of pediatrics (17th ed., pp. 2396-2427). Philadelphia: Saunders.

Pagana, K.D., & Pagana, T.J. (2005). *Mosby's diagnostic and laboratory test reference* (7th ed.). St. Louis: Mosby.

Poole, J.H., Sosa, M.E., Freda, M.C., Kendrick, J.M., Luppi, C.J., Krening, C.F., & Dauphinee, J.D. (2001). High-risk pregnancy. In K.R. Simpson & P.A. Creehan (Eds.), *AWHONN Perinatal Nursing* (2nd ed., pp. 173-296). Philadelphia: Lippincott.

Public Health Service Task Force. (2005). *Recommendations for using antiretroviral drugs in pregnant HIV-1 infected women for maternal health and interventions to reduce perinatal HIV-1 transmission in the United States.* Retrieved April 13, 2005, from http://AIDSinfo.nih.gov.

Public Health Service Task Force. (2005). *Safety and toxicity of individual antiretroviral agents in pregnancy.* Retrieved April 13, 2005, from http://AIDSinfo.nih.gov.

Resnik, R. (2004). The puerperium. In R.K. Creasy, R. Resnik, & J.D. Iams (Eds.), *Maternal-fetal medicine: Principles and practice* (5th ed., pp. 165-168). Philadelphia: Saunders.

Richard-Davis, G. (2002). Ovulation induction for in vitro fertilization: The role of gonadotropin-releasing hormone antagonists. *Infertility and Reproductive Clinics of North America, 13*(3), 437-444.

Riordan, J. (Ed.). (2005). *Breastfeeding and human lactation* (3rd ed., pp. 713-728). Boston: Jones and Bartlett.

Roberts, J.M. (2004). Pregnancy-related hypertension. In R.K. Creasy, R. Resnik, & J.D. Iams (Eds.), *Maternal-fetal medicine: Principles and practice* (5th ed., pp. 859-899). Philadelphia: Saunders.

Scoggin, J. (2004). Physical and psychologic changes. In S. Mattson & J.E. Smith (Eds.), *Core curriculum for maternal-newborn nursing* (3rd ed., pp. 371-386). St. Louis: Saunders.

Skidmore-Roth, L. (2004). *Mosby's handbook of herbs & natural supplements* (2nd ed.). St. Louis: Mosby.

Skidmore-Roth, L. (2005). *Mosby's nursing drug reference.* St. Louis: Mosby.

Spencer, J.W., & Jacobs, J.J. (2004). *Complementary and alternative medicine: An evidence-based approach* (2nd ed.). St. Louis: Mosby.

Stoll, B.J., & Kliegman, R.M. (2004). The high-risk infant. In R.E. Behrman, R.M. Kliegman, & H.B. Jenson (Eds.), *Nelson textbook of pediatrics* (17th ed., pp. 547-559). Philadelphia: Saunders.

U.S. Department of Health and Human Services. (2004). AIDS info: Approved medications to treat HIV infection. Retrieved April 1, 2004, from www.AIDSinfo.nih.gov.

U.S. Department of Health and Human Services and U.S. Department of Agriculture, (2005). *Dietary Guidelines for Americans* (6th ed.). Washington, DC: US Government Printing Office.

Weiner, C.P., & Buhimschi, C. (2004). *Drugs for pregnant and lactating women.* New York: Churchill Livingstone.

Index

A

Abdomen
  assessment of
    after cesarean birth, 327t
    during labor, 143t
  neonatal, 220t-221t
Abortion, 68-70
  assessing history of, 131t
  etiology/predisposing factors, 68
  medical, 393-394
  types of, 68-69
Abruptio placentae, 74-77
Abstinence, sexual, 348-349
  periodic, 358-359, 359t-360t
Abstinence syndrome, neonatal.
    See Neonatal abstinence
    syndrome
ACE inhibitors, use during
    pregnancy/breastfeeding, 493t
Acetaminophen, use during
    pregnancy/breastfeeding,
    485t-486t
Acquired immunodeficiency
    syndrome. *See* AIDS
Acrocyanosis, 215t
Adolescent pregnancy, 48-53
  assessment of, 49-50
  interventions in, 50-53
  intrapartal care in, 52
  maternal health implications, 48
  nutrition during, 46, 51-52
  parenting implications, 49
  socioeconomic implications,
    48-49
Adoption, management of, 64
Adrenal glands, adaptations to
    pregnancy, 27t
Affective disorders, postpartum,
    343-345
Afterpains, 303
  relieving, 320-321

AIDS
  maternal/fetal/neonatal effects
    of, 103t
  neonatal transmission/effects,
    294t
  signs/symptoms, diagnosis,
    management, 408t
Albuterol, use during pregnancy/
    breastfeeding, 489t
Alcohol use
  assessing, during labor, 135t
  maternal/fetal/neonatal effects
    of, 55t
  during pregnancy, 47
  as pregnancy risk factor, 37t
Allergies, assessing for, during
    labor, 134t
Alternative therapies during
    pregnancy, 41
Amebicides, use during
    pregnancy/breastfeeding,
    485t
Aminoglycosides, use during
    pregnancy/breastfeeding,
    495t
Amniocentesis, purpose of, 35t
Amniotic fluid
  assessing, 140t
  functions of, 19
Amniotic fluid embolism,
    characteristics and
    management, 201-203
Amniotic membranes, assessing,
    444-448, 445f-448f
Amniotomy, 168-169
Amphetamines,
    maternal/fetal/neonatal
    effects of, 57t
Analgesics, use during
    pregnancy/breastfeeding,
    485t-487t

519